Laboratory Animal Anaesthesia and Analgesia

T0383258

Laboratory Animal Anaesthesia and Analgesia

Fifth Edition

Paul Flecknell
Newcastle University, Newcastle-Upon-Tyne, United Kingdom
Flaire Consultants Ltd, Newcastle-Upon-Tyne, United Kingdom

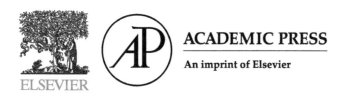

ELSEVIER

ACADEMIC PRESS
An imprint of Elsevier

Academic Press is an imprint of Elsevier
125 London Wall, London EC2Y 5AS, United Kingdom
525 B Street, Suite 1650, San Diego, CA 92101, United States
50 Hampshire Street, 5th Floor, Cambridge, MA 02139, United States
The Boulevard, Langford Lane, Kidlington, Oxford OX5 1GB, United Kingdom

Notices
Knowledge and best practice in this field are constantly changing. As new research and
experience broaden our understanding, changes in research methods, professional practices, or
medical treatment may become necessary.

Practitioners and researchers must always rely on their own experience and knowledge in
evaluating and using any information, methods, compounds, or experiments described herein.
In using such information or methods they should be mindful of their own safety and the safety
of others, including parties for whom they have a professional responsibility.

To the fullest extent of the law, neither the Publisher nor the authors, contributors, or editors,
assume any liability for any injury and/or damage to persons or property as a matter of products
liability, negligence or otherwise, or from any use or operation of any methods, products,
instructions, or ideas contained in the material herein.

ISBN 978-0-12-818268-0

For information on all Academic Press publications
visit our website at https://www.elsevier.com/books-and-journals

Publisher: Stacy Masucci
Acquisitions Editor: Linda Versteeg-Buschman
Editorial Project Manager: Pat Gonzalez
Production Project Manager: Sajana Devasi P K
Cover Designer: Christian J. Bilbow

Typeset by STRAIVE, India

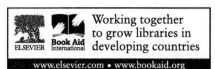

Contents

5.   Analgesia and postoperative care

6.   Anaesthesia of common laboratory species:
Special considerations

Preface

The art and science of anaesthesia and analgesia of laboratory animals continues to advance, but it is clear from reviewing the methods section of publications that only a very limited range of techniques are in widespread use. Research workers routinely review their laboratory methodologies to ensure they are the most appropriate for their research, so we should also evaluate our anaesthetic practices. Providing the most appropriate and effective anaesthetic regimen is an essential part of good experimental design. Reviewing our anaesthesia and perioperative care so that they are the most appropriate for a particular study will contribute to both reduction and refinement of animal use. This textbook aims to provide information and guidance to encourage this process.

Reporting of analgesic use in publications that describe work that involves the use of laboratory animals is improving. However, the methods used to assess postoperative pain are very rarely mentioned. This is almost certainly due to a failure to implement effective pain assessment, rather than an oversight in reporting. To provide greater emphasis on the need for effective pain assessment and pain management, additional information on this topic has been added to this new edition. To reflect the importance of this topic, the book's title has been changed.

My scientific colleagues constantly, and quite reasonably, ask for peer-reviewed publications to support recommendations of best practice in anaesthesia and analgesia, so the number of references has been increased and updated. I have tried where possible to include key publications that can speed the process of obtaining more detailed information on particular topics. Where older references continue to provide essential information they have been retained.

Despite my efforts to keep to the original concept for this book—the provision of an introductory text for new investigators—the length of the text has increased, but I hope it still represents an accessible source of information for all those involved in the anaesthesia and perioperative care of laboratory animals.

Paul Flecknell

Preface to the Fourth Edition

The front cover of this new edition displays a different molecule—buprenorphine. Unlike sevoflurane, which illustrated the cover of the previous edition, this isn't a new analgesic, but it is a compound that continues to shape strategies for managing pain in laboratory animals. The past few years have seen further data on the efficacy buprenorphine in alleviating postoperative pain in a range of species. New slow release formulations offer potential advances in providing long-term alleviation of severe pain, and the agent continues to be the most widely used analgesic in laboratory animals. It is a great disappointment, however, that reported use of postoperative analgesics continues to be very low, even though their use in veterinary clinical practice is now widespread. To try to address this problem, the section on pain assessment and pain management has been revised, updated and expanded to encourage not only greater use of analgesics but also more structured assessment of pain.

The anaesthetic methods used in many research facilities continue to improve as a result of the introduction of newer anaesthetic agents and new techniques. Sophisticated monitoring devices are widely available and their cost continues to fall. The introduction of newer techniques often represents significant refinements of research methodologies, but this is not invariably the case. Some research projects still benefit from the use of older agents because these may produce fewer interactions with the body systems being studied. For this reason, these older agents are still described in this new edition. The new edition continues to provide information on new methods and more complex procedures, but also emphasizes the basic principles of good anaesthetic practice for less experienced research workers. To emphasize these basic principles, the introductory chapters have been rearranged into a single section.

As in previous editions, the number of references has been increased and updated, and these are used, as in previous editions, to support contentious statements, to indicate conflicting opinions and to provide a starting point for searching the more specialist scientific literature. Where older references continue to provide essential information they have been retained.

Paul Flecknell

Preface to the Third Edition

The additions and amendments to this new edition reflect developments in anaesthetic practice and changes in our attitudes towards laboratory animal welfare. Standards of anaesthesia for laboratory animals have increased greatly since the publication of the second edition, and the use of technically demanding procedures have become much more widespread. This new edition attempts to balance the need for additional information in these areas with the main goal of the first edition: the provision of an introductory text for new investigators.

With the continued move towards evidence-based medicine, the number of references has been increased. It has never been my intention to provide a comprehensive anaesthesia textbook, so references have been used primarily to support contentious statements, to indicate conflicting opinions and to provide a starting point for searching the more specialist scientific literature. Whenever possible, recent papers that contain a good discussion of the literature have been selected for citation at appropriate points in the text.

Paul Flecknell

Preface to the Second Edition

Since writing the first edition of this book, there has been a welcome increase in concern for the welfare of laboratory animals. One result of this has been the introduction by a number of countries of formal training requirements for new research workers. This increased interest in animal welfare has also led to the improved dissemination of information regarding 'best practice' in many aspects of laboratory animal science. The second edition of 'Laboratory Animal Anaesthesia' has benefited from this exchange of information, and the additions and revisions which have been included owe much to comments from my colleagues from around the world. A major addition to this new edition is the inclusion of illustrations of techniques and equipment. The format of the book remains relatively unchanged, except for Chapter 7, which now incorporates some of the information previously included in the Appendices. This enables more of the information relating to a particular species to be accessed quickly and easily. Brief descriptions of anaesthetic techniques for fish, amphibia, reptiles and birds have also been included, to provide some basic guidance for dealing with these species.

Paul Flecknell

Preface to the First Edition

The majority of laboratory animals are anaesthetized by staff who have not received specialist training in this field. Unfortunately, most currently available textbooks of human or veterinary anaesthesia assume that the reader has a basic knowledge of the subject. Because of this, a good deal of published information has remained relatively inaccessible and this has limited the introduction of new techniques into the field of laboratory animal anaesthesia.

This handbook attempts to provide a basic guide to anaesthesia for research workers and animal technicians. It is not intended to be a comprehensive text on animal anaesthesia, but it concentrates on those areas that are of greatest practical importance when anaesthetizing laboratory animals.

The first sections of the book deal with the general principles of preoperative care, anaesthetic techniques, and anaesthetic management. The most important properties of the anaesthetic and other agents used are outlined, but a detailed description of their pharmacology has been deliberately excluded. These sections also provide details of some of the equipment which the author has found useful when anaesthetizing laboratory animals.

These general sections of the book should be read before using any of the anaesthetic regimes described in the final sections. In particular, it is hoped that the reader will study the sections on postoperative care and the provision of effective pain relief before carrying out any operative procedures on animals.

In order to provide rapid, easily accessible guidelines a list of recommended anaesthetic regimes for each of the common laboratory species is given in Appendix 1. For those research workers who require alternative techniques, a wider range of anaesthetic regimes is discussed together with an extensive list of dose rates for each species in Chapter 7.

In addition to providing guidance on basic anaesthetic technique, an introduction to more specialist procedures such as long-term anaesthesia and the use of neuromuscular blocking agents has been included. These sections provide only initial guidance, and it is recommended that, whenever possible, an experienced veterinary anaesthetist be consulted before attempting these techniques.

Paul Flecknell

List of Tables

List of Figures

Acknowledgements

This book has continued to develop in scope and content as a result of the advice and helpful comments and criticism from colleagues and readers of previous editions. I am also grateful to participants on the anaesthesia and pain management workshops run by myself and colleagues for their comments and questions which have helped shape the contents of this new edition.

As with previous editions, the content of this new edition has been enhanced by the many constructive comments and editorial corrections provided by Professor Eddie Clutton.

I am particularly grateful to Ruth, my wife, for her support and forbearance during all stages of the preparation of this book. Thanks also to our daughter, Laura, for the initial design of the new cover.

Glossary

Inevitably, a number of specialist terms are used throughout this book and these are defined below:

Anaesthesia A state of controllable, reversible insensibility in which sensory perception and motor responses are both markedly depressed.

Analgesia The temporary abolition or diminution of pain perception.

Analeptic Drug which stimulates respiration.

Anoxia Complete deprivation of oxygen for tissue respiration.

Apnoea Temporary cessation of breathing.

Arrhythmia (cardiac) Alteration in the normal rhythm of the heart.

Asystole Lack of cardiac muscle contractions.

Ataxia Lack of co-ordination, 'wobbliness'.

BMR Basal metabolic rate.

Bradycardia Slowing of the heart rate.

CNS Central nervous system.

CNS depressant Any agent which modifies function by depressing sensory or motor responses in the CNS.

Cyanosis Blue or purple colouring of the skin or visible membranes due to the presence of an increased concentration of reduced haemoglobin in capillary blood, symptomatic of hypoxia.

Dosages mg of drug per kg body weight (mg/kg) except for the neuroleptanalgesic combinations which are more conveniently expressed as mL of commercial or diluted premixed solution per kg body weight (mL/kg).

Dosage schedules u.i.d., once daily; b.i.d., twice daily; t.i.d., three times daily; q.i.d., four times daily.

Dyspnoea Laboured breathing.

ECG Electrocardiogram.

Hypercapnia Elevated blood carbon dioxide content.

Hyperpnoea Fast or deep breathing.

Hypertension Elevated (arterial) blood pressure.

Hypnotic A drug which induces a state resembling deep sleep, but usually with little analgesic effect.

Hypocapnia Reduced blood carbon dioxide content.

Hypopnoea Slow or shallow breathing.

Hypotension A fall in (arterial) blood pressure.

Hypothermia A fall in body temperature.

Hypovolaemia A fall in circulating blood volume.

Hypoxia Depressed levels of oxygen.

Induction (of anaesthesia) The initial establishment of a state of anaesthesia.

Injection routes iv, intravenous; im, intramuscular; ip, intraperitoneal; sc, subcutaneous.
Laryngospasm Spasm of the vocal cords, producing complete or partial obstruction of the airway.
Minute volume The volume of gas breathed in 1 min, that is, the product of tidal volume and respiratory rate.
Narcosis A state of insensibility or stupor from which it is difficult to arouse the animal.
Normovolaemic Having a normal circulating blood volume.
PCO$_2$ Partial pressure of carbon dioxide.
Per os By mouth.
PO$_2$ Partial pressure of oxygen.
Polypnoea Rapid, panting breathing.
Pulmonary ventilation The mechanical expansion and contraction of the lungs in order to renew alveolar air with fresh atmospheric air.
Tachycardia An increase in heart rate.
Tachypnoea Rapid respiration.
Tidal volume The volume of gas expired with each breath.

Chapter 1

Basic principles of anaesthesia

Anaesthesia in a research environment and the 3Rs

A requirement to comply with the principles set out by Russell and Burch (1959), of Reduction, Refinement, and Replacement, now forms part of the legislation controlling use of animals in research in the European Union and elsewhere. It might be considered that any use of anaesthesia would represent a 'refinement' of research procedures, contributing to a lessening in the degree of pain and distress caused to the animals that are still required, after replacement with nonsentient alternatives have been carefully considered. However, the use of inappropriate techniques and inadequate equipment can compromise efforts to minimize pain and distress. The effects of a poor choice of anaesthetic agent can be dramatic, for example, ileus (gut stasis) after administration of chloral hydrate, or muscle damage after injection of ketamine in small mammals. Failure to maintain body temperature effectively can greatly prolong recovery from anaesthesia, and failure to control pain has a clear detrimental effect on animal welfare.

Anaesthesia has profound effects on the physiological processes of animals and even if this does not cause pain or distress, it can have a marked influence on study outcomes. Effects can arise as a direct result of the anaesthetic agents used, for example, hyperglycaemia caused by dexmedetomidine or may be secondary to the depression of various body systems by anaesthetic agents. Some effects persist only during the period of anaesthesia, other effects may continue for hours or days. The effects often differ within animals in a study and increase variability in the data obtained. This increased variability can require an increased number of animals to be used to demonstrate treatment effects (Festing, 2002).

Providing the most appropriate and effective anaesthetic regimen is an essential part of good experimental design. Reviewing our anaesthesia and perioperative care so that they are the most appropriate for a particular study will contribute to both reduction and refinement of animal use.

When reviewing our current practice, it is important that attention is given to the anaesthetic agents used and to the measures adopted to minimize the unwanted side-effects of anaesthesia and surgery. This requires investment in appropriate equipment, and in effective training of personnel.

Laboratory Animal Anaesthesia and Analgesia. https://doi.org/10.1016/B978-0-12-818268-0.00016-4

Use of effective analgesia following surgical procedures is particularly important, and this is explained in detail in Chapter 5.

Almost all the analgesic and anaesthetic techniques currently used in humans were developed and assessed in laboratory animals, before being accepted for clinical use in people. We therefore have a very wide range of techniques and anaesthetic and analgesic agents available for use in laboratory animals. Careful consideration of the options available can lead to improvements both in the quality of scientific data obtained and in the welfare of the animals involved.

Introduction—What is anaesthesia and how do we produce it?

Anaesthesia means 'loss of sensation'. This can involve loss of consciousness (general anaesthesia), or the loss of sensation can be restricted to a small area of the body (local anaesthesia). Larger body areas can be anaesthetized by injecting drugs around nerve trunks, to produce regional anaesthesia. Each of these techniques can be used in laboratory animals, but general anaesthesia is the most common approach. This is because it provides a loss of awareness, as well as a loss of sensation, and so prevents any distress associated with the procedures that are to be undertaken during the anaesthetic period. It also ensures the animal remains largely immobile, produces muscle relaxation, and suppresses reflex activity. General anaesthesia is produced using either injectable or inhalational agents, or a combination of the two methods. Often a single drug can be given to produce all the required features of general anaesthesia: loss of consciousness, analgesia, suppression of reflex activity, and muscle relaxation. Alternatively, a combination of agents can be given, each contributing to the overall effect. The advantage of this approach is that the undesirable side-effects of anaesthetic agents can often be minimized. The side effects of anaesthetics are usually dose-dependent. Giving several drugs in combination, at relatively low dose rates, often has less effect on major body systems than when using a single anaesthetic agent. These combinations of agents are often administered as a single injection in small rodents. In larger species, sedatives and analgesics are usually given first, as preanaesthetic medication (or 'premeds'), followed by other drugs to produce anaesthesia. The initial onset of anaesthesia is termed 'induction', and its continuation is termed 'maintenance'. Injectable and inhalational agents can also be combined, for example, with anaesthesia being induced using an injectable agent, and then the period of anaesthesia prolonged or the depth of anaesthesia increased using inhalational agents.

Local anaesthesia is produced by infiltrating tissues with local anaesthetics, or by injecting these agents around specific nerves or nerve trunks. This technique can be combined with general anaesthetics, so that the local anaesthetic produces complete loss of sensation, and the general anaesthetic is given in a relatively low dose, to provide loss of consciousness.

The degree or depth of anaesthetic produced can vary, depending on the type of experimental procedures that are to be undertaken. If surgical procedures are to be carried out then pain perception must be completely suppressed. If the surgery involves relatively little trauma to tissues, then a medium plane of surgical anaesthesia may be sufficient. For more major surgery, especially if this involves traction and tearing of tissues, a deeper plane of surgical anaesthesia will be needed. In contrast, if anaesthesia is being induced simply to provide humane restraint while nonpainful procedures are carried out, then only light anaesthesia, with little pain suppression, will be required. Different general anaesthetic agents can appear to provide similar levels of hypnosis (sleep), but the degree of analgesia produced can vary widely.

Some agents are referred to as 'hypnotics', rather than anaesthetics, since they produce 'sleep' (hypnosis) but have no specific analgesic properties. This terminology causes some confusion since, at high doses, hypnotics (e.g. tribromoethanol) produce general anaesthesia. Different anaesthetics and hypnotics act in different ways to produce their effects. Surgical planes of general anaesthesia require both loss of consciousness and loss of pain sensation, and this can be produced by agents that have both analgesic and hypnotic properties. It can also be produced by hypnotics that have no specific analgesic effects, since if a high enough dose is given, even intense pain will not be perceived, because of the very marked depression of all brain activity. However, if no specific analgesic component is provided, this may result in increased postoperative pain (see Chapter 5) because of the effects of the surgical stimuli on the nervous system. For this reason, anaesthetic protocols using hypnotics often include use of analgesic agents, such as buprenorphine.

This introductory section outlines what equipment is needed to produce and maintain anaesthesia safely and effectively, what factors may influence your choice of anaesthetic, and what preparations should be made before anaesthesia. More detailed reviews of anaesthetic agents are available elsewhere (e.g. Grimm et al., 2015; Thomas and Lerche, 2022).

Anaesthetic equipment—Preparation and use

The factors influencing the choice of a particular anaesthetic are discussed in more detail later, but irrespective of the agent or combination of agents selected, it is important to establish that all the items of equipment that will be needed are available and in good working order. Check that sufficient anaesthetic drugs and anaesthetic gases are available not just for the anticipated period of anaesthesia but also to cover unexpected additional requirements (see Appendix 2 for guidance). Check the expiry date of all drugs and ensure they have been properly stored. For clear drugs stored in uncoloured glass bottles, check for unexpected turbidity or colour changes. In addition to the anaesthetic agents, drugs needed for coping with emergencies must also be readily available (see below).

Monitoring equipment

A wide range of different monitoring devices are available for use during an-aesthesia, and these are discussed in detail in Chapter 3. To use these devices effectively, they may need a period to stabilize after initially switching them on. It is also important to check they are functioning correctly. Alarm limits should be reset from the default settings (which may be values appropriate for human patients or larger animals) and then fine-tuned when the individual animal is connected. Heating pads and blankets should be switched on approximately 30–60 min before they are needed, to allow them to reach the correct operating temperature.

Incubators and recovery pens

If the animal is to recover from anaesthesia, check that a suitable area for post-operative recovery has been provided (see Chapter 5) and any incubator or heat pad needed in the recovery period is switched on well in advance.

Anaesthetic machines

If an anaesthetic machine is to be used to deliver a volatile anaesthetic or oxygen, then it is essential to check its components carefully before use. A simple preuse checklist for anaesthetic machines is given in Table 1.1. Anaesthetic machines appear complex, but their underlying design and operation is very simple. Most machines comprise a compressed gas source that, after pressure reduction, sup-plies gas that is passed through a flow meter and then to an anaesthetic vapor-izer. This delivers anaesthetic gases to the animal through a breathing system. If using an unfamiliar machine, ask a colleague who has used the apparatus or the equipment supplier to provide a demonstration. Very detailed descriptions of medical anaesthetic equipment are available (Davey and Diba, 2011; Al-Shaikh and Stacey, 2018). An excellent description of anaesthetic equipment together with animations to illustrate breathing systems can be found at http://www.ase-vet.com/resources/index.htm. Anaesthetic gases or oxygen are delivered from the anaesthetic machine to the animal using a breathing system. Irrespective of the anaesthetic breathing system selected, a face mask, nasal tube, or an en-dotracheal tube will be required to connect it to the animal. Alternatively, the anaesthetic gases can be used to fill an anaesthetic chamber (see below).

Compressed gas source

Gas is either supplied from cylinders on the anaesthetic machine or piped us-ing hoses from larger cylinders. If using hoses, a pressure reducing valve (see below) should be fitted to the large cylinder so that gas at lower pressure is sup-plied through the hose. The mounts on the anaesthetic machine for the hoses or cylinders have small pins that locate in corresponding holes in the cylinders to

TABLE 1.1 Preanaesthetic checks of anaesthetic equipment.

- Is only one oxygen cylinder marked as 'in use' and the other full?
- Check that the valve on the cylinder in use is opened fully to provide a free flow of gas (the reading on the pressure dial on an oxygen cylinder gives a reasonable indication as to how much oxygen it contains, Appendix 2).
- If you are using an oxygen generator, check that it is functioning correctly.
- Check that the cylinders are full and properly attached to the anaesthetic machine; ensure the flow meters are functioning correctly by opening the cylinder valves and the needle valves that control the flow of gas through the flow meters. The bobbins should rotate when gas is flowing (most are marked with a small white dot to assist in assessing this). The gas flow rate is measured from the top of the bobbin. Turn off the gas flow using the needle valve and check that the bobbin sinks smoothly back to zero and is not sticking and giving a false high gas flow rate.
- Check that the emergency oxygen button is functioning correctly.
- If a volatile anaesthetic is to be used, check that the vaporizer has been filled and that the control dial moves smoothly over the entire range of possible settings. If using a machine with several vaporizers, check that the correct one has been selected.
- If the anaesthetic machine has a built-in circle-type absorber, ensure that this is switched out of circuit (usually marked 'open') if the absorber is not to be used. Check that soda lime is not exhausted (indicated by a colour change from pink to white or white to violet).
- Attach the breathing system which will be used to the anaesthetic machine, turn on the oxygen supply and check the system for leaks by occluding the animal end of the tubing and fully closing any valves. Open the valves to check they are not sticking.
- If a mechanical ventilator is to be used, switch it on and observe it for a few respiratory cycles. If possible, check the tidal volume that is being delivered with a respirometer.
- Run through the manufacturer's recommended preuse check on any monitoring equipment.

These checks should be routine procedures since they will minimize the occurrence of anaesthetic accidents which could result in the death of the animal. A video illustrating the process is available at www.researchanimaltraining.com.

ensure that the correct gas (e.g. oxygen or nitrous oxide) is attached (Fig. 1.1). Gas cylinders are also colour coded (oxygen cylinders are green in the United States and black with a white shoulder in the United Kingdom; nitrous oxide cylinders are blue). A small metal and neoprene seal (Bodok seal) ensures a gas-tight fit between the cylinder and the mount block (Fig. 1.1). Under no circumstances should oil or grease be used around the seal because the pressurized gases give off heat as they are released from the cylinder and may cause explosions if oil is used. A pressure gauge (Fig. 1.2) indicates that gas is available. Oxygen cylinders contain oxygen under pressure, and the pressure gauge gradually falls as the cylinder is depleted. A full-size E cylinder (the size fitted to most

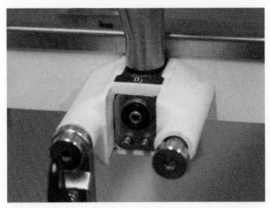

FIG. 1.1 Pin index system—the pins in the mounting block (left) fit into the holes in the gas cylinder (see Fig. 1.3).

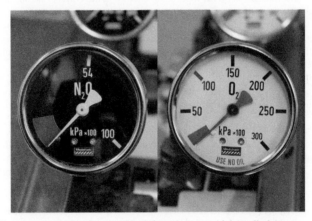

FIG. 1.2 Pressure gauges for nitrous oxide (left) and oxygen (right) cylinders.

anaesthetic machines) contains approximately 680 L of gas. Manufacturers label the cylinders to confirm this. Nitrous oxide cylinders contain liquid nitrous oxide, so, unlike an oxygen cylinder, the pressure reading will not fall until the cylinder is almost empty. Cylinders are either opened using a spanner or fitted with a hand-operated valve (Fig. 1.3). It is best to use a machine with two oxygen cylinders so that the supply can be switched from one cylinder to the other, if needed, during an anaesthetic. Most machines have check valves located with the cylinder mounting block so that the empty cylinder does not need to be turned off before turning on the full cylinder. Cylinders should be labelled 'full', 'in use', or 'empty' (and if empty, changed as soon as induction of anaesthesia is completed). When changing cylinders, handle them carefully, particularly full ones. If these are dropped, their 'neck' can fracture, leading to explosive decompression and injury to personnel. For this reason, cylinders

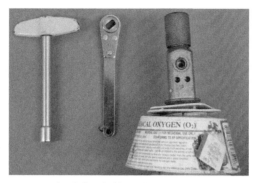

FIG. 1.3   Cylinders are opened and closed either using a ratchet spanner (left), cylinder key (centre) or hand-operated valve (right).

should always be secured to a wall or placed on special carts when not mounted on an anaesthetic machine.

Pressure-reducing valve

The pressure-reducing valve is sited between the cylinder and the rest of the anaesthetic machine. This reduces the pressure from approximately 134 bar (in a full-size E cylinder) to the 4 bar required in the anaesthetic machine. The valve also acts as a regulator to provide a constant pressure of gas. Using a pressure-reducing valve is therefore safer, allows the use of lower pressure pipework and connectors in the anaesthetic machine, and avoids having to constantly adjust the setting on the flow meter as the pressure in the cylinder falls as gas is used.

Oxygen concentrators

Oxygen concentrators (sometimes referred to as oxygen generators) can be used as an alternative to compressed gas cylinders. They produce 90%–95% oxygen from room air, by absorbing nitrogen. Portable units generally produce 4–10 L per minute (Fig. 1.4), and larger devices, producing up to 25 L per minute and capable of supplying several anaesthetic machines can also be obtained. All these devices are electrically operated, so a power failure will result in a failure of oxygen supply unless a standby generator, or a battery backup and power inverter are available. Alternatively, a cylinder of oxygen can be retained for emergency use. Since the flow of gas from a portable oxygen concentrator is relatively low, the emergency oxygen button on an anaesthetic machine will not function correctly but turning up the flow meter can rapidly flush anaesthetic vapour from a breathing system. The low flow and lower pressure of gas supplied from these units limits their use with some ventilators, and with larger animals. However, the small, relatively portable units are well-suited for use in small procedure rooms, where transport and storage of oxygen cylinders can be a problem. Newer devices are noticeably quieter than older models, and noise is not an issue if a larger unit is sited away from the immediate theatre area. The purchase cost of this equipment

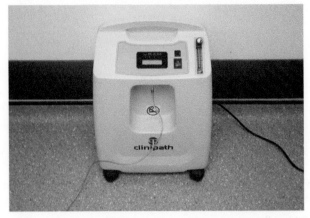

FIG. 1.4 Oxygen concentrator suitable for providing oxygen supplementation for small animal anaesthesia.

has fallen dramatically in recent years, and they can now be considered an economical and convenient alternative to compressed gas cylinders.

Flow meter

Separate flow meters are provided for each gas and a flow control valve controls the flow of gas. As the valve is opened, a bobbin or ball moves up the flow meter. The flow of gas is read from the position of the top of the bobbin or the middle of the ball (Fig. 1.5). The flow control valves are delicate and should only be opened and closed by hand. Some basic anaesthetic machines use turret-type flow meters (Fig. 1.6) in which the gas leaves the flow meter from the bottom of the unit. These can also be purchased combined with a pressure-reducing valve

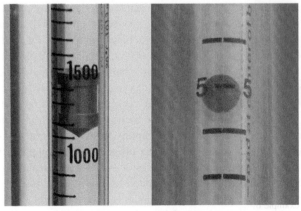

FIG. 1.5 The gas flow rate is read from the position of the top of the bobbin of the flow meter. In flow meters with a ball, rather than a bobbin (right), the reading is taken from the centre of the ball.

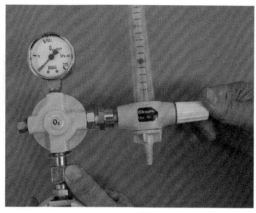

FIG. 1.6   Turret-type flow meters can be used as a simple means of providing a controlled source of oxygen, during both anaesthesia and recovery.

and regulator and used on a compressed gas cylinder as a simple and inexpensive means of supplying oxygen.

Vaporizers

Volatile anaesthetics are supplied as liquids that are vaporized (evaporated into a gas) before being mixed with oxygen or other gases and delivered to the animal. Vaporizers are designed for use with a specific anaesthetic agent, and many have a filling system that prevents them from inadvertently being filled with the wrong anaesthetic (Fig. 1.7). An agent-specific filler tube is used, one end

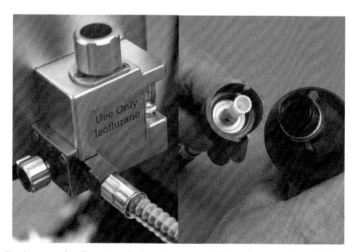

FIG. 1.7   An example of a system designed to prevent filling of a vapourizer with the incorrect anaesthetic agent. The end of the filling tube fits into a slot in the vapourizer (left), and the other end of the tube fits onto a collar on the bottle (right).

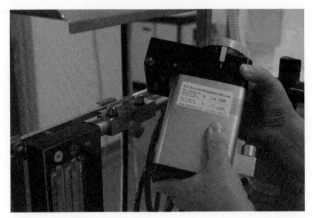

FIG. 1.8 Vapourizer mounting system (Selectatec) that allows vapourizers to be exchanged quickly and easily between machines.

of which slots into a fitting on the vaporizer and the other end slots into a collar on the bottle of anaesthetic. The fitting on the vaporizer and the collar on the bottle are specific to each agent, making it impossible to fill the vaporizer with the wrong agent. Modern vaporizers are usually fitted to the 'back bar' of the anaesthetic machine (Fig. 1.8). This may be via a special mounting system such as the 'Selectatec' mechanism that allows vaporizers to be exchanged quickly and easily between machines. Although more than one vaporizer may be fitted to the machine, for safety reasons most back bar systems prevent more than one vaporizer from being used at any one time.

Modern vaporizers are designed to deliver the designated concentration of anaesthetic and to compensate for changes in gas flow and the temperature drop that occurs as the agent is vaporized. They operate by splitting off a small proportion of the fresh gas flow and completely saturating it with anaesthetic. This is then remixed with the main gas flow. This requires that a pressurized gas is supplied, the vaporizer is correctly attached, and any locking mechanism is fully engaged to avoid leaks. Vaporizers must be serviced regularly to function correctly.

Pressure relief valve

Some anaesthetic machines have a pressure relief valve, usually situated on the back bar, to protect the flow meters and vaporizer from inadvertent over-pressurization, which can occur, for example, if the gas outflow is occluded. The valve usually operates at about 35 kPa.

Emergency oxygen flow

The emergency oxygen supply is operated by a spring-loaded button, usually located next to the gas supply to the animal. It provides a supply of oxygen at high flow (35 L/min) and bypasses the flow meters and vaporizers.

Oxygen failure alarm

Oxygen failure warning devices are now fitted to all anaesthetic machines designed for medical or veterinary clinical use. These are usually powered only by the oxygen pressure. When the oxygen pressure falls, they emit a loud whistle. They can only be reset by the return of the correct oxygen pressure.

Gas scavenging systems

A variety of hazards is reportedly associated with pollution of the operating room environment with anaesthetic gases (Varughese and Ahmed, 2021). The risk of explosion or fire associated with some older anaesthetic agents such as ether and cyclopropane is well recognized, and appropriate precautions must be taken to avoid these dangers. The risks to personnel which may arise from chronic exposure to low levels of certain inhalational anaesthetics are much more difficult to assess. The results of the many studies designed to determine these associated risks vary considerably, but at present, it would seem sensible to take appropriate steps to minimize operating theatre pollution. Measurements of trace anaesthetic concentrations in typical rodent operating areas have confirmed the need for modifying practices to reduce exposure of personnel.

Waste anaesthetic gases can be removed in various ways, and it should be possible to obtain equipment suitable for most applications. A scavenging system suitable for small laboratory animals was described by Hunter et al. (1984) and systems based on this design are available commercially. Note that systems that use activated charcoal are not effective in removing nitrous oxide. Many active scavenging systems require maintenance of relatively high fresh gas flows when using a face mask system (see below) and this can be significant practical problem when using these with small rodents. Even with an effective scavenging system, spillage of waste gas will occur when the lid of an anaesthetic chamber is removed to gain access to the anaesthetized animal. If this is considered a significant problem, then either the whole procedure can be carried out in a fume hood, or specially designed chambers can be used, which completely remove the anaesthetic gases before the chamber is opened (Fig. 1.9).

Anaesthetic chambers

When anaesthetizing small animals, it is often most convenient to use an anaesthetic chamber. Volatile anaesthetics are delivered from a precision vaporizer to the chamber and the waste anaesthetic gas removed in a controlled way and either ducted out of the room or adsorbed using activated charcoal. A particularly effective scavenging technique has been devised using a double-box system (VetTech Solutions) (Fig. 1.9). Since all anaesthetics cause some degree of respiratory depression, oxygen, either alone or in combination with nitrous oxide, should be used as the carrier gas, rather than air. A suitably sized (e.g. $30 \times 20 \times 20$ cm for rats) clear perspex box should be used so that the animal can be observed during induction. Chambers can either be purchased commercially

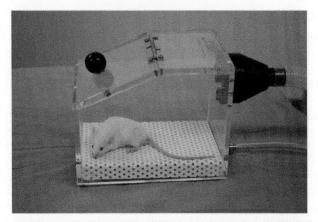

FIG. 1.9 Anaesthetic chamber for use with small mammals (VetTech Solutions)—the anaesthetic agent is piped in at the bottom of the chamber, and an exhaust port at the top is connected to a gas-scavenging device.

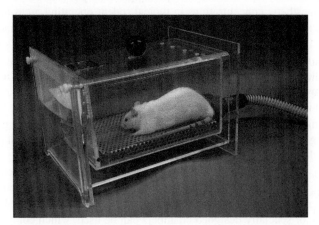

FIG. 1.10 A double-chamber system that is designed to minimize exposure of personnel to waste anaesthetic gases (VetTech Solutions).

(Fig. 1.10) or constructed 'in house'. Some chambers are provided with a metal grid in the base to separate the animal from any urine that it produces. Alternatively, a pad of towelling or dry bed (William Daniels, United Kingdom) or some paper towels should be placed on the floor of the chamber. The apparatus should be cleaned thoroughly after use.

Anaesthetic gases are denser than air, so should be filled from the bottom of the chamber, with waste gas scavenged from the top. To provide rapid induction, the entire chamber should be filled quickly. An appropriate gas flow can be estimated by measuring the chamber volume. The approximate time to completely fill the chamber can then be determined from the flow of anaesthetic:

$$\frac{\text{Chamber volume}}{\text{flow}} = \text{time constant for chamber}$$

The concentration of anaesthetic in the chamber will be close to the concentration supplied from the anaesthetic after twice the time constant has elapsed. For example, a chamber measuring $30 \times 20 \times 20$ cm will have a volume of 12 L, and with a flow rate of 4 L/min, the time constant would be 3 min. So, after 6 min (twice the time constant), with a vaporizer setting of 5%, the chamber would contain approximately 4.25% anaesthetic vapour.

When anaesthetizing animals in an anaesthetic chamber, the aim is to induce anaesthesia rapidly, but safely, and this can best be achieved by filling the chamber rapidly. Using smaller chamber sizes for smaller animals makes this easy to achieve, but filling times for larger chambers (e.g. those designed for use in rabbits and cats), with volumes exceeding 50 L, can be considerable, since most flow meters have a maximum flow of 10–12 L/min. Occasionally, it may be necessary to induce anaesthesia using a volatile anaesthetic in a larger animal, and in these circumstances, the entire cage may be enclosed in a polythene bag and anaesthetic vapour piped in. A quick calculation using the formula above shows that this inevitably results in very slow induction of anaesthesia, with animals undergoing a very prolonged period of semi-consciousness and involuntary excitement. A better alternative is to use a vapour wand (Hodgson, 2007) that provides much more rapid delivery of anaesthetic vapour, and consequently more rapid induction of anaesthesia.

'Ether jars'

In the past, it was common practice to anaesthetize small rodents by placing them in a glass receptacle containing a pad of gauze or cotton wool soaked in liquid anaesthetic. Direct contact with the liquid anaesthetic is extremely unpleasant for the animal, as it is irritant to mucous membranes. Even if the gauze is separated from the animal by a metal grid, liquid anaesthetic is often spilt onto areas that are in contact with the animal. The concentration of anaesthetic that can be achieved in such containers is unpredictable and is invariably dangerously high if potent, easily vaporized anaesthetics such as isoflurane are used. For example, the concentration of isoflurane produced at 20°C is approximately 32%, more than six times the safe induction concentration (Table 2.1). If ether is used, there will be a significant risk of fire or explosion. Whichever volatile anaesthetic is used, it is frequently impossible to prevent contamination of the environment with anaesthetic vapour, and this may present a hazard to staff. The use of such an anachronistic technique has no advantage other than the low cost of the apparatus. However, it may still be necessary to use if no alternative is available, or when anaesthetizing wild animals under field conditions. In these circumstances, attempts can be made to reduce the concentration of anaesthetic vapour produced by mixing the anaesthetic with propylene glycol (Itah et al.,

2004). If 'field' anaesthesia is being undertaken regularly, it may be worthwhile investing in a mobile anaesthetic system, as described by Mathews et al. (2002).

Anaesthetic breathing systems

Anaesthetic chambers are useful for inducing anaesthesia in small animals that may be difficult to restrain, but the animals must be removed from the chamber to enable surgical manipulations to be carried out. Unless the procedure is of extremely short duration (30–60 s), some method of maintaining anaesthesia must be provided. The simplest system is a face mask connected directly to the anaesthetic machine. This is easy to use but requires relatively high fresh gas flows to prevent the animal rebreathing expired gases. Alternative arrangements of the mask and the fresh gas supply can reduce the fresh gas flow needed, simplify the removal of waste anaesthetic gases, and make assisting ventilation easier, should this become necessary. These advantages become more significant when working with larger species (>400 g).

General considerations

All anaesthetic breathing systems aim to deliver sufficient anaesthetic gases to meet the animal's requirements and to remove exhaled gases, which contain carbon dioxide. It is an advantage if these exhaled gases can be removed from the operating area, as trace concentrations of anaesthetic gases may have adverse effects on operating theatre personnel. An additional consideration when selecting a breathing system is the ease and efficiency with which assisted ventilation can be controlled.

Different types of breathing systems produce different degrees of resistance to breathing and have different volumes of dead space. The dead space of a breathing system is the part of the system that remains filled with expired gas at the end of expiration. This carbon dioxide-rich gas is then re-inhaled by the animal. If a significant amount of expired gas is rebreathed, the blood carbon dioxide concentration will rise and produce a range of adverse effects (see Chapter 3). The resistance of an anaesthetic breathing system influences the effort that must be made by the animal to move gas in and out of, or around, the breathing system. Breathing systems with narrow or sharply angled components and those with valves will provide a greater resistance to gas flow and so will require a greater respiratory effort by the animal. This is important since excessive effort to breathe can cause fatigue of the respiratory muscles and depress respiration. It also increases the oxygen needs of the animal.

Tidal volume and minute volume

Two measures of an animal's respiratory function also influence the choice of breathing system—the 'tidal volume' and the 'minute volume'. The tidal volume is the volume of gas drawn into the respiratory tract with each breath. The minute volume is the volume of gas drawn into the respiratory tract in 1 min and so is calculated by multiplying the tidal volume by the respiratory rate. The minute volume is not always equivalent to the flow of gas that needs to be delivered to the animal by the breathing system. During each respiratory cycle, gas is only drawn into the lungs for approximately one-third of the time, that is, during inspiration but not during expiration or during any pauses between expiration and inspiration. This means that the animal's minute volume is inhaled in approximately 20 s, so using a simple face mask system, a fresh gas flow of three times this volume per minute is required. Occasionally, an even greater flow is required to meet the most rapid rate at which gas is drawn into the lungs, the peak inspiratory flow rate. Using this type of breathing system is clearly very uneconomical, so various breathing systems have been designed to reduce the fresh gas flows required, by providing a reservoir for the unused gas delivered by the anaesthetic machine.

Open breathing systems

As mentioned earlier, the most widely used breathing system is an open face mask (Fig. 1.11), which is a simple and convenient way of delivering anaesthetic

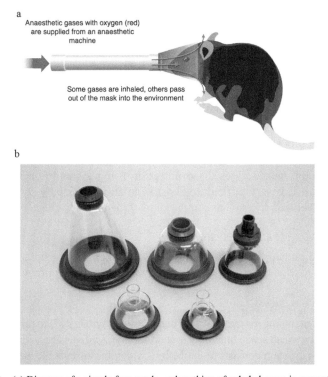

FIG. 1.11   (a) Diagram of a simple face mask—rebreathing of exhaled gases is prevented by use of relatively high fresh gas flow rates. (b) Face masks for use with a range of laboratory species. The rubber diaphragm helps provide a seal around the animal's nose to prevent breathing of room air around the mask.

gases to an animal. Expired gases pass around the edges of the mask. Provided the gas flow is sufficiently high, rebreathing of exhaled gases will be small and the dilution of the anaesthetic gases by breathing room air will be avoided. If the gas flow is too low, the animal will breathe in room air from around the edges of the mask. This will result in a reduction in the depth of anaesthesia if volatile anaesthetics are being used. As mentioned above, to meet inspiratory flow requirements, the gas flows must be three times the animal's minute volume. Typical flows are shown in Table 1.2.

This simple method of delivery has several drawbacks. The gas flow must be relatively high for larger animals, for example, flows of 15–20 L/min for a 20-kg minipig. Removing waste anaesthetic gases is difficult since gas escapes all around the mask. To avoid this, with smaller animals (<1 kg), a concentric mask system can be used (see Fig. 1.12). The concentric mask system appears to resemble the Bain coaxial breathing system described below, but it must be stressed that the outer tube does not act as a gas reservoir, so gas flows appropriate to an open system must be used (Table 1.2).

One problem with currently available concentric systems of this type is that the gas extraction rate is often too high, which results in dilution of the fresh gas intended to supply the animal. As a result, when flows calculated based on minute volume are employed, the animal may be inadequately anaesthetized. To avoid this, minimum flows of 500–1000 mL/min may be required. This wastes a considerable volume of anaesthetic gases, something that may represent a significant economic loss when using more expensive agents such as sevoflurane. An alternative is to use a low flow mask (Fig. 1.13) with a passive scavenging system, or to combine use of this with use of a down-draft table to remove any waste anaesthetic gases. Several systems are available commercially, including those that incorporate heating devices that help maintain the animal's body temperature during anaesthesia (Fig. 1.14).

Perhaps the most serious disadvantage in using a simple open breathing system is that it is very difficult to assist ventilation artificially should this be required, other than by manual compression of the animal's chest.

Semi-closed breathing systems

Semi-closed breathing systems are systems in which some rebreathing of expired gases may occur and in which no carbon dioxide absorption is used.

The T-piece system

The T-piece breathing system was first described by Ayre (1937) to provide a low-resistance, low-dead space breathing system for use in infants and young children. The breathing system consists of a tube into which the anaesthetic gas mixture is introduced through a small inlet tube at right angles to the main limb (Figs. 1.15 and 1.16). One end of the T-piece is connected to the animal, while the other is left open to the air. A length of tubing is attached to this open end, providing a small reservoir for anaesthetic gases that would otherwise escape into the outside air.

TABLE 1.2 Recommended fresh gas flow rates for different anaesthetic breathing systems.

Body weight	Estimated tidal volume (mL)	Minute volume (L)	Flow rate (L/min)			
			Open system	T-piece or Bain's system	Magill	Closed circuit[a]
30g	0.3	0.015	0.045	0.03	–	–
200g	2	0.1	0.3	0.2	–	–
500g	5–7.5	0.4–0.6	1–2	1–1.5	–	–
1kg	10–15	0.5–1	1.5–3	1.5–2.5	–	–
3kg	30–45	1–1.5	3–4.5	2.5–3.5	–	–
6kg	60–90	1.5–3	4.5–9	3.5–7.5	–	0.2
10kg	100–150	3–6	9–18	6–12	3–6	0.3
20kg	200–300	5–9	15–27	10–18	5–9	0.5

[a] See text.

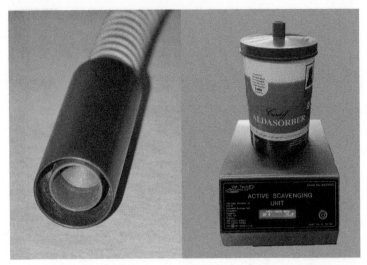

FIG. 1.12   Concentric mask system for rodents and rabbits that combine delivery of anaesthetic gases with removal of waste gas through an outer tube. An extraction fan and activated charcoal absorber are used to remove the anaesthetic gases and prevent exposure of personnel (Vet Tech Solutions, UK).

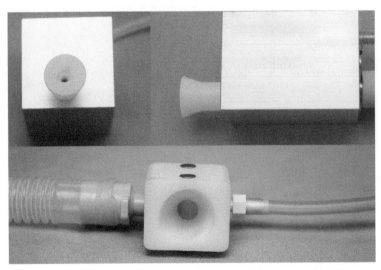

FIG. 1.13   Low flow face masks: side view right top and end-view of mask left (AAS), and below, low flow mouse mask (Flair designs)

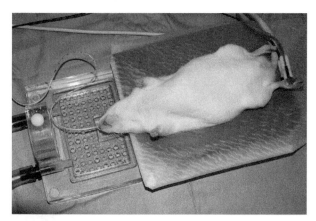

FIG. 1.14   Down-draft operating table—a heating blanket has been added to maintain the animal's body temperature. Anaesthetic is being delivered via a nasal catheter, and a pulse oximeter is in use.

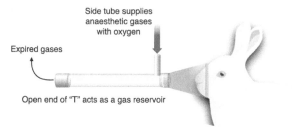

FIG. 1.15   Ayre's T-piece to show gas flow pattern. Exhaled gas is blown out through the open-ended reservoir tube, which then fills with fresh gas from the side port and is inhaled by the animal. The breathing system can be connected to a face mask or an endotracheal tube.

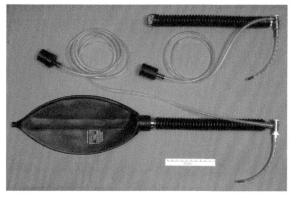

FIG. 1.16   T-pieces with low-dead space connectors. Above, standard T-piece; below, Jackson Rees modified T-piece.

The presence of this reservoir enables the fresh gas flow to be reduced to about twice the animal's minute volume, without rebreathing (see Table 1.2).

During inspiration, fresh gas is drawn in both from the sidearm and from the reservoir. During expiration, exhaled gas fills the reservoir limb, and during the pause before the next inspiration, this is washed out by the fresh gas from the sidearm. The volume of the reservoir limb is unimportant so long as it exceeds one-third of the animal's tidal volume and does not impose any appreciable resistance to expiration. Ventilation can be controlled simply by intermittently occluding the end of the reservoir limb, but if carried out manually, the anaesthetist has very little idea of the pressure being delivered to the animal's lungs. It is preferable to attach an open-ended reservoir bag to the expiratory limb: the Jackson Rees modification. Squeezing the bag with the end occluded inflates the lungs, and exhalation occurs through the open end of the bag (Fig. 1.16). No increase in fresh gas flow is required when assisting ventilation in this way. It is easy to attach a mechanical ventilator to the reservoir limb and ventilate the limb with air. Provided the reservoir is of sufficient volume, little or no mixing of the anaesthetic gases and the ventilating gas occurs.

To use the T-piece effectively, it should be connected directly to an endotracheal tube or to a close-fitting face mask. The volume of the side of the T-piece that is connected to the animal should be low to reduce equipment dead space. Similarly, the volume of endotracheal tube connectors should be minimized. This is best achieved by using connectors produced for use in human babies and infants. These connectors contribute a dead space of approximately 0.2 mL compared to 1.5 mL when using a conventional type of connector (Fig. 1.17). The dead space of a T-piece designed for use in human infants is approximately 1 mL. If a face mask is used, it is essential that this fits closely around the animal's muzzle. If it does not, gas will be drawn in around the edges of the mask and the anaesthetic gas mixture will be diluted with room air. If ventilation is assisted, gas will escape around the mask, and the degree of lung inflation produced will be inadequate. For these reasons, it is preferable to intubate the animal's trachea whenever possible. A simple T-piece for very small mammals can be constructed from Luer adaptor 'Y' connectors and plastic tubing (Fig. 1.18).

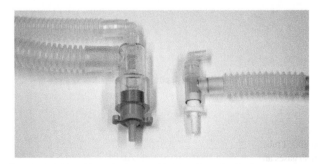

FIG. 1.17 Standard (left) and low-dead space (right) endotracheal tube connectors and T-pieces.

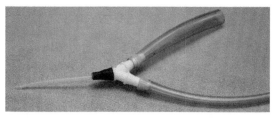

FIG 1.18 Low dead space T-piece for use with small rodents, constructed from a disposable Y connector and 'Bubble-tubing'.

The T-piece is an ideal breathing system for small laboratory animals since it offers low resistance to breathing and has a small dead space. It is not always necessary to purchase commercially produced T-pieces, as the apparatus can be constructed easily from plastic 'T' connectors (Portex Ltd., Appendix 4) and rubber tubing.

The Bain coaxial breathing system

The Bain breathing system is a coaxial version of a T-piece, in which the fresh gas inflow tubing runs inside the reservoir limb (Figs. 1.19 and 1.20). The breathing system was designed to provide a light-weight breathing system in which any valves or breathing bags were situated some distance from the patient and close to the anaesthetic machine (Bain and Spoerel, 1972). The light-weight construction reduces the tendency for the breathing system to pull on the endotracheal tube and so reduces the risk of accidental extubation. Positioning the expiratory port well away from the animal allows ventilation to be assisted easily without interfering with sterile drapes or the activities of the surgeon. In addition, anaesthetic gases can be scavenged easily and do not accumulate at the surgical site. The breathing system has a low dead space (<2 mL) and so is suitable for use in small animals. The Bain breathing system functions similarly to a T-piece. During inspiration, gas is drawn in from the central fresh gas supply and from the outer reservoir tube. During expiration, exhaled gas fills the

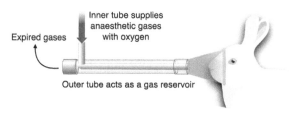

FIG. 1.19 Bain's breathing system to show gas flow patterns. Exhaled gas is blown out through the outer, open-ended tube. Fresh gas is supplied through the inner tube, which also fills the outer tube and the fresh gases are inhaled by the animal. The breathing system can be connected to a face mask or an endotracheal tube.

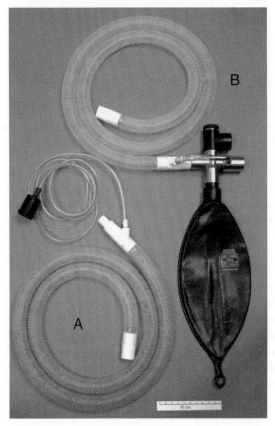

FIG. 1.20   Bain's breathing system (A) and modified Bain breathing system (B).

reservoir tube, and during the pause before the next inspiration, this is replaced with fresh gas, provided the fresh gas flow is adequate.

Two modifications of the basic breathing system have been described. The expiratory limb may terminate with a 'pop-off' valve and a reservoir bag (Fig. 1.20), or an open-ended reservoir bag may be mounted at the end of the expiratory limb. Adding a 'pop-off' valve is unsuitable for small animals (<10 kg body weight), since the valve increases breathing system resistance. When used in larger animals, the valve and the reservoir bag allow ventilation to be assisted easily by partially closing the valve and intermittently squeezing the reservoir bag. The open-ended reservoir bag is equivalent to the Jackson Rees modified T-piece and serves a similar function by allowing easy control of ventilation. Mechanical ventilators can be connected to the reservoir limb, as with a T-piece.

The gas flows required to prevent rebreathing have been quoted as ranging from 100 mL/kg body weight/min (Manley and McDonell, 1979) to 200–300 mL/kg body weight/min (Ungerer, 1978). The use of the lower flows can be explained by the animal responding to changes in blood carbon dioxide concentration by altering its rate and depth of respiration. When the fresh gas flow is low, some rebreathing of exhaled carbon dioxide from the reservoir limb will occur. This will result in an increase in the blood carbon dioxide concentration that stimulates respiration. This moderate hyperventilation results in blood carbon dioxide tensions being maintained at acceptable levels. It is not certain whether the additional respiratory effort produced is deleterious to the animal, but the conventional view has always been that rebreathing should be minimal during spontaneous respiration. For this reason, it is recommended that fresh gas flow rates of 2–2.2 times minute volume should be used (see Table 1.2). During mechanical ventilation, some degree of rebreathing of carbon dioxide can be advantageous, since it may help to avoid the production of hypocapnia. Fresh gas flow rates of 70–100 mL/kg/min allow the maintenance of normal carbon dioxide concentrations (normocapnia) during mechanical ventilation (Manley and McDonell, 1979), but inaccuracies in flow meter settings limit the usefulness of this technique in small animals (Hird and Carlucci, 1977).

Magill breathing system

The Magill breathing system is widely used in human anaesthesia, and this probably accounts for the frequency with which it is used in animal anaesthesia. While the advantages that have assured its popularity in human anaesthesia are applicable to similar-sized animals, it is generally unsuitable for use in animals with a body mass below 10 kg.

This breathing system consists of a reservoir bag connected by a length of corrugated tubing to the animal (Figs. 1.21 and 1.22). An expiratory 'pop-off' valve is situated as close to the patient as possible, to reduce equipment dead space. During expiration, the first portion of expired gas is from the animal's anatomical dead space (the trachea and the bronchi), and since no gas exchange occurs in this region, it contains no carbon dioxide. The expired gas travels up the corrugated tubing towards the reservoir bag that fills; then, as the pressure in the breathing system rises, the expiratory valve lifts and the remaining expired

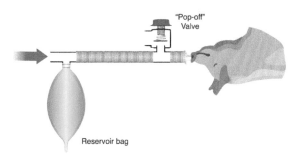

FIG. 1.21   Magill breathing system—fresh gas is supplied from the anaesthetic machine and is breathed in from the reservoir bag and the connecting tubing. During exhalation, as pressure rises in the system, the pop-off valve lifts allowing the escape of exhaled gases.

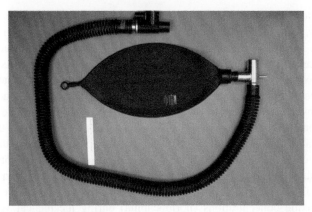

FIG. 1.22 Magill breathing system.

gas passes out of the breathing system. The continuous flow of fresh gas down the breathing system flushes out any remaining carbon dioxide-rich alveolar gas during the pause before the next inspiration. Because of the preferential elimination of carbon dioxide-rich alveolar gas, significant rebreathing does not occur in humans until the fresh gas flow falls below 70% of the minute volume (Kaïn and Nunn, 1967). The breathing system is therefore extremely economical in its fresh gas requirements. It is important to realize that during controlled ventilation achieved by manual compression of the reservoir bag, this preferential elimination of alveolar gas is lost. Under these conditions, fresh gas flows of three times minute volume may be required to prevent rebreathing.

The major problem in using the breathing system in small animals is that it imposes a significant resistance to expiration. In addition, the dead space of a typical breathing system is 8–10 mL, which is likely to represent a significant proportion of the tidal volume of a small animal. If it is to function effectively, the Magill breathing system must be attached to the animal by an endotracheal tube or a close-fitting face mask. It is common practice to connect this system to small animals with a badly fitting mask. Under these circumstances, the breathing system functions as an open system so that fresh gas flows more than three times minute volume are required to prevent either rebreathing or the dilution of the inspired gas mixture by room air, which will be drawn in around the face mask. When used correctly, waste anaesthetic gases can be scavenged by means of a suitable attachment on the expiratory valve. If a badly fitting face mask is used, the same problems of pollution arise as occur with open breathing systems.

Lack breathing system

The Lack breathing system is also widely used in human anaesthesia. It is a modification of the Magill system, with an expiratory tube that either runs parallel to the inspiratory tube (Parallel Lack) or within the inspiratory tube

(Co-axial Lack). The expiratory tube connects to the expiratory valve close to the reservoir bag. This is a much more convenient arrangement if the valve needs to be partly closed to assist ventilation. It is also very economical in its fresh gas requirement, usually requiring only 0.8–1.0 times the minute volume. Similar, to the Magill system, it is generally unsuitable for use in animals with a body mass below 10 kg.

Closed breathing systems

Closed breathing systems are systems in which the expired carbon dioxide is absorbed, usually by means of a soda lime canister. Because of the considerably lower fresh gas flows required, closed breathing systems are often used when anaesthetizing larger animals (body weight > 20–30 kg). The use of such breathing systems can pose considerable problems for the less experienced anaesthetist, and expert advice and assistance should be obtained before attempting to employ these techniques. The most widely used closed breathing system is the circle system (Figs. 1.23 and 1.24). In a circle system, two unidirectional valves control the flow of gas. These direct expired gases to pass through a soda lime canister, where carbon dioxide is absorbed, before the gases pass around the circuit, to be breathed in again by the animal.

When using a closed breathing system, it would be possible to supply only the animal's metabolic oxygen requirements (approximately $10 \times$ body weight$^{0.75}$, i.e. 6–9 mL/kg/min for a 3-kg animal) (Brody, 1945), but for practical reasons, it is more usual to operate the circle system as a low flow rather than completely closed system. Typically, fresh gas flows of 100 mL/kg/min are used for small animals (> 10 kg) and 20–30 mL/kg/min for larger animals. This represents a major advantage of circle systems in comparison with other breathing systems in controlling anaesthetic costs. The newer anaesthetic agents such

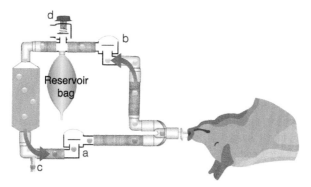

FIG. 1.23   Circle system to show gas flow patterns. Gases pass around the circuit directed by one way valves (a and b), a 'pop-off' valve (d) allows excess gas to escape. Exhaled gas containing carbon dioxide (*blue*) is absorbed by soda lime (es) before passing back around the circuit to the animal. Fresh gas is supplied from the anaesthetic machine (c).

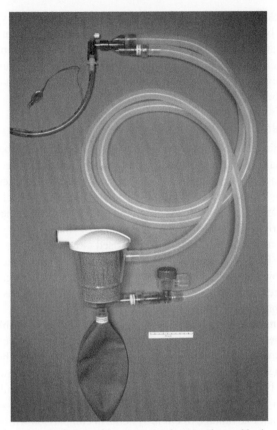

FIG. 1.24 Circle system. Both disposable systems (as shown) and re-usable circuits are available.

as sevoflurane are expensive, and in larger animals, the use of a closed system, where appropriate, can reduce costs very significantly (Appendix 2).

Although circle systems have been more frequently used for larger animals, the introduction of light-weight disposable systems with low-resistance valves has increased their use in smaller animals. Despite advances in breathing system construction, the system still offers more resistance to breathing than a T-piece or Bain breathing system, and it is advisable not to use these breathing systems on small (<5 kg) animals unless mechanical ventilation is used. As mentioned earlier, less experienced users are strongly advised to seek assistance before using closed breathing systems. Two important points should be noted. If nitrous oxide is used, the concentration of this gas can build up in the breathing system, resulting in a dangerously low concentration of oxygen. Either nitrous oxide should not be used, or an oxygen content monitor should be included in the breathing system. When using a closed breathing system, the concentration of volatile anaesthetic in the breathing system will not be the same as that shown by the vaporizer setting. This can result in a failure to maintain adequate depths of anaesthesia. As experience is gained, the vaporizer setting can be increased to compensate for the dilution of anaesthetic in the breathing system, and uptake by the animal. A more reliable technique is to purchase an anaesthetic gas analyser. The cost of these monitors has fallen considerably, and they simplify the use of rebreathing systems.

Besides economic considerations, another advantage of closed or low flow breathing systems is that heat and moisture are conserved. A detailed comparison of the advantages and disadvantages of rebreathing and nonrebreathing systems has been given by Brouwer and Snowdon (1986).

The diagram of the circle system in Fig. 1.23 has the vaporizer placed outside the main breathing system. In-circle vaporizers can also be used, and a full discussion of the relative merits of each arrangement can be found in standard veterinary anaesthesia texts (e.g. Grimm et al., 2015; Dugdale et al., 2020).

Breathing systems—Recommendations

Although open-mask techniques are best used only for short procedures in large animals, they may often be the most convenient system for small rodents, when the higher fresh gas flows required by these breathing systems will be of little significance. If nitrous oxide or volatile anaesthetic agents are used, the provision of effective gas scavenging is essential. For larger animals such as the cat, rabbit, and nonhuman primate, the advantage of lower fresh gas flow requirements, ease of gas scavenging and ability to assist ventilation favour the selection of a more sophisticated breathing system. If an Ayre's T-piece is used, it is strongly recommended that either a human paediatric model with a low dead space is obtained or one with similar features is constructed. The Bain breathing system offers several advantages for use in small animals, particularly in respect of its low weight and small dead space. The ease with which controlled ventilation can be carried out from a point remote from the surgical field is a further distinct advantage. In addition, it is suitable for use both in small animals such as guinea pigs and rabbits and in larger species such as pigs. The Magill and Lack breathing systems are not suitable for use in animals with a body mass of less than 10 kg, but it may be used as an alternative to the Bain breathing system in larger animals such as dogs, sheep, and pigs. Prolonged anaesthesia of larger animals (>10 kg), particularly when using relatively expensive agents such as sevoflurane, is best provided using a circle system. If an anaesthetic agent monitor is not available to measure the concentration of anaesthetic in the circuit, then rather than using a fully closed system, a moderate fresh gas flow of 500–1000 mL/min should be delivered, as this will simplify the use of the breathing system (see above).

All the commonly used anaesthetic breathing systems are now available as light-weight single-use items for human anaesthesia (Appendix 4). Many of these disposable systems can be re-used on numerous occasions without difficulty, but it is essential that a careful check is made of the condition of the system each time it is used. Ensure that any pressure-relief valves are functioning correctly and, when using a Bain breathing system, that the inner, fresh gas tube has not become disconnected at the anaesthetic machine end of the breathing system. Anaesthetic breathing systems and reservoir bags should be washed in hot soapy water and either pasteurized or rinsed with a chlorine disinfectant. Metal components can be autoclaved after washing.

Face masks

The face masks manufactured for veterinary use are cone shaped and will be found suitable for sheep, pigs, dogs, cats, and rabbits, provided the appropriate size is used. Face masks should fit snugly around the muzzle and must not obstruct the mouth or nose. If too large a mask is used, then the space around the animal's nose and mouth (the equipment dead space) may trap exhaled gas, high in carbon dioxide, and this may be rebreathed unless very high gas flows are used to remove it. However, since even the lowest flow that can be provided accurately by many anaesthetic machines are higher than those required by small rodents, most systems that use a face mask act as open systems and the dead space in the face mask becomes relatively unimportant.

A set of small, transparent masks fitted with flexible rubber diaphragms are useful for a range of animals and birds (Fig. 1.11). A mask design that incorporates a removal of waste anaesthetic gas to prevent exposure of the operator has been described (Hunter et al., 1984), and is available commercially (VetTech Solutions, Harvard Apparatus) (Fig. 1.12). Several alternative systems that combine gas scavenging with anaesthetic delivery are also available. Masks for small rodents that allow use of low flows of anaesthetic gases are also available (Figs. 1.13). Face masks should be cleaned after use by washing in warm soapy water, followed by drying. Most cannot be autoclaved, but some may be sterilized using ethylene oxide.

Delivering anaesthetic gases or oxygen using a face mask can cause practical difficulties, especially when anaesthetizing small rodents or birds. Masks can easily become displaced, and may interfere with access to the animal, for example, when carrying out surgery on the head or neck. Several techniques to prevent masks becoming displaced have been described. Fig. 1.25 illustrates one approach using an elastic band and the plastic mounts from a protective face mask. If an animal is placed in a stereotaxic frame, it becomes impossible to use a standard face mask, and a specialized mask must be purchased or constructed. These problems can be resolved by intubating the animal's trachea (see below), but this can be technically difficult. As an alternative, a catheter can be passed up one nostril and used to deliver anaesthetic gases (see below).

Endotracheal tubes

Endotracheal tubes are passed through the larynx into the trachea and are used to maintain a clear airway and enable breathing to be assisted if necessary. They

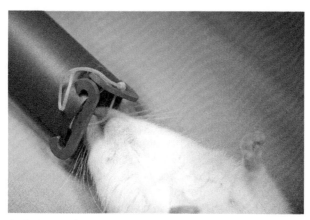

FIG. 1.25   Elastic band used to help maintain the position of a rat or mouse in a face mask. The attachment is made from the components of a protective face mask (Segre, Sweden) (concentric mask supplied by VetTech Solutions).

also protect the airway when the swallowing and coughing reflexes are sup-pressed, so that material such as saliva does not enter the trachea. Endotracheal tubes are available from many manufacturers and are provided either as plain tubes or with an inflatable cuff that seals the gap between the wall of the tube and the trachea (Fig. 1.26). The cuff can be inflated either with a syringe (2–5 mL) or with a specially designed inflator. The cuff is prevented from de-flating either by means of a nonreturn valve (present on most disposable tubes), by use if an attached stopper or by clamping with a pair of haemostats. Tubes may be reusable or be intended only for single use. Reusable tubes are generally constructed of rubber and are opaque. They deteriorate gradually, becoming brittle and easily kinked. The cuff often becomes distorted and may leak, so it is preferable to purchase single-use tubes and allow a limited amount of reuse. Clear polyethylene tubes have the advantage in that condensation appearing in the tube with each breath provides an immediate indication that the tube is

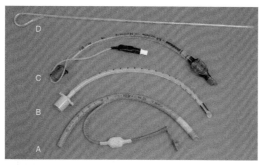

FIG. 1.26   Endotracheal tubes of different sizes and designs. (A) Re-usable cuffed tube, (B) dis-posable uncuffed tube, (C) disposable armoured, cuffed, tube and (D) introducer.

correctly positioned in the airway. Most commercially available tubes are excessively long for animal use, and they should be shortened to reduce unnecessary dead space. When animals are intubated and the head and neck are flexed excessively (e.g. when placed in some positions in a stereotaxic frame), there is a greater risk of the tube kinking. This can be prevented by using an armoured tube that is reinforced with a wire coil (Fig. 1.26C). Note that these types of tubes should not be used during an MRI examination.

Tubes should be inspected carefully before use to ensure they have not begun to deteriorate. The cuff should be inflated to make sure there are no tears and that it inflates evenly. They should be cleaned after use by washing in hot soapy water, then thoroughly rinsed and dried. If apparatus for pasteurization is available, tubes can be pasteurized. Some types do not withstand autoclaving, although some may be autoclaved a limited number of times at lower temperatures (121°C for 15 min) or sterilized using ethylene oxide. If ethylene oxide is used, it is critically important that all traces of the gas are eliminated before subsequent use of the tube. Since disposable tubes are readily available at low cost, if there are concerns relating to infection, then it is better simply to dispose of the tube. Endotracheal tubes suitable for use in small rodents and other small laboratory species can be purchased commercially but can also be constructed from 'over-the-needle' intravenous catheters (Fig. 1.27).

Endotracheal intubation

Endotracheal intubation of large animals such as dogs, sheep, pigs, old-world primates, and large birds (>1 kg) is relatively straightforward, provided a suitable size and shape of laryngoscope is available. Laryngoscopes are used to obtain a clear view of the larynx so that an endotracheal tube may be passed

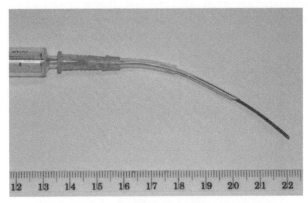

FIG. 1.27 Endotracheal tubes for rodents and other small mammals can be constructed from intravenous catheters. A small piece of Silastic tubing is placed approximately 1.5–2 cm from the tip, and acts as a seal on the larynx to reduce leakage of gas around the tube. A flexible wire (from a Seldinger catheter) is used to guide the tube into the trachea.

easily and atraumatically. A variety of designs are available commercially, and a list of recommended blades is given in Table 1.3 and illustrated in Fig. 1.28. The handle, besides usually containing the batteries, acts as a counterbalance to the blade. For this reason, it will be found most convenient to purchase handles of the appropriate size for each range of blade sizes. Replacement bulbs should also be purchased so that they are always available. After use, the handle should be separated from the blade and wiped clean. The blade should be washed in hot soapy water and dried thoroughly. A range of MacIntosh or Soper laryngoscope blades can be used for cats (size 1) and dogs (sizes 1–4) and a MacIntosh blade

TABLE 1.3 Endotracheal intubation, equipment required.

Species	Body weight	Endotracheal tube diameter	Laryngoscope
Cat	0.5–1.5 kg	2.0–3 mm O/D[a]	MacIntosh size 1
	>1.5 kg	3–4.5 mm O/D	
Dog	0.5–5 kg	2–5 mm O/D	MacIntosh size 1–4
	>5 kg	4.0–15 mm O/D	
Guinea pig	400–1000 g	16-12 G plastic catheter	Purpose-made laryngoscope[b]
			Otoscope
Hamster	120 g	0.9–1.5 mm—22-18 G plastic catheter	Purpose-made laryngoscope[b]
Mouse	25–35 g	0.7–0.9 mm—25-23 G plastic catheter	Purpose-made laryngoscope[b]
Primate	0.35–20 kg	2–8 mm O/D (or purpose-made tube for smallest animals)	MacIntosh or Wisconsin size 1–3
Pig	1–10 kg	2–6 mm O/D	Soper or Wisconsin size 1–4
	10–200 kg	6–15 mm O/D	
Rabbit	1–3 kg	2–3 mm O/D	Wisconsin size 0–1 or otoscope
	3–7 kg	3–6 mm O/D	
Rat	200–400 g	1.3–2.4 mm—18-14 G plastic catheter	Purpose-made laryngoscope[b]
			Otoscope
Sheep	10–90 kg	5–15 mm O/D	MacIntosh size 2–4

[a] O/D, outside diameter.
[b] See text.

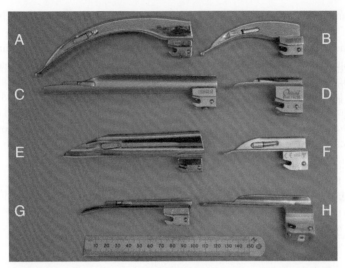

FIG. 1.28 Laryngoscope blades of various designs. Macintosh (A, B), Wisconsin (C, D), Soper (E, F) and Miller (G, H).

(sizes 2–4) for sheep. When anaesthetizing pigs, Soper (sizes 1–3) or Wisconsin (sizes 1–4) blades are preferable, although large pigs may require the use of a purpose-made laryngoscope blade. Rabbits can be successfully intubated using a Wisconsin blade (size 1 or 0) (Table 1.3).

If intubation of a particular species is planned, a careful examination of the pharynx and the larynx should first be carried out on a postmortem specimen. This will enable an appreciation of the anatomical relationships within this area, particularly that of the soft palate and the epiglottis. Once the normal anatomy of the region has been reviewed, a suitable-sized endotracheal tube should be prepared. Most commercially available tubes are excessively long; therefore, their length should be reduced so that it approximates to the distance from the external nares to just anterior to the thoracic inlet. If a small (<4 mm outside diameter) tube is to be used, an uncuffed tube is preferable, as this enables the largest possible diameter tube to be passed. It is advisable to lubricate the tube with a small quantity of lidocaine gel.

The animal should be anaesthetized to a sufficient depth to abolish the cough and swallowing reflexes. It is possible to intubate lightly anaesthetized animals, but while this may be desirable under some circumstances, it is advisable to gain some proficiency in the technique of intubation before attempting this. Before intubating any animal, oxygen should be administered for approximately 2 min. If the larynx is inadvertently obstructed during attempted intubation, it will usually take over 60 s for hypoxia to develop if the animal has been breathing oxygen. If the animal has been breathing air, hypoxia will develop much more rapidly.

Dog, cat, and sheep

The animal is placed in sternal recumbency, with its jaws opened as widely as possible by an assistant. The tongue is drawn forwards and the laryngoscope advanced over the tongue towards the pharynx. The larynx is usually masked by the epiglottis. Gentle upward pressure on the soft palate with the end of the endotracheal tube will disengage the epiglottis, allowing it to fall forwards, providing an unobstructed view of the larynx. In cats and sheep, the larynx should be sprayed with a local anaesthetic, to prevent laryngospasm. Disposable 'insulin' syringes with a preattached 25-SWG (Standard Wire Gauge) needle, with the needle bevel cut off, are ideal. The endotracheal tube can then be advanced through the larynx into the trachea. Then the tube should be connected to the anaesthetic breathing system, the cuff (if present) inflated, and the tube tied in place to the animal's jaw, using a 1-cm-wide cotton tape. It is preferable at this stage to assist ventilation (as described earlier) and observe that there is movement of both sides of the thorax. This ensures that the tube has not been inadvertently positioned in one of the two mainstem bronchi. In addition, manual inflation of the chest will enable an appreciation of the degree of resistance to gas flow. Increased resistance may indicate twisting or kinking of the tube, or its partial obstruction due to positioning close to the bifurcation of the trachea. If any uncertainty exists about tube placement, use a stethoscope to check that breath sounds can be heard on both sides of the thorax.

Pig

Intubation in the pig is complicated by the difficulty of obtaining an unobstructed view of the larynx. The animal is best positioned on its back or chest, with the ventro-dorsal position reported to allow most rapid intubation (Theisen et al., 2009). As with other species, care must be taken when the tongue is extended to avoid damaging its surface on the teeth, particularly the canines in boars. Intubation is easier if an introducer is used (Fig. 1.26D). This is a blunt stilette that is placed inside the tube to straighten it and make it easier to direct into the larynx. Introducers can be purchased commercially (Portex, Smiths Medical International, Appendix 4), and this ensures that the tip is soft and atraumatic.

The laryngoscope is advanced over the tongue and the epiglottis disengaged from the soft palate, if necessary, by pushing on the soft palate using the tip of the introducer. Once the larynx has been located, it should be sprayed with lidocaine. The introducer and the endotracheal tube can then be gently advanced into the larynx and the introducer withdrawn. The tube should then be gently advanced; at this stage, its progress is usually arrested by the laryngeal wall. If this occurs, the tube should be withdrawn very slightly, rotated through 90 degrees and reinserted. This should be repeated as necessary until no resistance is experienced. Under no circumstances should attempts be made to pass the tube forcibly through the larynx, as this is likely to result in severe trauma, oedema, haemorrhage, and consequent asphyxiation.

Rabbit

Visualization of the larynx in the rabbit is difficult, and it is necessary to use a purpose-designed laryngoscope blade, a Wisconsin laryngoscope blade (2- to 5-kg animal, size 1; 1- to 2-kg animal, size 0) or an otoscope if intubation is to be carried out under direct vision.

Intubation using an otoscope or laryngoscope: The rabbit is positioned on its back as shown (Fig. 1.29). To view the larynx, the tongue is gently grasped and pulled forwards and to one side, taking care to avoid the sharp edges of the incisor teeth. The otoscope or laryngoscope is introduced into the mouth and advanced until the larynx is visible. It is possible to advance the instrument into the oesophagus if the tip of the epiglottis is positioned on the nasal aspect of the soft palate. To avoid this, the soft palate can be pushed with the otoscope or laryngoscope tip, or the introducer can be passed down the otoscope and pushed against the soft palate to reposition it and provide a clear view of the larynx.

As the speculum is advanced, the paler triangle of the epiglottis can often be seen through the end of the soft palate, alerting the anaesthetist to the need to manipulate the structure. In many cases, the larynx is immediately clearly visible. At this point, the larynx can be sprayed with lidocaine, although this is often unnecessary. An introducer can now be passed through the otoscope into the larynx and on into the trachea. If a purpose-made introducer is not available, then a bitch or cat urinary catheter can be used, depending upon the size of the rabbit. If a catheter is used, then the Luer fitting should be removed before use, since this will not pass through the tip of the otoscope. After placing the introducer, the otoscope or laryngoscope is removed, taking care not to change the position of the introducer. An endotracheal tube (2.5–3 mm for 2- to 3-kg rabbits) is then threaded onto the end of the introducer and advanced into the trachea. When the endotracheal tube reaches the larynx, some resistance is often felt. Gently rotating the tube as it is advanced may ease its passage into the

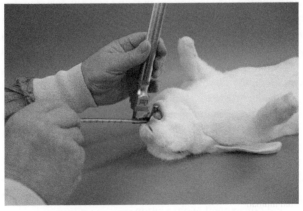

FIG. 1.29   Intubation of the rabbit by using a laryngoscope with a modified Wisconsin blade.

trachea. Prior application of lubricating gel (e.g. lidocaine gel) can also aid the passage of the tube. Take care at this stage not to remove the introducer until the tube is in the trachea, or intubation will be unsuccessful. As the tube is advanced further into the trachea, the introducer is removed, and the tube tied in place.

'Blind' intubation: An alternative technique for intubation does not require visualization of the larynx. The rabbit is placed in sternal recumbency, and the head gripped firmly and extended, and the animal lifted so that its forelegs are just touching the operating table (Fig. 1.30). The endotracheal tube is advanced through the gap between the incisors and the premolars, over the tongue and towards the larynx. The operator listens for breath sounds at the end of the tube or alternatively, if a clear polyethylene tube is used, looks for the presence of condensation. A loud breath sound or condensation indicates that the tube tip is close to the larynx. As the rabbit breathes in, the tube is gently advanced. If it fails to enter the larynx, as indicated by cessation of breath sounds and loss of condensation, then the tube is withdrawn, the head repositioned either by tilting it further backwards or slightly forwards and another attempt made. Giving a quarter turn to the endotracheal tube as it enters the larynx can help its passage.

In some instances, intubation can be eased by use of a local anaesthetic spray. This can be delivered onto the larynx by positioning the endotracheal tube at the point of maximal breath sounds, and then spraying lidocaine into the end of the tube or injecting a small (0.1 mL) quantity of lidocaine into the end of the tube. The local anaesthetic is drawn down the tube as the rabbit inhales, and some reaches the larynx. After waiting a minute or two to allow the drug to act, another attempt at intubation can be made. If problems arise, oxygen should be administered every 2–3 min to ensure the animal does not become hypoxic.

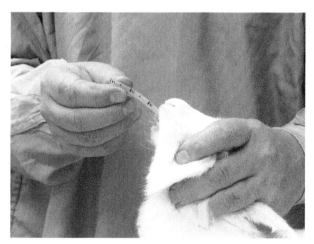

FIG. 1.30 Blind intubation of a rabbit. Listening to the animal's breathing as the tube is advanced aids correct placement.

Although this technique sounds challenging, it is relatively easy to become proficient and has the advantage of requiring no additional equipment. In small rabbits (<1 kg), it is not always possible to hear breath sounds or observe condensation in the small endotracheal tube (2–2.5 mm) that is needed. For this reason, it is best to intubate larger rabbits when first attempting this technique.

With both techniques, the confirmation of successful placement is based on observing condensation of breath on a cold surface (e.g. the end of the otoscope handle), or movement of a piece of tissue paper placed at the end of the tube. Alternatively, as in other species, a capnograph can be attached to confirm the tube is in the trachea.

Rat

Intubation of the rat is possible using a number of different purpose-made intubation devices (e.g. Costa et al., 1986) or using an otoscope. The rat is positioned on its back, and the tongue pulled gently forward and to one side. The laryngoscope or otoscope is then inserted until the larynx can be visualized. The animal can then be intubated using a suitably sized (14-18 G) arterial cannula (e.g. Abbocath, Abbott Laboratories). Some modification of the Luer fitting is needed to provide connections to an appropriate anaesthetic breathing system, and care must be taken to ensure that these connectors introduce only a minimum of dead space into the breathing system. To avoid inadvertent intubation of one bronchus, and to provide a seal around the larynx, a small piece of rubber tubing can be positioned around the catheter, about 0.75–1 cm from the tip. Alternatively, some 'Micropore' tape (3M) can be applied to make a similar cuff. This will reduce the leakage of gas around the tube, making ventilation more effective, and will also improve the efficacy of positive end expiratory pressure (PEEP) if this is required. A final modification that can be helpful is to superglue a silk ligature onto the base of the Luer mount of the catheter, to enable it to be anchored to the rat's jaw.

When using an otoscope, it is necessary to use an introducer, since the cannula will not pass through the lumen of the otoscope. A guide wire from a Seldinger catheter makes an ideal introducer since its tip is soft and flexible. The wire is passed through the otoscope and through the larynx under direct vision, the otoscope carefully removed, and the endotracheal tube threaded over the wire into the trachea. These wires can be purchased separately, and a 0.7-mm-diameter wire will fit through both 16- and 18-gauge catheters. Alternatively, the neck may be transilluminated using a powerful light source and the mouth opened using a small gag. The tongue is pulled forwards and a bright spot of light seen, which flashes as the rat breathes; this indicates the opening of the larynx.

A final option is to purchase one of the commercially available systems that usually combine a small table for positioning the animal with a system for visualizing the larynx. The apparatus shown (Figs. 1.31 and 1.32) can be used for intubation of both rats and mice. An alternative approach using a fibre optic

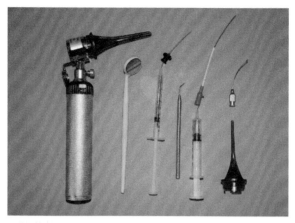

FIG. 1.31   Apparatus for intubation of rats and mice, available from Hallowell instruments.

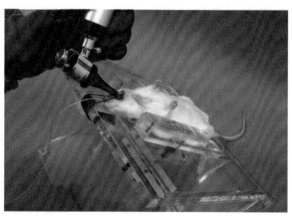

FIG. 1.32   Rat positioned for intubation. (Tilting table and modified otoscope from Hallowell instruments.) Oxygen is being supplied through a nasal catheter during the procedure.

system has also been described (Rivera et al., 2005), and a commercially produced instrument is also available (Fig. 1.33).

Guinea pig, mouse, gerbil, and hamster

Intubation of the mouse, gerbil, and hamster is more difficult than in larger species and requires especial skill and purpose-made apparatus (Hamacher et al., 2008). A suitable set of laryngoscope blades has been described by Costa et al. (1986), and the apparatus shown in Figs. 1.31 and 1.32 can be used in mice and other small rodents. The guinea pig can also be intubated using a purpose-designed laryngoscope blade, or the technique employing an otoscope, as described above for the rat. As with the rat, the use of an otoscope in combination with transillumination of the neck provides optimal conditions for intubation.

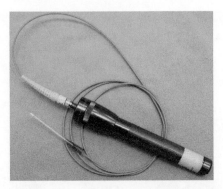

FIG. 1.33 Fibreoptic system for illuminating the larynx during intubation. An intravenous catheter which will be used as the endotracheal tube has been placed over the tip of the illuminated guide (Kent Scientific).

Positioning of the otoscope is more difficult in the guinea pig than in the rat, and a narrow speculum is needed to pass between the cheek teeth. The pharynx narrows markedly at the junction of larynx with the oesophagus, and considerable care must be taken to avoid inserting the speculum too far and occluding the larynx. As with the rat, intubation is achieved by passing a Seldinger guide wire through the larynx, removing the otoscope and then passing a 12- to 16-gauge catheter over the wire into the trachea.

Birds

Intubation of birds is relatively simple, since the opening to the airway is positioned much further forwards, compared to mammals. Opening the beak enables the opening to be seen at the base of the tongue. Intubation is assisted by pulling the tongue forwards. Larger birds (poultry) can be intubated using standard paediatric tubes (2.5 mm upwards), but small birds require the use of either intravenous or urinary catheters cut to a suitable length as necessary. Uncuffed endotracheal tubes should always be used, since it has been suggested that the use of cuffed tubes can cause pressure necrosis of the tracheal mucosa because of the presence of complete tracheal cartilage rings in these species (Briscoe and Syring, 2004).

Intranasal intubation

Placement of a catheter in one nostril allows delivery of oxygen or anaesthetic gases and can be a useful alternative to a face mask, for example, when using a stereotaxic frame. A variety of catheters can be used, including vascular catheters, nasogastric feeding tubes, flexible oral-dosing catheters, and urinary bladder catheters (Fig. 1.34). The catheter should be lubricated before insertion and, in most species, should be directed medially and ventrally. The nostrils of most small animals are surrounded by muscle, and this restricts the diameter of the nasal opening, but gentle pressure from

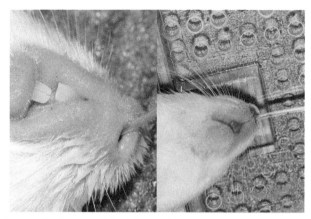

FIG. 1.34 Intranasal catheters used for delivery of anaesthetic agents or oxygen (guinea pig, left, with cat urinary catheter; rat, right, with paediatric nasogastric tube).

the catheter tip will usually dilate the nostril slightly, allowing passage of the catheter. Slight rotation of the catheter can aid insertion. The diameter of the passage through the nasal chamber is often significantly larger than the external nasal opening. Occasionally, there may be slight trauma to the nasal mucosa, resulting in a small amount of haemorrhage, but this is usually minor and stops rapidly.

The fresh gas flows needed are similar to those when using a face mask, approximately three times the animals' minute volume. Some air will be drawn in through the other nostril, and this will dilute the supplied gas. However, increasing the vaporizer setting (e.g. by 0.5%–1% when using isoflurane) will compensate for this. Gas scavenging can be accomplished using a down-draft table. The catheter can be connected to the anaesthetic machine using a Luer adapter and oxygen bubble tubing (Fig. 1.35). This tubing is extremely useful for adapting anaesthetic breathing systems, as its internal diameter varies along its length from 3 to 8 mm, allowing it to be cut at a convenient point to connect different-sized connectors.

Laryngeal masks

As an alternative to endotracheal intubation, a laryngeal mask (Fig. 1.36) can be used to maintain a patent airway and assist ventilation if required. These masks are designed to slide into the mouth and to be positioned over the larynx. The large cuff is then inflated to seal them in place. Laryngeal masks are produced to fit a human larynx, but the anatomy of some species is sufficiently similar to allow them to be used successfully (Wemyss-Holden et al., 1999). In rabbits and pigs, the use of a laryngeal mask has been reported to be more easily mastered by inexperienced anaesthetists than intubation, and to provide effective control of the rabbit's airway (Fulkerson and Gustafson, 2007).

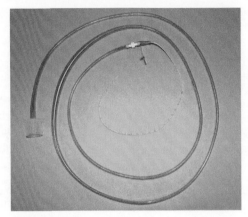

FIG. 1.35   Oxygen bubble tubing used for connecting a nasal catheter to an anaesthetic trolley, for delivery of oxygen or anaesthetic agents.

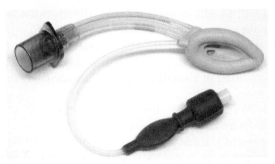

FIG. 1.36   Laryngeal mask

V-gel airways

An alternative airway management system has been introduced into veterinary clinical practice, the 'V-gel' airway. The device has a soft, noninflatable cuff that rests over the larynx, and is claimed to be easier to place than a laryngeal mask and to cause less tracheal mucosal damage than an endotracheal tube (Oostrom et al., 2013; Uzun et al., 2015). The devices are marketed for cats and rabbits.

Administration of anaesthetics by injection

Equipment

Although the equipment required for injection of anaesthetics consists basically of a syringe and a needle, some attention should be given to the range of syringe and needle sizes available and to the use of indwelling catheters, cannulae, extension tubing, and infusion devices.

Syringes

Plastic disposable syringes are almost universally used for delivering anaesthetics. These single-use syringes should not be resterilized for further use. Ensure that an appropriate-volume syringe is used so that the required dose of anaesthetic can be administered accurately. The syringes designed for insulin administration to human patients are particularly useful for administering small doses of drugs to rodents (Fig. 1.37). Select a syringe design that is comfortable to hold and that enables a firm grip to be maintained even when the barrel is wet. Avoid using syringes that have been stored for a length of time that exceeds the period recommended by the manufacturers, as the plastic may have become brittle and can fracture during use.

Needles and cannulae

Disposable hypodermic needles should be used, and an appropriate gauge selected for each purpose. Needles should never be resterilized, as they rapidly become blunt when used and injection with a blunt needle can cause considerable discomfort. Successful venepuncture of small vessels is particularly difficult to achieve if the needle has been blunted. For this reason, it is advisable to replace the needle after drawing up liquid from a rubber-capped vial.

Often it is preferable to use a butterfly type infusion set, rather than a simple hypodermic needle. These infusion devices provide a short length of flexible catheter between the needle and the syringe so that movements of the animal during injection are less likely to result in the needle becoming dislodged from the vein (Fig. 1.37). This is particularly important when inducing anaesthesia with short-acting anaesthetic agents since the administration of an inadequate dose of drug may produce involuntary excitement. If the ensuing limb movements result in displacement of the needle from the vein, its replacement may be virtually impossible.

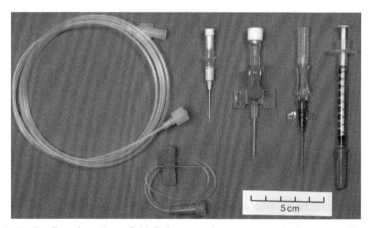

FIG. 1.37   Insulin syringe, 'butterfly' infusion set, catheters and anaesthetic extension line.

Even more useful for intravenous induction are indwelling catheters since these enable successive intravenous injections of anaesthetics and other drugs to be made easily and reliably. A flexible catheter will not pierce the vessel wall should movements of the animal occur, so accidental extravascular injection will be avoided. Several types of catheters are available, but they can be broadly grouped as 'over-the-needle' designs in which the flexible catheter is placed on the outside of a needle which acts as an introducer and 'through-the-needle' designs in which the catheter runs through the needle. A further variation that is often used for placing catheters in deeper vessels, or for placing larger catheters, is 'over-the-wire' designs. A needle is placed into the blood vessel, and a flexible wire passed down the needle into the vessel. The needle is then withdrawn, and the catheter threaded along the wire and into the vessel. The wire is then withdrawn.

In most circumstances, 'over-the-needle' catheters are preferable for use in small animals since they allow the largest possible catheter to be inserted into the vessel (Fig. 1.37). In large animals, the skin may offer significant resistance to passage of the catheter and may damage an 'over-the-needle' type, but this does not occur when using a 'through-the-needle' design. An alternative solution is to make a very small skin incision with a scalpel blade to allow easy passage of an 'over-the-needle' catheter.

Simple 'over-the-needle' catheters are relatively inexpensive, and the advantages of maintaining a secure route for intravenous drug administration can be considerable. In addition to the administration of anaesthetics, other drugs and intravenous fluids can be administered rapidly, even by relatively unskilled assistants. It is important that the catheter is securely anchored in place. This can be achieved as illustrated in Fig. 1.38. When anchoring catheters in the marginal ear vein in species such as the rabbit or sheep, it is helpful to cut off one wing to reduce the risk of dislodging the catheter (Fig. 1.38).

Extension lines

It is often inconvenient to require access to the catheter site for repeated drug administration, and this can be avoided by using a plastic tubing of suitable length (Fig. 1.37). Extension lines that are equipped with a Luer-locking fitting are preferable, as they are less likely to become disconnected. A problem with many of the extension lines produced for human use is their large volume, which can cause problems if different drugs are to be administered successively to a small animal. It is often undesirable to administer a bolus of 4–5 mL of saline to a small animal to flush an infusion line. Small-volume extension lines (<1 mL) are available from Vygon Ltd. (Appendix 4). A useful compromise is to select an indwelling catheter with a side-injection port (Fig. 1.38). Routine infusion of anaesthetic can be carried out through an extension line and administration of other drugs through the side-injection port. Extension lines are also useful when administering large volumes of drugs by the intramuscular route to larger animals such as pigs. Use of an extension between the needle and the

a

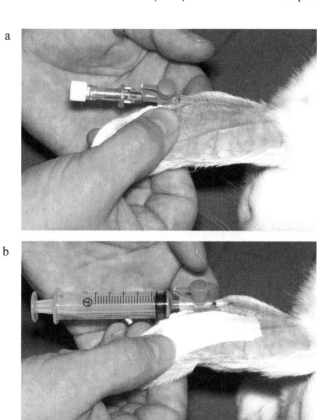

b

c

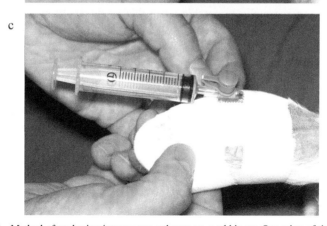

FIG. 1.38   Method of anchoring intravenous catheters on a rabbit ear. One wing of the catheter is removed (a), a piece of tape is laid along the ear across the remaining wing (b) and two further pieces of tape are wrapped around the ear (c).

syringe enables placement of the needle, followed by controlled injection without the need to restrain the animal.

Infusion pumps

It is often convenient to administer intravenous anaesthetics by continuous infusion. A range of infusion pumps is available commercially, and the cost of sophisticated microprocessor-controlled models has fallen rapidly. Pumps designed for clinical use in humans generally operate using a 50-ml syringe. Although this syringe size is somewhat excessive for use in small animals, the rate at which drugs can be delivered can be as little as 0.1 mL/h.

Smaller volume pumps, particularly those designed for insulin infusion, are suitable for use in small animals. Purpose-designed infusion pumps that allow the use of different syringe sizes are more versatile and are a worthwhile investment if total intravenous anaesthesia is to be employed.

If an infusion pump is not available, drugs can be administered using an intravenous infusion set and a burette to allow better control over the volumes administered. The use of such gravity feed devices has the obvious disadvantage that changes in the position of the cannula, or movements of the limb, can greatly affect the infusion rate. Nevertheless, such simple devices can be used successfully, particularly if a central venous cannula, which is less susceptible to occlusion, is used. Further details of infusion techniques and equipment are given in Chapter 4.

Routes of administration

Injectable anaesthetics can be administered by a variety of routes. Intravenous administration is usually preferable since this produces the most predictable and rapid onset of action. This enables the drug to be administered 'to effect' to provide the desired depth of anaesthesia. Practical considerations, such as the absence of suitable superficial veins or difficulty in providing adequate restraint of the animal, may limit the use of this route in some laboratory species. Administration by intramuscular, intraperitoneal, or subcutaneous injection is relatively straightforward in most species, but the rate of drug absorption and hence its anaesthetic effects may vary considerably. A relatively high failure rate has been reported with intraperitoneal dosing (Das and North, 2007; Laferriere and Pang, 2020), with injection of some of the anaesthetic into the viscera, fat, or the subcutaneous tissues. There is also a very great variation in response to anaesthetics between different strains, ages, and sex of animals. The magnitude of these effects is illustrated with pentobarbital in mice in Fig. 1.39, but this variation must be anticipated in all species and with all anaesthetics. Similar major differences in response were noted with ketamine/medetomidine in response between male and female animals (Cruz et al., 1998), and similar effects have been observed with other anaesthetics in other species, including humans (Ciccone and Holdcroft, 1999). When using an anaesthetic technique for the

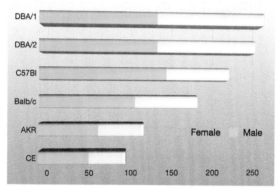

FIG. 1.39 Sleep time (min) in different strains of mice given pentobarbital. *(Data redrawn from Lovell, D.P., 1986. Variation in pentobarbitone sleeping time in mice. 2. Variables affecting test results. Lab. Anim. 20 (2), 91–96; Lovell, D.P., 1986. Variation in pentobarbitone sleeping time in mice. 1. Strain and sex differences. Lab. Anim. 20 (2), 85–90.)*

first time, it is essential to assess its effects on one animal, before beginning to anaesthetize the remainder of the group. This will enable the recommended doses to be adjusted to suit the responses of the particular animals being used. As mentioned above, this variability in response can be a particular problem in small rodents, since most injectable anaesthetics are administered to these species by the intraperitoneal route as a single dose. When administering anaesthetics in this way, it is impossible to adjust the dose according to the individual animal's response, so accidental over- and under-dosing will frequently occur, until experience is gained with a particular strain, age and sex of the animal. Variation in response to anaesthetics, administered by any route, also occurs with changes in environmental factors. Standardization of all these variables will not only simplify anaesthetic dose calculations but also constitute good experimental designs. When selecting anaesthetics for intramuscular, intraperitoneal or subcutaneous administration, it is also advisable to select those that have a wide safety margin.

A further disadvantage of the intraperitoneal, subcutaneous, or intramuscular routes is that relatively large doses of anaesthetic must be given to produce the required effect. Absorption is slow relative to intravenous administration; residual drug effects can persist for prolonged periods and so full recovery can be very prolonged (Fig. 1.40).

An additional consideration with intramuscular or subcutaneous injection is that administration of an irritant compound can cause unnecessary pain or discomfort to the animal. This is a particular concern with intramuscular injection in small rodents. The problem often arises because commercial formulations of anaesthetics (e.g. ketamine) are designed to provide a convenient volume for injection into a particular species (e.g. cats). Small rodents require very much higher dose rates of some anaesthetics per unit of body mass than do larger

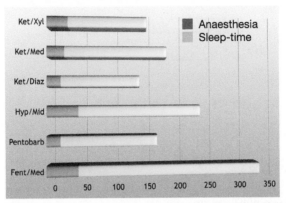

FIG. 1.40 Duration of anaesthesia and sleep time (min) in rats with different anaesthetics. *Ket/Xyl*, ketamine and xylazine; *Ket/Med*, ketamine and medetomidine; *Ket/Diaz*, ketamine and diazepam; *Hyp/Mid*, hypnorm and midazolam; *Pentobarb*, pentobarbital; *Fent/Med*, fentanyl and medetomidine. Sleep times can be reduced for some anaesthetic regimens by use of specific antagonists (see text). *(Data from various studies.)*

species, for example, 75 mg/kg ketamine in rats compared to 10 mg/kg in a non-human primate. Since the concentration of the agent is fixed, this results in a major increase in the volume given—0.75 mL/kg in rats compared to 0.1 mL/kg in a primate in the example given. Not surprisingly, there are a number of reports of tissue reactions and myositis following anaesthetic administration in small mammals (Smiler et al., 1990; Beyers et al., 1991). For this reason, it is recommended that the intramuscular route is avoided in small rodents.

Intravenous administration avoids the problems discussed above, and the technical problems associated with intravenous injection in small mammals are often more imagined than real. Research workers may avoid intravenous anaesthesia and yet administer other compounds by the intravenous route as part of their research protocol. Before discounting intravenous administration, consider whether the necessary expertise is already available, or if developing this expertise would be worthwhile. In rats, for example, placement of an 'over-the-needle' catheter allows both intravenous anaesthesia and administration of other drugs and fluids as necessary. Several short-acting anaesthetics can be used to provide 5- to 10-min periods of anaesthesia (see Chapter 2), and some are suitable for continuous infusion to provide long-term anaesthesia. When carrying out venepuncture in animals, consider using a local anaesthetic cream (e.g. EMLA cream, Astra) to produce local anaesthesia of the skin.

Preparations for anaesthesia—People and animals

Personnel

If personnel are allocated to assist with anaesthesia, check that they have been properly briefed about the research protocol and are familiar with the equipment and techniques to be used. Ensure that they are aware of the time for which they are required, including attendance for postoperative observation and care, which may be outside the normal working day.

Animals

The single most important factor that can reduce the risks associated with anaesthesia is the use of animals of high health status. It is most important to ensure that any animal that is to be anaesthetized is at least in overt good health and free from clinical disease. Whenever possible, animals of defined health status should be obtained so that the occurrence of respiratory and other diseases can be eliminated. Anaesthetizing animals that have spontaneous disease, even if it causes no overt clinical signs, usually results in increased mortality and morbidity. Aside from the wasted resources and animal welfare implications, spontaneous disease increases variability in research data and so requires use of a larger number of animals to detect significant differences between different treatment groups.

Acclimatization

Animals should be obtained at least 7 and preferably 14 days before their intended use, so that an appropriate period is allowed for acclimatization to their new environment. Requirements vary in different establishments, and research workers should check on local practices. During this period, the metabolic and hormonal changes caused by the stress of transportation will return to normal (Obernier and Baldwin, 2006), and the animal can be monitored for any signs of ill health. Animal care staff and research workers will have the opportunity to familiarize themselves with the behaviour and characteristics of the particular group of animals, and body weight, growth rate, and food and water consumption can be recorded. This information is invaluable if animals are intended to recover from anaesthesia after undergoing a surgical procedure. Many of the pain assessment schemes that are under development rely on knowledge of these variables, and it is important that such information is obtained and recorded (see Chapter 5). Even when planning nonrecovery procedures, an assessment of food and water intake or growth rate will provide some reassurance that the animal is in a normal physiological state.

Acclimatization of species that can rapidly develop a relationship with their handler (e.g. dogs, cats, and pigs) has the advantage of reducing avoidable distress during induction and recovery from anaesthesia. Regular handling of most species, including small rodents, will habituate the animals to the procedure. Consequently, the animals will be easier to restrain and more co-operative, and induction of anaesthesia will be safer for both the animals and the staff involved (Krall et al., 2019).

If animals are to be housed singly after a surgical procedure, it is preferable to acclimatize them to this environment beforehand. This will allow them to adapt to the stress of social isolation (Hurst et al., 1998) and therefore be better able to cope with the stress of anaesthesia and surgery. It will also allow assessment of their normal behaviour when housed singly. Reduction of postoperative stress and anxiety can contribute to pain management, and this is discussed in more detail in Chapter 5.

Clinical examination

Whatever the health status of the animal, a general clinical examination should be carried out before induction of anaesthesia. Although many investigators may not be familiar with signs of disease or ill health in animals, they are often very familiar with the behaviour and appearance of normal animals. If there is any deviation from the normal, further advice can be sought from experienced animal technicians and veterinarians. The presence of discharges from the eyes or nose, matting of the fur around these regions, or soiling of the perianal region with faeces requires further investigation. If the overall appearance of the animal is abnormal or any of the clinical signs mentioned is present, anaesthesia should be delayed until expert advice is obtained. As mentioned above, it is helpful to monitor food and water intake and body weight for a few days preoperatively. This will allow assessment that the intake is normal and will be of use in monitoring the postoperative recovery of the animal.

Preanaesthetic fasting

Cats, dogs, ferrets, primates, and pigs should receive no food during the 8–12 h before anaesthesia to minimize the risk of vomiting during induction of anaesthesia or during recovery. Withholding food from ruminants has virtually no effect on the volume of ingesta that remain in the rumen, unless excessive periods of starvation are employed (3–4 days), but a short period of starvation (12–24 h) may help reduce the incidence of ruminal tympany or bloat (the accumulation of gas in the stomach).

Preanaesthetic fasting of rabbits and small rodents is unnecessary since vomiting during induction does not occur in these species. Problems may occasionally be seen with guinea pigs since they may retain food in their pharynx after being anaesthetized. If this occurs in a significant number of animals, then a short period of preanaesthetic fasting (3–4 h) should be introduced. It has been claimed that fasting helps in accurate anaesthetic dosing in rabbits and guinea pigs. This might have been relevant when anaesthetics with a narrow therapeutic margin (i.e. the anaesthetic dose is close to the lethal dose, e.g. pentobarbital) were in use, but is less important when more modern agents are used. It is also important to note that rabbits and guinea pigs are particularly susceptible to gastrointestinal disturbances following surgery. This can lead to serious consequences as it can predispose to the development of enterotoxaemia. For this reason, the author almost never withholds food from these species. An exception is if gastrointestinal tract surgery is to be undertaken and a reduction in the volume of gut contents is required. In these circumstances, fasting may be required in all species, but it is important to note that rodents and rabbits are coprophagic, so measures to prevent them ingesting their faeces may be necessary to provide a completely empty stomach.

An additional complication arises because of the diurnal rhythms of some species. Although food may be provided immediately postoperatively, it may not be eaten until the onset of the dark phase of the animal's photoperiod. In addition, if the animal's appetite is depressed because of pain, surgical stress, or delayed recovery from anaesthesia, food and water intake may be severely depressed for at least 24 h postoperatively. The metabolic consequences of this, especially when coupled with preoperative fasting, can be severe and can compromise both the research data obtained and animal welfare. It is therefore preferable to withhold food only when required by a particular research protocol. If a short period of fasting is needed, this can be achieved by providing a limited amount of food in the food hopper. Rodents don't plan ahead and will eat normally until the food is exhausted, so food can be withdrawn for part of the night, without the need for attendance by animal care staff.

Withholding food from pregnant animals of all species, but especially in ruminants and guinea pigs, can produce severe metabolic disturbances that may prove fatal. Large or medium-sized birds (e.g. ducks, chickens, pigeons) may be fasted for 6–12 h to reduce the risk of regurgitation of the contents of the crop. Smaller birds should not be fasted for longer than 2 h to avoid the risk of inducing hypoglycaemia. Fasting of reptiles, amphibians, and fish is generally unnecessary.

All animals should be provided with drinking water until approximately 60 min before induction of anaesthesia. If the animal has a reduced fluid intake, or if vomiting, diarrhoea, or haemorrhage has occurred, then some preoperative fluid therapy will be necessary. The basic principles are outlined in Chapter 3, but whenever possible veterinary advice should be obtained. Whenever practicable, animals should be weighed before anaesthesia, both to allow accurate calculation of drug dosages and to enable assessment of any postoperative weight loss.

Chapter 2

Anaesthetic and analgesic agents

Preanaesthetic agents

Preanaesthetic medication is often included in anaesthetic protocols for larger species. The advantages of this are

- Administering sedatives or tranquillizers can reduce aggression and fear or apprehension and aid stress-free induction of anaesthesia.
- Use of analgesics can reduce pain, especially in the immediate postoperative period, and may provide more effective pain relief through 'preemptive analgesia' (see Chapter 5).
- Atropine or glycopyrrolate can be given to reduce bronchial and salivary secretions and to protect the heart from vagal inhibition caused by some procedures (e.g., endotracheal intubation, manipulation of the viscera during surgery). It is advisable to use glycopyrrolate in rabbits, as atropine is often relatively ineffective in this species (Harrison et al., 2006).
- Use of sedatives, tranquillizers, and analgesics can reduce the amount of anaesthetic needed to produce the desired level of anaesthesia. These agents also provide smoother induction of anaesthesia and a smoother recovery.

Although the advantages listed above apply to all animal species, preanaesthetic medication is used most often in larger animals, where sedation and tranquillization are required to aid humane restraint and minimize the risk of injury to the animal and its handler. Preanaesthetic medication should be used in a wider range of species, since even when restraint is not a problem, the use of sedatives and tranquillizers may be advantageous. In humans, many of the drugs used have been shown to reduce fear and allay anxiety, and similar effects occur in animals. In addition to the use of drugs, careful and expert handling of laboratory animals is an essential part of their management before and after anaesthesia.

Consideration of the techniques used and their possible stressful effects upon the animal should enable modification of anaesthetic protocols to minimize pain or distress. For example, administration of a sedative/analgesic to an animal still housed in its pen or cage, followed by removal to the operating theatre or research laboratory only after the drug has taken effect, can considerably reduce the stress that might otherwise be caused.

Laboratory Animal Anaesthesia and Analgesia. https://doi.org/10.1016/B978-0-12-818268-0.00006-1

If an intravenous induction agent is to be used, then it is helpful to apply a local anaesthetic cream (e.g., EMLA, Astra) to the skin overlying the vein, about 30–60 min before intravenous injection. This eliminates the pain or discomfort of venepuncture and has the added advantage of eliminating any movement in response to the procedure, since the skin is completely anaesthetized (Flecknell et al., 1990b; Keating et al., 2012). The selection of a preanaesthetic drug regime will depend on the animal species to be anaesthetized; the anaesthetic agents to be used; the particular requirements of the research protocol; and the personal preferences of the anaesthetist. The characteristics of the major groups of drugs available are listed below, and more detailed recommendations for each species are given in Chapter 6.

Antimuscarinics (or anticholinergics)

Anticholinergics have been used primarily to reduce bronchial and salivary secretions, but current opinion is that this is rarely necessary with healthy laboratory animals and modern anaesthetic agents.

Atropine

Desirable effects: These include reduction of bronchial and salivary secretions that might partially occlude the airways. Atropine protects the heart from vagal inhibition, which can occur during endotracheal intubation or during surgical procedures, particularly if the viscera are handled. Atropine may also be used to correct any slowing of the heart caused by opioids such as fentanyl.

Undesirable effects: These include increased heart rate. In ruminants, atropine does not completely block salivary secretions, which become more viscous.

Special comments: Avoid the use of atropine if the heart rate is already elevated; also avoid if tachycardias are likely to be produced (e.g., during cardiac surgery). Atropine is rapidly metabolized in some strains of rabbits and so its effects may be unpredictable in this species (Harrison et al., 2006).

Glycopyrrolate

Desirable effects: These include reduction of salivary and bronchial secretions, protection of the heart from vagal inhibition.

Undesirable effects: These include increased heart rate, although less pronounced than atropine in some species.

Special comments: Glycopyrrolate has a longer duration of action than atropine and has been reported to be the more effective agent in rodents and rabbits (Olson et al., 1994). It is the antimuscarinic agent of choice in rabbits since its duration of action is less affected by the high levels of atropinase that may be present in this species. Glycopyrrolate does not cross the blood–brain barrier, and in people produces fewer visual disturbances than atropine. This may be advantageous in some animal species.

Tranquillizers and sedatives

Tranquillizers produce a calming effect without causing sedation. At high doses, they produce ataxia (lack of co-ordination), and animals become much less alert, but are readily roused, particularly in response to painful stimuli, since these drugs have no analgesic properties. Sedatives produce drowsiness and appear to reduce fear and apprehension in animals. There is considerable overlap in the action of many agents and a good deal of species variation in their effects, making definitive classification of drugs as either sedatives or tranquillizers difficult.

Phenothiazines: Chlorpromazine, acepromazine, and promazine

Desirable effects: These agents produce sedation; potentiate the action of anaesthetics, hypnotics (agents that produce sleep), opiates (morphine and morphine-like) analgesics; and so reduce the dose of these drugs required to produce surgical anaesthesia. Sedation may extend into the postoperative period, so that recovery from anaesthesia is smooth.

    Undesirable effects: Moderate hypotension (reduction in blood pressure) may occur because of dilatation of peripheral blood vessels. Temperature regulation is depressed and moderate falls in body temperature may occur.

    Special comments: The undesirable effects noted above are well tolerated by normal animals, but the drugs should not be used in animals with any form of fluid deficit, for example, dehydration or haemorrhage. This group of drugs has no analgesic action, but they potentiate the action of opiates.

Butyrophenones: Droperidol, fluanisone, and azaperone

Desirable effects: These drugs have effects similar to those of phenothiazines (above) but are more potent.

    Undesirable effects: The hypotensive effects of these drugs are generally less severe than those caused by phenothiazines.

    Special comments: Butyrophenones such as droperidol and fluanisone are most widely used as components of neuroleptanalgesic combinations (see below).

Benzodiazepines: Diazepam, and midazolam

Desirable effects: These include sedation, but there is considerable species variation in effect: sedation is very variable in dogs, but marked in rabbits, rodents, sheep, and pigs. Benzodiazepines potentiate the action of most anaesthetics and opioid (morphine-like) analgesics. They produce good skeletal muscle relaxation (NB: not muscle paralysis). A specific antagonist, flumazenil, is available, so that sedation can be reversed if necessary.

    Undesirable effects: In some species (dog and cat), benzodiazepines may cause mild excitement and disorientation rather than sedation. Injection of some preparations of diazepam into small blood vessels can cause irritation pain and damage to the vessel.

Special comments: Benzodiazepines (e.g., diazepam, midazolam) have both potent tranquillizing and sedative actions. Diazepam is the agent most frequently used, although some injectable formulations in organic solvents cannot be mixed with other water-soluble agents. An emulsion formulation of diazepam (Diazemuls, Pharmacia, and Upjohn) is not irritant to blood vessels and so avoids the problem mentioned above. Midazolam has effects similar to those of diazepam but has a shorter duration of action. Unlike diazepam, it is water soluble and so can be mixed with other agents (see below). The hypnotic (sleep-inducing) effects of these agents in animals, unlike humans, are generally minimal. When administered alone, benzodiazepines have a hyperalgesic effect in humans in some circumstances (i.e., they increase the degree of pain which is perceived). This may also occur in animals, so they should not be used for postoperative sedation unless effective analgesia is also provided, for example, by the administration of opioids.

Alpha-2-adrenergic agonist tranquillizers: Xylazine, medetomidine, and dexmedetomidine

Desirable effects: Xylazine and medetomidine are potent sedatives and are hypnotics in some species. Their analgesic effects vary in different species, but in most animals, mild to moderate analgesia is produced. Xylazine and medetomidine markedly potentiate the action of most anaesthetic drugs. Their action can be reversed by administration of specific antagonists such as yohimbine and atipamezole. Medetomidine is an equal mixture of two optical enantiomers, dexmedetomidine and levomedetomidine. Dexmedetomidine, the active component in this mixture, is now available as a veterinary product. The majority of studies utilizing this single enantiomer has so far been undertaken in companion and farm animals (Kästner et al., 2006); but data are becoming available in laboratory species (Franken et al., 2008). These studies indicate that, as would be predicted, it has double the potency of an equal dose of medetomidine. This suggests that it can be used at 50% of the medetomidine doses listed in Tables 6.3–6.26 in laboratory species (Burnside et al., 2013).

Undesirable effects: These drugs produce cardiovascular and respiratory depression, and when high doses are given, these side-effects can be significant. Cardiac arrhythmias may occur following administration of xylazine in some species. Xylazine may cause severe respiratory depression if administered in combination with barbiturates or alphaxalone. In species that vomit, medetomidine and xylazine often trigger this reflex. All of these agents produce a diuresis both due to inhibition of ADH and as a result of the production of marked hyperglycaemia (Greene and Thurmon, 1988; Saha et al., 2005). This can result in significant fluid loss in small rodents, especially during prolonged anaesthesia. These agents also depress thermoregulatory mechanisms. Xylazine can also cause temporary (Calderone et al., 1986) (Fig. 5.12) or permanent corneal injury in mice (Koehn et al., 2015) and rats (Turner and Albassam, 2005).

Special comments: Xylazine is a useful sedative in cattle, sheep, goats, horses, cats, and primates. It may also be a valuable (but relatively short acting) analgesic in sheep and goats (Grant and Upton, 2004). Xylazine, medetomidine, and dexmedetomidine should be used with caution in sheep, since they can produce severe hypoxia (Kästner, 2006; Kästner et al., 2007). The major use of xylazine in laboratory animal anaesthesia is in combination with ketamine to produce surgical anaesthesia (see below). Medetomidine and Dexmedetomidine have similar effects to xylazine, but are much more specific aplah-2 agonists and therefore have a lower incidence of side-effects (Virtanen et al., 1988a,b). They can be used to provide deep sedation with complete immobilization in many species, avoiding the need for general anaesthesia, and can be rapidly and completely reversed using the specific antagonist, atipamezole (Virtanen et al., 1988). Atipamezole is preferable for use as a reversing agent for dexmedetomidine, medetomidine, xylazine, and other related agents, as it has fewer side-effects and is more rapidly effective (Janssen et al., 2017) than older antagonists such as yohimbine. It can be given by the subcutaneous, intraperitoneal, intramuscular or intravenous routes. Absorption following subcutaneous injection is rapid, generally acting within 5–10 min. Dose rates of 0.5–1.0 mg/kg are required in small laboratory animal species, although less is required in larger species, for example, 25 µg/kg in sheep. The required dose also depends upon the dose of the Alpha-2-agonist that has been administered. Other drugs of this group, for example, detomidine, are available for use in horses and ruminants, but there is only limited information available concerning their effects in small mammals (Virtanen and MacDonald, 1985; Cox et al., 1994).

Morphine and morphine-like analgesics (opioids)

Morphine, pethidine (meperidine), buprenorphine, butorphanol, nalbuphine, pentazocine, methadone, fentanyl, alfentanil, sufentanil, remifentanil, etorphine, oxymorphone, hydromorphone.

Opioids are widely used postoperatively to provide pain relief, but they are most effective when given preoperatively. More details of the timing of analgesic administration are given below ('Analgesic agents').

Desirable effects: Opioids profound analgesia, and either moderate sedation or hyperactivity and excitement, depending upon the species, dose, and the degree of pain present. Further details of the effects of each agent are given below (Analgesic agents).

Undesirable effects: These drugs may produce respiratory depression, although generally only at high-dose rates and in combination with other central nervous system (CNS) depressants. Nausea and vomiting can be caused in some species (dog, primates). A more detailed discussion of side-effects can be found in Chapter 5.

Special comments: These analgesics can be used both to provide analgesia and if given preoperatively, then they will reduce the dose of anaesthetic agents needed to produce surgical anaesthesia. The preoperative administration may also provide more effective postoperative pain relief (see below, 'Preventive analgesia'). Opioids are also widely used as components of neuroleptanalgesic combinations (see below) and other multimodal analgesic regimens. Several commercial preparations that combine a potent opioid with a sedative or tranquillizer have been developed, such as 'Hypnorm' (Vetapharma, UK) (fentanyl and fluanisone) in Europe and 'Innovar-Vet' (fentanyl and droperidol) in the USA. It is also possible to produce other combinations. For example, a mixture of acepromazine and butorphanol is useful when blood sampling in rabbits, as it provides some sedation, analgesia, and dilates the ear veins. Buprenorphine combined with acepromazine provides excellent restraint for procedures such as radiography in dogs. Dose rates for these combinations are included in Tables 6.3–6.19. Short acting opioids such as fentanyl and remifentanil are used as continuous infusions as components of balanced anaesthetic techniques (see below).

Dissociative agents

Ketamine and tiletamine

Desirable effects: Ketamine produces immobility in most species and can be administered by the intramuscular, intraperitoneal, and intravenous routes. It causes only moderate respiratory depression in most species and increases blood pressure.

Undesirable effects: Skeletal muscle tone is increased. The degree of analgesia produced is very variable. Recovery can be prolonged and may be associated with hallucinations and mood alterations (Amornyotin, 2014). Ketamine has a low pH (commercial solutions have a pH of 3.5–4.1) and is irritant when administered by intramuscular injection. In small species, the relatively high doses of ketamine that need to be injected into a relatively small muscle mass can cause muscle damage (Smiler et al., 1990; Beyers et al., 1991).

Special comments: Ketamine produces a state of cataleptic sedation with apparent lack of awareness of the surroundings (White et al., 1982; Amornyotin, 2014; Mion and Villevieille, 2013). In those species in which profound analgesia appears to be produced (e.g., old-world primates), spontaneous movements often occur, but these are usually unrelated to painful stimuli. In some species, the corneal blink reflex is lost for prolonged periods, and drying of the cornea may occur unless the eyes are filled with a bland ophthalmic ointment as a preventive measure. Laryngeal and pharyngeal reflexes are maintained at all, except very high, dose rates, although salivary secretions are increased and airway obstruction remains a significant hazard. Ketamine is the drug of choice for immobilization of large primates; it is an effective chemical restraining agent in cats and pigs and, to a lesser extent, in rabbits. Its effects in rodents are variable, and high-dose rates may be necessary to produce immobilization (Green et al., 1981a). It is extremely useful when administered in combination with medetomidine, xylazine, or diazepam to produce surgical anaesthesia in sheep, primates, cats, dogs, pigs, rabbits, and small rodents (see below and Chapter 6). In all species, it may be necessary to use atropine or glycopyrrolate together with ketamine to reduce the otherwise excessive bronchial and salivary secretions that are produced. Long-term administration of ketamine can result in bladder irritation (Morgan and Curran, 2012), and these effects have been reported after 2–3 week administration to rats (Chuang et al., 2013). Repeated administration of ketamine results in tolerance (Douglas and Dagirmanjian, 1975).

Ketamine is widely used in old-world primates and produces immobility and some analgesia. It has the advantage that even at light levels of sedation, the bite reflex is lost. It is usually administered intramuscularly, but it can also be given by mouth if intramuscular injection is not possible. It is most effective if applied to the mucous membranes of the mouth, once in the stomach it undergoes some first-pass liver metabolism, and both the onset of action and the peak effect are markedly reduced compared to administration by injection (4–10 times the intramuscular dose is required). It can, however, be injected into foods such as bananas, to sedate animals that have escaped from their cages.

Tiletamine is rarely used alone and is available commercially combined with zolazepam (a benzodiazepine). More details of the use of dissociative agents are given below.

Anaesthetic agents

Inhalational agents

A range of different inhalational agents are available for use in animals. The features of each agent are outlined below. Most agents are volatile liquids that are vapourized, and the vapour is inhaled to produce anaesthesia. The potency of each drug is indicated by its minimum alveolar concentration $(MAC)_{50}$ value. MAC_{50}, most commonly referred to simply as MAC, is the alveolar concentration of an anaesthetic required to block the response to a specified painful stimulus, for example, clamping a haemostat onto a digit, in 50% of a group of animals. The lower the MAC value, the lower the concentration required to maintain anaesthesia (Table 2.1). The concentration of anaesthetic that can be delivered to the animal is influenced by the drug's boiling point. The lower the boiling point of an anaesthetic, the easier it is to vapourize, and so the higher the concentration that can be delivered. This is of considerable practical importance when selecting an anaesthetic agent and deciding how to vapourize it. A very potent drug, that is, one with a low MAC value and a low boiling point, which makes it easy to vapourize, must be used with great care. There will be a considerable risk of over-dosing the patient unless vapourization is carried out in a controlled way, using a calibrated vapourizer. Less potent anaesthetics, that is, ones with higher MAC values and higher boiling points, can be used with

TABLE 2.1 Induction and maintenance concentrations of inhalation anaesthetic agents.

Anaesthetic	Concentration for induction of anaesthesia (%)	Concentration for maintenance (%)	Minimum alveolar concentration (indicates relative potency of different agents) (in rat)
Desflurane	18	11	6.5–8
Enflurane	3–5	3	2.2
Ether	10–20	4–5	3.2
Halothane	4	1–2	0.95
Isoflurane	5	1.5–3	1.38
Methoxyflurane	3	0.4–1	0.22
Nitrous oxide	–	–	250
Sevoflurane	8	3.5–4.0	2.7

Data shown for rat; some species variation occurs; data from Mazze, R.I., et al., 1985. Halothane, isoflurane, and enflurane MAC in pregnant and nonpregnant female and male mice and rats. Anesthesiology 62 (3), 339–341; Steffey, E.P., et al., 1974. Anesthetic potency (MAC) of nitrous oxide in the dog, cat, and stump-tail monkey. J. Appl. Physiol. 36, 530–532; Kashimoto, S., et al. 1997. The minimum alveolar concentration of sevoflurane in rats. Eur. J. Anaesthesiol. 14 (4), 359–361; Gong, D., et al., 1998. Rat strain minimally influences anesthetic and convulsant requirements of inhaled compounds in rats. Anesth. Analg. 87 (4), 963–966; and Brosnan, R.J., et al., 2007. Anesthetic properties of carbon dioxide in the rat. Anesth. Analg. 105 (1), 103–106.

greater confidence in simple apparatus, since dangerously high concentrations will not usually be produced.

The speed of induction of anaesthesia and the rate of recovery are affected by the concentration of anaesthetic delivered, the anaesthetic potency (MAC value) and the blood–gas partition coefficient. The partition coefficient influences the rate at which the concentration of anaesthetic in the brain approaches that necessary for anaesthesia to be produced. The higher the partition coefficient, the slower the rate of induction of anaesthesia and the slower the recovery rate. These properties are summarized in Table 2.2. The MAC values of anaesthetics are relatively constant between species (Table 2.3), apart from nitrous oxide (see below). MAC also varies relatively little with different genotypes (Sonner, 2002), for example MAC of isoflurane ranged from 0.99 to 1.59 (Mogil et al., 2005) and 1.23 to 1.77 (Sonner et al., 2000) between different inbred strains.

Of particular concern to some research workers is the fate of inhalation anaesthetics once absorbed into the animal. A common misconception is that all of the agent that is inhaled is exhaled from the body. Many inhalation anaesthetics undergo significant metabolism, and this can result in induction of liver enzyme systems, as may occur following the use of injectable

TABLE 2.2 Physical characteristics and relative potency (MAC$_{50}$) of different volatile anaesthetics.

	Desflurane	Enflurane	Halothane	Isoflurane	Methoxyflurane	Nitrous oxide	Sevoflurane
Molecular weight	168	184.5	197.4	184.5	163.9	44.0	200.1
Vapour pressure (mmHg at 20°C)	669	172	240	240	23	Gas at room temperature	157
Vapour concentration (% saturated at 20°C)	89.6	23	32	32	3	100	22.4
MAC (in dog)	7.2	2.2	0.87	1.28	0.23	188–222	2.1–2.36
Stability in soda lime	Stable	Stable	Slight decomposition	Stable	Slight decomposition	Stable	Decomposition to compound A
Blood–gas partition coefficient	0.42	1.9	2.3	1.4	15	0.47	0.69
Rubber–gas partition coefficient	19	74	120	62	630	1.2	14
Percentage of anaesthetic recovered as metabolite (in humans)	0–0.02	0–2	15–40	0–0.2	50	0.004	5–8

Data adapted from Steffey, E.P., et al., 1974. Anesthetic potency (MAC) of nitrous oxide in the dog, cat, and stump-tail monkey. J. Appl. Physiol. 36, 530–532 and Preckel, B., Bolten, J., 2005. Pharmacology of modern volatile anaesthetics. Best Pract. Res. Clin. Anaesthesiol. 19 (3), 331–334.

TABLE 2.3 Minimum alveolar concentration (MAC$_{50}$) values (%) for inhalation anaesthetics in different species.

	Ether	Desflurane	Halothane	Enflurane	Isoflurane	Nitrous oxide	Sevoflurane
Human	1.92	6.6	0.75	1.63	1.17	104	1.8
Primate	–	–	1.15	1.84	1.28	200	2.0
Dog	3.04	7.2	0.87	2.20	1.28	188–222	2.1–2.36
Pig	–	8.3	1.25	–	1.45	277	3.5
Sheep	–	9.5	–	–	1.58	–	3.3
Cat	2.10	10.3	0.82	1.20	1.63	255	3.4
Rat	3.20	5.7	1.10	2.21	1.38	150	2.7
Mouse	3.20	6.5–8.8	0.95	1.95	1.41	275	2.5
Rabbit	–	8.9	1.39	2.86	2.05	–	3.7

Data from Barter, L.S., et al., 2004. Animal dependence of inhaled anaesthetic requirements in cats. Br. J. Anaesth. 92 (2), 275–277; Drummond, J.C., 1985. MAC for halothane, enflurane, and isoflurane in the New Zealand white rabbit: and a test for the validity of MAC determinations. Anesthesiology 62 (3), 336–338; Eger, E.I.I., Johnson, B.H., 1987. Rates of awakening from anesthesia with I-653, halothane, isoflurane, and sevoflurane: a test of the effect of anesthetic concentration and duration in rats. Anesth. Analg. 66 (10), 977; Lukasik, V.M., et al., 1998a. Minimal alveolar concentration and cardiovascular effects of desflurane in sheep. Vet. Surg. 27, 167; Lukasik, V.M., et al., 1998b. Minimal alveolar concentration and cardiovascular effects of sevoflurane in sheep. Vet. Surg. 27, 168; Mazze, R.I.,et al., 1985. Halothane, isoflurane, and enflurane MAC in pregnant and nonpregnant female and male mice and rats. Anesthesiology 62 (3), 339–341; Martin-Cancho, M.F., et al., 2006. Relationship of bispectral index values, haemodynamic changes and recovery times during sevoflurane or propofol anaesthesia in rabbits. Lab. Anim. 40 (1), 28–42; Nickalls, R.W.D., Mapleson, W.W., 2003. Age-related iso-MAC charts for isoflurane, sevoflurane and desflurane in man. Br. J. Anaesth. 91 (2), 170–174; Moeser, A.J., et al., 2008. Determination of minimum alveolar concentration of sevoflurane in juvenile swine. Res. Vet. Sci. 84 (2), 283–285; Piriou, V., et al., 2002. Pharmacological preconditioning: comparison of desflurane, sevoflurane, isoflurane and halothane in rabbit myocardium. Br. J. Anaesth. 89 (3), 486–491; Puig, N.R., et al., 2002. Effects of sevoflurane general anesthesia: immunological studies in mice. Int. Immunopharmacol. 2 (1), 95–104; Scheller, M.S., et al., 1988. MAC of sevoflurane in humans and the New Zealand white rabbit. Can. J. Anaesth. 35 (2), 153–156; Steffey, E.P., et al., 1974. Anesthetic potency (MAC) of nitrous oxide in the dog, cat, and stump-tail monkey. J. Appl. Physiol. 36, 530–532; and Sonner, J.M., et al., 2000. Naturally occurring variability in anesthetic potency among inbred mouse strains. Anesth. Analg. 91 (3), 720–726.

anaesthetics. This can be of significance if the animal is to be used subsequently in a study which involves assessing the in vivo effects of a novel pharmaceutical or another compound. Although information is available concerning long-term exposure to inhalation anaesthetics (Linde and Berman, 1971; Brown et al., 1974), there is little information concerning the effects on liver enzyme systems of brief periods of exposure. One means of avoiding the effects is to use isoflurane, an anaesthetic which undergoes virtually no metabolism (Eger, 1981). If other agents are used, it seems reasonable to suggest that brief ($\geqslant$5 min) periods of anaesthesia are unlikely to cause significant effects, but more prolonged exposure to anaesthetizing concentrations may result in induction of enzyme systems.

Properties of specific agents

Isoflurane

Desirable effects

Isoflurane produces very rapid induction and recovery from anaesthesia, and the depth of anaesthesia can be altered easily and rapidly. It is nonirritant, nonexplosive, and nonflammable.

Undesirable effects

Isoflurane produces moderate respiratory and cardiovascular system depression. Its pungent odour has been reported to cause breath holding during induction in children, but this does not seem a significant problem in most animal species, except for the rabbit and the guinea pig (see Chapter 6).

Special comments

Isoflurane is a safe and effective anaesthetic in all species provided it is delivered in a controlled way, using a calibrated vapourizer (Preckel and Bolten, 2005). It undergoes less biotransformation than any other agent and is almost completely eliminated from the body by exhalation from the lungs. This suggests that there will be little effect on liver microsomal enzymes and, hence, minimal interference in drug metabolism or toxicology studies (Eger, 1981). This characteristic, together with the rapid induction and recovery from anaesthesia, has resulted in the widespread adoption of isoflurane in many research establishments (Stokes et al., 2009).

Sevoflurane

Desirable effects

Sevoflurane produces even more rapid induction and recovery from anaesthesia than does isoflurane, and the depth of anaesthesia can be altered very easily and rapidly (Preckel and Bolten, 2005; Brioni et al., 2017). It is nonexplosive and nonflammable. Sevoflurane is much less pungent than other agents and has been shown to be less aversive in mice than isoflurane (Guedes et al., 2017). Mask induction is well tolerated in many species (apart from rabbits and guinea pigs).

Undesirable effects

Sevoflurane is unstable in the presence of soda lime, the carbon dioxide absorber used most commonly in closed-breathing system anaesthesia. The breakdown products can cause renal injury, but the concentrations produced are very low in normal circumstances (O'Keeffe and Healy, 1999). It is highly unlikely that significant toxicity will be encountered during use in laboratory animals.

Special comments

The main advantage of sevoflurane is the even greater ease of matching the depth of anaesthesia to the degree of surgical stimulation, coupled with very rapid and smooth recovery. If undisturbed, many animals recover from sevoflurane without a period of involuntary excitement. In the author's institute, it has been used with great success for very prolonged procedures and also for very brief procedures when rapid induction and recovery are needed.

Desflurane

Desirable effects

Induction of and recovery from anaesthesia with desflurane is the most rapid of any of the volatile anaesthetics (Eger, 1992; Caldwell, 1994). Desflurane undergoes the least degree of metabolism (Koblin, 1992). It is relatively nonirritant.

Undesirable effects

Desflurane is relatively expensive and requires a pressurized, temperature-controlled vapourizer because of its very low boiling point.

Special comments

Desflurane has not been widely used in either veterinary clinical practice or laboratory species, however, the very rapid recovery can make it particularly suitable for some procedures, especially those requiring very long-term anaesthesia (e.g., see Bertrand et al., 2018).

Halothane

Desirable effects

Halothane is easy to vapourize, and induction and recovery are rapid (1–3 min). It is a potent anaesthetic, is nonirritant and is neither flammable nor explosive.

Undesirable effects

Halothane has a depressant effect on the cardiovascular system. Moderate hypotension is produced at surgical levels of anaesthesia because of a reduction in cardiac output and peripheral vasodilatation. A dose-dependent depression of respiration also occurs. Some hepatic metabolism of halothane occurs, and marked liver microsomal enzyme induction may follow anaesthesia (Wood and Woad, 1984).

Special comments

The desirable effects listed above have made halothane a popular agent for maintaining anaesthesia in most species. However, it is now rarely used in medical anaesthetic practice in Europe and North America, and as a result, the manufacture of this agent has been discontinued. However, it will still be available from specialist sources and will continue to have an important role, particularly as an anaesthetic for neurophysiological studies (Murrell et al., 2008).

Nitrous oxide

Desirable effects

Nitrous oxide causes minimal cardiovascular and respiratory system depression.

Undesirable effects

Nitrous oxide has very low anaesthetic potency and cannot be used alone to produce anaesthesia, or even unconsciousness, in most species (e.g., (Mahmoudi et al., 1989). It reacts with vitamin B12, producing vitamin depletion after prolonged (>6 h) anaesthesia and can cause bone marrow depression.

Special comments

Nitrous oxide is extensively used for anaesthesia in animals and humans, although the mechanisms of its anaesthetic and analgesic effects are still not fully characterized (Maze and Fujinaga, 2000). Since nitrous oxide has minimal effects on the respiratory and cardiovascular systems, it can be used to reduce the required concentration of other agents and so to reduce the overall degree of depression of blood pressure or respiration at a particular depth of anaesthesia. It is usually administered as a 50:50 or a 60:40 mixture with oxygen. Following the cessation of prolonged nitrous oxide administration, 100% oxygen should be administered to prevent so-called diffusion hypoxia. This phenomenon causes lowered alveolar oxygen tension due to the rapid diffusion of nitrous oxide from the blood to the alveoli. Because of its low anaesthetic potency, nitrous oxide must never be used as the sole anaesthetic agent in association with neuromuscular blocking (NMB) agents such as pancuronium. Its main value lies in reducing the required concentration of other more potent agents which have more marked side-effects. It is important to note that nitrous oxide is not absorbed by the activated charcoal used in some gas-scavenging systems. If nitrous oxide is used, then an active scavenging system that ducts expired gases directly to the room ventilation extract must be used.

A common misconception is that it is necessary to administer nitrous oxide in order to administer other inhalation anaesthetics. This is not the case, and all the other agents mentioned above can safely be administered in 100% oxygen. It is only necessary to avoid this if prolonged periods of anaesthesia are planned (>12–24h) (Thomson and Paton, 2014), when the inspired oxygen concentration should be reduced (to approximately 40%) to avoid the possible development of oxygen toxicity (del Portillo et al., 2014). This can be achieved without the use of nitrous oxide by using an air/oxygen or nitrogen/oxygen mixture, the other gas being supplied from an appropriate compressed gas cylinder. If the gases are mixed at the outlet from the anaesthetic machine, then the delivered concentration of anaesthetic vapour will be reduced, and the vapourizer setting should be increased accordingly.

Older agents

Several other anaesthetics have been developed, but they are primarily only of historical interest. Chloroform vapour has numerous side-effects which resulted in it being discarded from human and veterinary clinical practice, and which make it unsuitable for laboratory use.

Trichlorethylene vapour produces good analgesia and is inexpensive, noninflammable, and nonexplosive. It also causes only minimal cardiovascular system depression, but it has poor muscle relaxant properties, low anaesthetic potency, and decomposes in the presence of soda lime to form toxic and explosive products, so that it must never be used in closed breathing systems. Trichlorethylene undergoes extensive hepatic metabolism and has been established as a hepatic carcinogen in some species (Rusyn et al., 2014). It is rarely used for animal anaesthesia.

Ether was one of the most widely used anaesthetics for laboratory rodents but has been largely superseded by more modern anaesthetic agents. It was popular because it is easy to vapourize in simple apparatus. It is difficult to kill an animal with high ether concentrations, so it is a relatively safe agent for inexperienced anaesthetists. Unfortunately, induction is unpleasant and stressful for the animal, and the irritant properties of ether can cause coughing, profuse bronchial and salivary secretions and occasionally laryngospasm. Ether can cause preexisting chronic respiratory disease to develop into an acute severe infection, following recovery from anaesthesia, and this may be particularly important in rodents and rabbits. Ether is flammable and forms explosive mixtures with both oxygen and air. Anaesthetic ether is now difficult to obtain, although the agent can still be purchased from chemical manufacturers and suppliers. Induction of and recovery from anaesthesia are relatively slow. This is advantageous for inexperienced anaesthetists, as it makes accidental overdose less likely. Conversely, a prolonged induction period can present problems in restraining the animal, particularly as most animals strongly resent inhaling the vapour.

Administration of ether stimulates catecholamine release (Carruba et al., 1987), which counteracts the depressant effect that this anaesthetic exerts on the heart, so that blood pressure is maintained at near-normal levels at all except deep levels of anaesthesia. The catecholamine release also results in a moderate rise in blood glucose concentrations, and in a wide range of other metabolic changes, which may interfere with particular research protocols. Ether is not, as commonly believed, an inert compound. It undergoes extensive metabolism and exposure to ether results in induction of liver enzyme activity (Linde and Berman, 1971).

Although ether has been a popular anaesthetic, its use for induction is unpleasant for the animal and hazardous in several species, particularly guinea pigs. Its explosive properties make it a significant safety hazard: animals should not be killed with ether, as the carcasses may be stored in refrigerators which are not spark-proof, and an explosion may result. In summary, it should be replaced with other more appropriate modern anaesthetic agents.

Enflurane is a volatile anaesthetic with similar properties to halothane, but which undergoes less liver metabolism. It is now rarely used for anaesthetizing either humans or animals.

Methoxyflurane is now rarely used as an anaesthetic, but because of its potent analgesic effects it is used to provide immediate pain relief for emergency trauma patients. Methoxyflurane is now very difficult to obtain in North America and Europe, although it is still available in Australia. In small animals, it can safely be used in anaesthetic chambers, using simple vapourizers, where its slow induction and the low vapour concentration produced can be an advantage in reducing the risk of inadvertent overdose.

Injectable anaesthetic agents

Properties of specific agents

Barbiturates

Pentobarbital

Desirable effects: Pentobarbital can be administered either by intravenous or by intraperitoneal injection and can be used in a wide range of animal species.

Undesirable effects: Pentobarbital causes severe cardiovascular and respiratory system depression and has poor analgesic activity. Recovery can be prolonged, particularly after the administration of an additional dose to prolong anaesthesia.

Special comments: Pentobarbital has been the most widely used laboratory animal anaesthetic. Surgical anaesthesia is attained in most small laboratory animals only when dosages close to those which cause respiratory failure have been administered. At these dose rates, severe cardiovascular depression and respiratory depression are produced. Slow intravenous administration of a dose sufficient to produce basal narcosis, followed by further incremental doses, usually achieves surgical levels of anaesthesia reasonably safely. Intraperitoneal administration of the calculated amount of drug as a single bolus is often associated with high mortality not only because the anaesthetic dose is very close to the lethal dose, but because there is also considerable between-strain variation. Pentobarbital is probably best used to provide hypnosis rather than anaesthesia, and in most circumstances, safer and more effective agents are available.

Pentobarbital is no longer commercially available as an anaesthetic in several countries; however, the agent can be purchased from specialist suppliers (e.g., Sigma) if needed for specific research projects. It has relatively low solubility, and commercial preparations may include propylene glycol or other agents. Aqueous solutions of 50 mg/mL can be prepared from pentobarbital powder.

Like other barbiturates, pentobarbital solution has a very high pH, so intraperitoneal injection can cause pain (Svendsen et al., 2007). When used as a euthanasia agent, the addition of a local anaesthetic can prevent pain on intraperitoneal injection.

Thiopental

Desirable effects: Thiopental produces smooth and rapid induction of anaesthesia following intravenous injection and can be used in virtually all species.

Undesirable effects: Thiopental has poor analgesic activity and causes transient apnoea after intravenous injection. It is irritant if injected perivascularly. Repeated administration results in very prolonged recovery time (see Chapter 4).

Special comments: Thiopental is a short-acting barbiturate which is useful for rapid induction of anaesthesia when administered intravenously. It is unstable in aqueous solution, so once reconstituted, it should be used within 7–10 days. Its duration of action depends upon both the amount of drug injected and the rate of injection. The doses quoted in Chapter 6 should be administered as follows: half the calculated dose should be given rapidly, followed by the remainder to effect over 1–2 min. This will result in 5–15 min of anaesthesia. Transient apnoea usually follows administration, but assisted ventilation is rarely required. Thiopental solution is extremely irritant if injected perivascularly and should be diluted as much as practicable (preferably to enable the use of a 1.25%–2.5% solution). If extravascular administration occurs, then the area should be infiltrated with a solution of 1 mL of lidocaine 2% in 4 mL normal saline. Since thiopental is highly irritant, primarily because of its high pH, it should not be administered by the intraperitoneal, intramuscular, or subcutaneous routes. The drug's major use is by intravenous injection to provide rapid induction of anaesthesia, followed by maintenance using inhalational agents.

Methohexital

Desirable effects: Methohexital produces smooth and rapid induction of anaesthesia after intravenous administration and can be used in a wide range of species.

Undesirable effects: Like other barbiturates, methohexital has poor analgesic activity, and transient apnoea often occurs after induction. Recovery is frequently accompanied by muscular tremors unless suitable preanaesthetic medication has been administered.

Special comments: This agent is now rarely used as an anaesthetic and is unavailable as a commercial product in many countries. Methohexital has a shorter duration of action than thiopental and is about twice as potent. It should be administered as described above for thiopental. Anaesthesia lasts for 2–5 min, and several incremental doses can usually be given without unduly prolonging the rate of recovery. Methohexital is suitable for the induction of anaesthesia, provided intravenous administration is possible. Although intraperitoneal administration has been reported, the use of this route of administration often has less predictable effects, with some animals failing to become anaesthetized.

Inactin

Desirable effects: 'Inactin' (sodium thiobutabarbital) produces smooth induction of anaesthesia after intravenous administration and has a prolonged duration of action.

Undesirable effects: It has variable analgesic activity.

Special comments: Inactin is a thiobarbiturate which has been reported to produce prolonged anaesthesia in rats following intraperitoneal (Buelke-Sam et al., 1978) or intravenous (Walker and Buscemi-Bergin, 1983) administration. Whilst it appears to be a satisfactory induction agent when given intravenously (resembling thiopental in its effects), its effects when given by the intraperitoneal route may vary. In the author's experience, some rats remain lightly anaesthetized for several hours, whereas others appear completely recovered within 60 min. Provided that an appropriate dose rate has been established in the particular strain of rat which is to be anaesthetized, Inactin can be used to produce prolonged anaesthesia.

Steroid Anaesthetics.

Alphaxalone

Desirable effects: Alphaxalone produces smooth induction of anaesthesia following intravenous administration. It is relatively noncumulative so that administration of repeated doses of the drug has little effect on recovery time. The solution is nonirritant.

Undesirable effects: Moderate cardiovascular depression, moderate respiratory depression.

Special comments: This steroid anaesthetic was originally formulated as a mixture of alphaxalone/alphadolone together with a solubilizing agent, Chremophor EL (polyoxyethylated castor oil). This solubilizing agent caused side-effects, notably histamine release and the original formulation is no longer available. A new formulation, of alphaxalone alone is now available. This has very similar properties to the older product, but does not cause histamine release as the original solubilizing agent is not present. Much of the information relating to the older formulation is still relevant to the new agent ('Alfaxan', Jurox Pty. Ltd.).

Following intravenous administration, it produces rapid-onset anaesthesia followed by rapid recovery. The agent is nonirritant, and accidental extravascular injection does not appear to be associated with any adverse effects.

The effects of administration by the intramuscular or intraperitoneal routes vary between species. In some cases, light surgical anaesthesia is produced; but small rodents the volume of drug required precludes intramuscular administration, and absorption following intraperitoneal injection is very unpredictable (Green et al., 1978). It is an effective agent for immobilizing small primates when administered intramuscularly, however.

As the drug is rapidly metabolized, it is an excellent agent for maintenance of long-term anaesthesia, although moderate hypotension may occur (Child et al., 1972a; Dyson et al., 1987). Continuous intravenous infusion can be used to provide safe and stable anaesthesia in sheep, pigs, primates, cats, and rodents, although in larger species economic considerations may limit its usefulness. In rabbits, the degree of analgesia produced is insufficient for major surgery until high doses have been administered, and at these dosages, respiratory arrest often occurs. However, including opioids or an alpha$_2$ agonist such as medetomidine can result in surgical planes of anaesthesia.

Although structurally related to the steroid hormones, alphaxalone has no significant endocrine effects (Child et al., 1972b). Much of the published data on the combination and its effects are still relevant to the newer, single steroid, formulation (e.g., Child et al., 1971, 1972a, b) which has similar properties to the older product in all species (Keates, 2003; Rodríguez et al., 2012; Goodchild et al., 2015; Siriarchavatana et al., 2016).

Dissociative anaesthetics

Ketamine

Desirable effects: Ketamine produces immobility in most species and can be administered by the intramuscular, intraperitoneal, and intravenous routes. It causes only moderate respiratory depression in most species (NB: rodents, see below) and increases blood pressure. Although the degree of analgesia produced may vary, ketamine is an NMDA (N-methyl-D-aspartate) antagonist and has been shown to prevent sensitization to noxious stimuli during surgery (see Chapter 5).

Undesirable effects: Skeletal muscle tone is increased. The degree of analgesia produced is very variable, and in small rodents, severe respiratory depression is produced following administration of the high-dose rates needed for surgical anaesthesia. Recovery can be prolonged and may be associated with hallucinations and mood alterations.

Special comments: Ketamine produces a state of cataleptic sedation with apparent lack of awareness of the surroundings (White et al., 1982; Mion and Villevieille, 2013; Amornyotin, 2014). In those species in which profound analgesia appears to be produced, spontaneous movements often occur, but these are usually unrelated to surgical stimuli. In some species, the corneal blink reflex is lost for prolonged periods, and drying of the cornea may occur unless the eye is filled with a bland ophthalmic ointment as a preventive measure. Laryngeal and pharyngeal reflexes are maintained at all, except very high-dose rates, although salivary secretions are increased, and airway obstruction remains a significant hazard. In all species, it may be necessary to use atropine or glycopyrrolate together with ketamine to reduce these otherwise excessive bronchial and salivary secretions. Ketamine is the drug of choice for immobilization of large primates and is an effective chemical restraining agent in cats and pigs and, to a lesser extent, in rabbits. Its effects in rodents are variable, and high-dose rates may be necessary to produce surgical anaesthesia (Green et al., 1981a).

It is extremely useful when administered in combination with medetomidine, xylazine, or diazepam to produce surgical anaesthesia in sheep, primates, cats, dogs, pigs, rabbits, and small rodents (see Chapter 6). It is important to appreciate that the stimulatory effects of ketamine on the cardiovascular system do not offset the depressant effects of drugs such as xylazine, and the use of these combinations almost invariably results in significant hypotension (Middleton et al., 1982; Allen et al., 1986). Ketamine can be mixed with medetomidine, xylazine, or acepromazine and the combination administered as a single injection. Long-term administration of ketamine can result in bladder irritation (Morgan and Curran, 2012), and these effects have been reported after 2–3 week administration to rats (Chuang et al., 2013). Repeated administration of ketamine results in tolerance (Douglas and Dagirmanjian, 1975).

Neuroleptanalgesics

Fentanyl/fluanisone,   fentanyl/droperidol,   etorphine/methotrimeprazine, etorphine/acepromazine.

Desirable effects: Neuroleptanalgesic combinations produce profound analgesia and can be administered by the intramuscular, intraperitoneal, or intravenous routes to most species. The effects of these drug combinations can be reversed by administration of mu-opioid antagonists such as naloxone or nalbuphine or partial agonists such as butorphanol and buprenorphine (see below).

Undesirable effects: Neuroleptanalgesic combinations produce moderate or severe respiratory depression and a poor degree of muscle relaxation (NB: see below). Hypotension and bradycardia may also be produced.

Special comments: Neuroleptanalgesic combinations consist of a potent opioid analgesic, which can abolish the perception of pain, and a neuroleptic— a tranquillizer/sedative (e.g., acepromazine or fluanisone)—which suppresses some of the undesirable side-effects of the narcotic such as vomiting or excitement. The analgesics used in commercially available neuroleptanalgesic combinations are fentanyl and etorphine. When neuroleptanalgesic combinations are used alone, the adverse effects mentioned above can be marked, and the poor degree of muscle relaxation produced makes them unsuitable for anything other than superficial surgery. When given in combination with a benzodiazepine (e.g., midazolam or diazepam), the dose of the commercial neuroleptanalgesic mixtures can be reduced by 50%–70%, and the benzodiazepine produces good skeletal muscle relaxation. Used in this way, combinations such as fentanyl/fluanisone and midazolam are often the anaesthetic method of choice for rodents and rabbits (Flecknell and Mitchell, 1984). Although pharmacologically similar, fentanyl/fluanisone (Hypnorm) and fentanyl/droperidol (Innovar-Vet, Thalamanol) differ in their effects in animals. As mentioned above, fentanyl/fluanisone in combination with diazepam or midazolam produces good surgical anaesthesia. The effects of a comparable mixture of fentanyl/droperidol and midazolam are much less predictable, and this latter combination cannot be recommended (Flecknell, unpublished observations (Marini et al., 1993). Another commercially available combination, etorphine/methotrimeprazine (Immobilon SA), has been evaluated in combination with midazolam. Although surgical anaesthesia is produced, respiratory depression can be severe (Whelan and Flecknell, 1995).

An important advantage of these drug combinations is that their action is readily reversible by the administration of opioid antagonists such as naloxone or partial mu agonists such as buprenorphine or butorphanol (Flecknell et al., 1989b) (see Chapter 5). Fentanyl/fluanisone and fentanyl/droperidol are useful for providing restraint and analgesia for minor procedures, and the combination of fentanyl/fluanisone/midazolam is recommended for surgical anaesthesia in rodent and rabbits. The use of other neuroleptanalgesic combinations has been described (Green, 1975).

Other opioid combinations

Because of their potent analgesic action, short-acting opioids such as fentanyl and alfentanil can be used in combination with a variety of compounds to produce balanced anaesthesia. Mixtures of fentanyl or alfentanil and a benzodiazepine produce effective surgical anaesthesia in dogs (Flecknell et al., 1989a) and pigs, and they can be added to anaesthetics in which analgesia would otherwise be inadequate (e.g., alphaxalone or propofol) (Michalot et al., 1980; Flecknell et al., 1990a). The use of opioids often enables the production of profound analgesia, without major effects on the cardiovascular system, although bradycardia can be produced if the drugs are given rapidly. Opioid-induced bradycardia can rapidly be reversed with atropine, without affecting the analgesia produced by these drugs. Severe respiratory depression can occur when using high doses of opioids, although this can be overcome using intermittent positive pressure ventilation (IPPV).

Fentanyl/medetomidine and sufentanil/medetomidine: Fentanyl and medetomidine can be combined to produce anaesthesia in dogs, rabbits, guinea pigs, and rats (Hu et al., 1992) and similar effective anaesthesia can be produced using sufentanil in combination with medetomidine in rats (Ter Horst et al., 2018). The combination is most effective in dogs and rats. In the dog, the drugs are given by intravenous injection, and in the rat, the two compounds are combined and given as a single intraperitoneal injection. Several other opioid combinations have been described, and these are discussed in more detail in Chapter 6.

Desirable effects: The combination reliably produces surgical anaesthesia with good muscle relaxation in some species (see Chapter 6). Anaesthesia is completely reversible by administering specific antagonists (nalbuphine or butorphanol together with atipamezole).

Undesirable effects: Mild to moderate respiratory depression is produced. In the rat, the relatively large volume for injection is inconvenient for the operator but does not appear distressing to the animal. In the mouse, the combination can cause urinary retention which may result in rupture of the bladder, and so should not be used in this species.

Special comments: The rapid and complete reversal of anaesthesia avoids the problems that may be associated with managing animals during the prolonged recovery that can be associated with other injectable anaesthetic techniques. Reversal of the fentanyl component with a mixed opioid agonist/antagonist results in maintenance of postoperative analgesia.

Other hypnotics

Etomidate and metomidate

Desirable effects: Etomidate and metomidate are short-acting hypnotics with minimal effects on the cardiovascular system.

Undesirable effects: Etomidate and metomidate have little analgesic action when used alone and suppression of adrenocortical function following prolonged infusion of etomidate has been reported (Kruse-Elliott et al., 1990).

Special comments: Etomidate has been shown to cause little cardiovascular depression in animals (Nagel et al., 1979; Kissin et al., 1983), and so may be useful as part of balanced anaesthetic regimens. Metomidate and etomidate are useful for providing unconsciousness (and therefore restraint) in many mammals, birds, reptiles, and fish (Janssen et al., 1975). Metomidate in combination with fentanyl, administered as a subcutaneous injection, is an effective anaesthetic combination for small rodents (Chapter 5) (Green et al., 1981b).

Propofol

Desirable effects: Propofol produces rapid induction of a short period of anaesthesia in a wide range of species. Recovery is smooth and rapid with little cumulative effect if additional doses are administered.

Undesirable effects: Insufficient analgesia for major surgery in some species, a short period of apnoea, may occur after induction if propofol is administered rapidly, and respiratory depression can occur with high doses of propofol. Prolonged infusion causes lipaemia because of the formulation (see below). A rare adverse reaction to propofol in people, associated with progressive bardycardia has been described (Fudickar and Bein, 2009) and a similar syndrome associated with prolonged infusion of high doses of propofol has been described in rabbits (Ypsilantis et al., 2007, 2011).

Special considerations: Propofol (2,6-di-isopropyl phenol) is an alkyl phenol (Glen, 1980; Adam et al., 1980) which, because of its poor water solubility, is prepared as an emulsion formulation in soya bean oil and glycerol. Intravenous administration of this compound produces rapid-onset anaesthesia in a wide range of species, with a sleep time similar to thiopental. In contrast to thiopental, animals recover more rapidly following propofol administration, and sleep times are not greatly prolonged following repeated dosing (Glen, 1980).

Because of its rapid redistribution and metabolism, propofol is best given by intravenous injection to be effective; otherwise, the rapid redistribution to body tissues that occurs will prevent anaesthetic concentrations being achieved in the brain. Propofol should be administered relatively slowly, as this avoids causing transient apnoea. Typically, the dose needed to produce unconsciousness and sufficient relaxation to allow intubation should be given over 1–2 min in small animals (1–10 kg). Propofol produces a moderate fall in systolic blood pressure, and a small fall in cardiac output (Sebel and Lowdon, 1989). Propofol causes significant respiratory depression in most species, manifested either as a reduction in respiratory rate (Glen, 1980), or as little change in rate but a fall in arterial oxygen tension, suggesting a fall in tidal volume (Watkins et al., 1987). It is therefore advisable to provide supplemental oxygen. Propofol is believed to have no significant effects on hepatic (Robinson and Patterson, 1985) or renal function (Stark, 1985), nor on platelet function or blood coagulation (Sear et al., 1985). In humans, propofol causes a fall in intraocular pressure (Vanacker et al., 1987), has limited effects in sheep (Torres et al., 2012) and in dogs it causes a small increase in pressure (Hasiuk et al., 2014). The pain on injection of propofol which has been reported in humans does not appear to be a significant problem in animals (Michou et al., 2012; Flecknell et al., 1990a). Propofol is nonirritant when injected perivascularly (Morgan and Legge, 1989).

Propofol can be administered by the intraperitoneal route in small rodents at high-dose rates (see Chapter 6, Tables 6.2 and 6.5). When administered by this route it usually only produces light anaesthesia, but the depth of anaesthesia can be increased by the addition of medetomidine or fentanyl (Alves et al., 2009).

Tribromoethanol

Desirable effects: Tribromoethanol ('Avertin') produces surgical anaesthesia in rats and mice, with good skeletal muscle relaxation and only a moderate degree of respiratory depression.

Undesirable effects: If incorrectly stored, or administered more than once, tribromoethanol is irritant to the peritoneum (see below). Even freshly prepared solutions can cause undesirable side-effects (see below).

Special comments: Tribromoethanol is a popular anaesthetic for mice, and it produces 15–20 min of anaesthesia with rapid recovery (Papaioannou and Fox, 1993). It has been known for some time that decomposition of stored solutions can result in severe irritation and peritoneal adhesions following its use. Even if a freshly prepared solution is used, administration of a second anaesthetic at a later date was associated with high mortality in gerbils (Norris and Turner, 1983). More recently, it has been established that the use of freshly prepared solutions can be associated with postanaesthetic mortality and that tribromoethanol causes low-grade peritonitis (Zeller et al., 1998). Analysis of different batches of tribromoethanol by using a range of analytical techniques indicated that it contains several impurities and that the concentration and the identity of these may vary (Lieggi et al., 2005). This may account for the varying incidences of side-effects. This study also established that monitoring of the pH of tribromoethanol stock solution, to try to detect breakdown products, was ineffective. Tribromoethanol has also been reported to have variable anaesthetic effects in mice (Hill et al., 2013). Use of an alternative formulation in cyclodextrin slightly reduced the variation in anaesthetic effect (McDowell et al., 2014). Given the unpredictable adverse effects, tribromoethanol use should be avoided and alternative anaesthetics used.

Chloral hydrate

Desirable effects: Chloral hydrate produces medium-duration (1–2h), stable, light anaesthesia (Field et al., 1993). The drug has minimal effects on the cardiovascular system and on baroreceptor reflexes.

Undesirable effects: Chloral hydrate has poor analgesic properties, and the high doses required for surgical anaesthesia can produce severe respiratory depression. Intraperitoneal administration to rats has been associated with a high incidence of postanaesthetic ileus (dilation and stasis of the bowel) (Fleischman et al., 1977). Although the use of low concentrations of chloral hydrate (36 mg/mL) may reduce the incidence of this effect, it may not completely solve the problem.

Special comments: Chloral hydrate can often be replaced by more effective anaesthetics if surgical procedures are to be undertaken. As with many other anaesthetics, there is considerable strain variation in the response to chloral hydrate in rodents, and it is important to evaluate the drug's efficacy and safety in the particular strain of animals that will be used. Chloral hydrate has also been used in combination with magnesium sulphate and pentobarbital ('Equithesin') (Bo et al., 2003) as an anaesthetic for a number of species. It has been particularly widely used in pharmacological studies, because of the limited effects on a number of receptor systems. Although the concentration of chloral hydrate in 'Equithesin' is low, it can still produce ileus in some strains of rat (Deacon and Rawlins, 1996).

Alpha-chloralose

Desirable effects: Alpha-chloralose produces stable, long-lasting (8–10h) but light anaesthesia. It produces minimal cardiovascular and respiratory system depression (Holzgrefe et al., 1987; Svendsen et al., 1990).

Undesirable effects: Alpha-chloralose has poor analgesic properties, although this varies considerably between different species and strains of animals. Both induction and recovery can be very prolonged and associated with involuntary excitement.

Special comments: Alpha-chloralose is useful for providing long-lasting light anaesthesia for procedures involving no painful surgical interference. A more potent but short-acting anaesthetic can be administered to produce a depth of anaesthesia sufficient to allow surgical procedures to be undertaken, following which unconsciousness can be maintained with alpha-chloralose. Recovery is prolonged and associated with involuntary excitement, so alpha-chloralose is best used for nonrecovery studies. A more detailed discussion of this anaesthetic can be found in Chapter 4.

Urethane

Desirable effects: Urethane produces long-lasting (6–10h) anaesthesia, with minimal cardiovascular and respiratory system depression (Field et al., 1993; Maggi and Meli, 1986c and e).

Undesirable effects: Urethane is carcinogenic (Field and Lang, 1988) and produces peritoneal effusion (Severs et al., 1981) and haemolysis.

Special comments: Urethane resembles chloralose in producing long-lasting, stable anaesthesia, but unlike chloralose, the degree of analgesia produced is sufficient to allow surgical procedures to be undertaken in small rodents. It is a useful agent for long-term anaesthesia (see Chapter 4), but it is also a carcinogen, so its use should be avoided whenever possible. If it is necessary to use urethane, precautions appropriate to the handling of a known carcinogen should be adopted. Animals should not be allowed to recover after being anaesthetized with urethane. A more detailed discussion of this anaesthetic can be found in Chapter 4.

Local and regional anaesthesia

Local anaesthetics act directly on nervous tissue to block the conduction of nerve impulses. For example, they can be applied to the surface of the cornea and the conjunctiva to produce local anaesthesia of that part of the eye, or they can be used to anaesthetize mucous membranes to ease the passage of catheters or an endotracheal tube.

Local anaesthetics (e.g., bupivacaine or lidocaine) can also be injected into tissues to provide a localized area of anaesthesia. Infiltration of the skin and underlying connective tissue will usually provide sufficient anaesthesia to suture minor wounds or to take a biopsy of skin. Infiltration of more extensive areas and the different tissue planes can be used to provide sufficient anaesthesia to carry out surgical procedures such as laparotomy. When injecting local anaesthetics for this purpose, a fine (e.g., 26 gauge), long needle should be used, to minimize the discomfort associated with the injection. The syringes used in human dentistry, which are loaded with a local anaesthetic cartridge, are ideal for this procedure. Discomfort on injection can also be reduced by warming the solution to body temperature and by buffering the solution with sodium bicarbonate (8.4% solution). A 1:10 ratio with 0.5–2% lidocaine, and a 1:30 ratio with 0.25% bupivacaine, buffers the solution without affecting the solubility of the local anaesthetic (Bigeleisen and Wempe, 2001). Although the toxicity of local anaesthetics is similar in different laboratory mammals, the small size of rodents makes inadvertent overdose more likely. To avoid this, calculate an appropriate safe dose. In most larger species, recommendations are that no more than 2–4 mg/kg of lidocaine or 1–2 mg/kg of bupivacaine are administered. In rodents, doses of up to 10 mg/kg lidocaine, or 3 mg/kg bupivacaine appear both safe (de Jong and Bonin, 1980) and effective. The doses required to produce significant adverse reactions are. When using these agents in small rodents, it is advisable to calculate the dose and prepare the agents for injection in advance. When using local anaesthetics in small rodents, the volume of solution for injection can be increased by diluting the mixture. The author's preference is to mix 1% lidocaine with 0.25% bupivacaine, as a 50:50 mixture, and to dilute this mixture with no more than an equal volume of water for injection. Greater dilution reduces the duration of local anaesthesia (Grant et al., 2000). Toxicity of these two agents is additive, so the dose limits suggested here should be reduced. However, in mice, 3 mg/kg bupivacaine **plus** 10 mg/kg lidocaine has proved safe and effective in our laboratory (see Chapter 5). Using local anaesthetics as part of a multimodal analgesic regimen (see below) is a very effective means of improving the quality of postoperative pain relief.

Care must be taken to infiltrate all the tissue planes that will be involved in the surgical procedure. If reinsertion of the needle is necessary, this should be done through a previously anaesthetized area, so that discomfort to the animal is minimized. Considerable experience is necessary to ensure that complete blockage of the nerve supply to the surgical field is achieved, and expert practical advice should be obtained before carrying out this technique.

If the nerve supply to the operative site is well defined, regional anaesthesia can be produced by infiltration of local anaesthetics around the major sensory nerves. This may involve a single nerve or blockade of several nerves, for example, in producing a paravertebral block by infiltration of the lumbar spinal nerves as they emerge from the vertebral column, and so desensitizing the abdomen.

More extensive effects of local anaesthetics can be produced by injection of the drug into the spinal canal. The site of injection may be into the fat-filled space between the dura mater and the wall of the vertebral canal (epidural anaesthesia), or directly into the cerebrospinal fluid (subarachnoid or spinal anaesthesia). The techniques for injection have been described in both large animals such as the cow, sheep, and dog (see (Grimm et al., 2015), for a review) and laboratory species such as the rabbit (Hughes et al., 1993) and the guinea pig (Thomasson et al., 1974). In attempting to become proficient in the technique, it is advisable to first practice injecting a dye, such as Methylene Blue, into the spinal canal of a recently killed animal.

A major problem associated with the use of local anaesthetic techniques in laboratory species is that it is often difficult to provide humane, stress-free restraint of the animal during the surgical procedure. It is possible, however, to produce effective surgical anaesthesia, with these techniques and combine this with low doses of hypnotics or anaesthetics, to provide effective restraint. In some animals, the use of a tranquillizer or sedative, together with the careful attention of an expert handler, may provide sufficient restraint to enable local anaesthesia to be used safely and humanely. When contemplating using local anaesthetic techniques, the likely behaviour of the animal, the type of surgical procedure involved and the expertise of the operator and his or her assistants should be carefully considered.

Analgesic agents

Nonsteroidal antiinflammatory drugs (NSAIDs)

Traditionally, NSAIDs have been considered low-potency analgesics, suitable for the control of mild pain, or as agents primarily for use in conditions such as arthritis, where the inflammatory component of the disease process was responsible for some or all of the pain. The perception of NSAIDs has changed with the introduction of a number of compounds that have been shown to have considerable analgesic potency (Gaynor and Muir, 2014). In laboratory species, data from a number of nociceptive tests provide a basis for estimating appropriate dose rates for clinical use in these species (Liles and Flecknell, 1992), and some investigations of their use for postoperative pain control are now available. Estimating the frequency of administration is much more difficult, since there are very considerable variations in elimination times for NSAIDs in different species (Lees et al., 1991; Busch et al., 1998; Baert and De Backer, 2003; Turner et al., 2006; Shukla et al., 2007). Despite these problems, there are now a range of NSAIDs with clear indications for use in alleviating pain in animals (Lees et al., 2004; Papich, 2008).

NSAIDs exert their main effects by inhibiting the action of the enzyme cyclooxygenase (COX). COX is an enzyme that catalyses the conversion of arachidonic acid to prostaglandin H2, the first step in the synthesis of prostanoids. The prostanoids are important mediators of inflammation, and both directly and indirectly influence the degree of pain associated with tissue injury and other inflammatory processes. COX exists in two isoforms: COX-1 and COX-2. A third isoform, COX-3, has now been described (Chandrasekharan et al., 2002; Botting and Ayoub, 2005). COX-1 mediates essential physiological responses in a wide range of body tissues; in contrast, COX-2 is expressed by cells that are involved in inflammation (e.g., macrophages), and it has emerged as the isoform primarily responsible for the synthesis of prostanoids involved in acute and chronic inflammatory states. It was initially thought that developing NSAIDs with effects only on COX-2 would avoid any undesirable side-effects; however, this relatively simple view of the functions of COX and the effects of COX-1 and COX-2 inhibition is now outdated (Hotz-Behofsits et al., 2010).

One of the problems that arise when trying to interpret information about new and older NSAIDs is the wide variation of assays used to determine COX-1 and COX-2 inhibitory effects. This is further compounded by the use of both EC_{50} and EC_{80} for comparison, and the failure in some studies to link these data to the tissue concentrations that are likely to be produced when the drug is used clinically. A further problem is that the drug concentration produced, the relative COX-1–COX-2 inhibition and the duration of action of the drug are likely to vary between species. It is therefore important to balance an enthusiasm to provide the most effective pain management, with the need for caution when using drugs in different species. It is clear, however, that the new generation of highly selective COX-2 NSAIDs, in particular the coxibs such as deracoxib and firocoxib, are likely to provide effective pain relief with a reduced risk of side-effects, particularly those involving the gastrointestinal tract (McCann et al., 2004), although systematic reviews of clinical veterinary data have been inconclusive (KuKanich et al., 2012; Monteiro Steagall et al., 2013). Information is also becoming available on the use of these agents in less familiar species (e.g., birds; Baert and De Backer, 2003). The most significant problems associated with NSAID administration are gastrointestinal disturbances, notably ulceration and haemorrhage, nephrotoxicity, and interference with platelet function (Mathews, 2000; Bongiovanni et al., 2021). Other problems such as blood dyscrasias and liver toxicity can also occur (Lees et al., 1991). These side-effects are seen primarily following prolonged administration and are rarely of significance when treatment is for 2 or 3 days postoperatively. It should be noted that some NSAIDs (e.g., aspirin) have been reported to cause foetal abnormalities, so it is often recommended that they should not be administered to pregnant animals, although the likelihood of adverse effects may be low (Cook et al., 2003). In the research environment, the nonspecific effects of NSAIDs may preclude their administration in certain research protocols. For example, carprofen and other NSAIDs have been shown to increase the risk of leakage after intestinal anastomoses in rats (van der Vijver et al., 2013). Consideration of the nature of the research study and potential interactions with analgesics allows a logical choice of analgesic agent to be made.

Drugs available

Aspirin Aspirin can be used to alleviate mild pain. It is most effective in humans for musculoskeletal pain and is less effective for visceral pain. Water soluble and enteric-coated tablets are available. Injectable formulations are generally available only for research use. There are few reports of the use of aspirin for the control of postoperative pain in animals, although it appeared to have some positive effects in rats (Jablonski and Howden, 2002).

A wide range of preparations that combine aspirin with other analgesics [e.g., paracetamol (acetaminophen), codeine, and dextropropoxyphene] are available for use in humans, but their efficacy in animals for use in postoperative pain has not been evaluated.

Paracetamol (acetaminophen) Paracetamol has similar analgesic efficacy as aspirin but has little antiinflammatory activity. It causes less gastrointestinal irritation, but overdosage causes liver toxicity. These analgesics should not be administered to cats, because of problems of toxicity. Tablets and oral suspensions are available for human use, and these may be used in a wide range of laboratory species, although very little data concerning efficacy in postoperative pain in animals are available. In acute pain models in mice and rats, paracetamol has clear analgesic effects (Mickley et al., 2006; Miranda et al., 2008), and its use for postoperative pain relief has been suggested (Bauer et al., 2003). Assessment of its analgesic efficacy in mice, indicated that it had very limited effects after surgery (Dickinson et al., 2009; Matsumiya et al., 2012). An injectable formulation of paracetamol is available, recommended for intravenous infusions in people, however it may be effective when administered by the sc or ip routes in rodents (Minville et al., 2011; Viberg et al., 2014).

Ibuprofen Ibuprofen is effective against mild pain in human beings, but very few controlled clinical trials in animals have been undertaken (Hayes et al., 2000). Both tablets and suspensions are available for human use.

Phenylbutazone Phenylbutazone has been widely used for controlling mild pain in larger species. Nociceptive testing enables initial estimates of dose rates for small rodents, but no clinical trials have been carried out in these smaller laboratory species. Injectable (intravenous only) and oral preparations (tablets and powder) are available.

Flunixin Flunixin has been reported as being effective in controlling postoperative pain in dogs (Reid and Nolan, 1991), and it has been widely used as an analgesic in larger species (cattle and horses). It also appears to be an effective analgesic in pigs, sheep and cats, but no controlled trials have been undertaken in these species. It has been reported to have little efficacy in mice (Goecke et al., 2005; Tubbs et al., 2011) Both injectable and oral preparations are available. The most significant problem reported has been nephrotoxicity either when administered together with a known nephrotoxic agent (Mathews et al., 1987), or in circumstances when renal blood flow was likely to have been compromised (McNeil, 1992). The mechanism of action has been suggested to be inhibition of the normal prostaglandin regulation of renal blood flow, resulting in a failure of renal perfusion during periods of hypotension. Good anaesthetic practice, appropriate fluid therapy, and administration of flunixin after the completion of surgery are likely to minimize this risk. Administration to conscious, healthy animals appears not to be associated with any significant risk, but more recently developed NSAIDs should be used when practicable.

Carprofen Carprofen can provide effective postsurgical pain relief in the dog, cat, and rat (Nolan and Reid, 1993b; Slingsby and Waterman-Pearson, 2000; Roughan and Flecknell, 2001) and has also been used in a number of different species with apparent success (Allison et al., 2007; Paull et al., 2007). Both oral and injectable preparations are available. Recent studies have demonstrated efficacy following surgery in mice (Jirkof et al., 2010), but relatively high-dose rates were needed to produce significant changes in the mouse grimace scale (MGS, see Chapter 5) (Matsumiya et al., 2012).

Ketoprofen Ketoprofen is a nonselective COX inhibitor that provides moderate pain relief in rats, dogs, cats, and horses. Its efficacy in other species is uncertain, although likely effective dose rates can be suggested from analgesiometric data. Both oral and injectable formulations are available. However, significant side effects have been reported at clinically effective dose rates in rats (Lamon et al., 2008; Shientag et al., 2012), so its use in this species should be avoided.

Ketorolac Ketorolac is used in humans to control moderate to severe postoperative pain, and it may be effective in the dog (Mathews et al., 1996) and rat (Martin et al., 2004) for the control of postoperative pain. Data on its pharmacokinetic properties in a number of species are available (Mroszczak et al., 1987). Both injectable and oral formulations are available (Mroszczak et al., 1990). As with other NSAIDs, ketorolac is best not administered to animals with preexisting renal disease or fluid deficits.

Meloxicam Meloxicam is available in the UK as an oral suspension and an injectable preparation for use in dogs, cats, and cattle. It has been shown to be effective for alleviating postoperative pain in rats (Roughan and Flecknell, 2003), mice (Wright-Williams et al., 2007; Tubbs et al., 2011; Rätsep et al., 2013), dogs, cats, and cattle. It is effective against mild to moderate pain, and the palatable oral preparation makes it particularly useful when additional doses of drugs are required. Relatively high doses may be necessary in mice ((Wright-Williams et al., 2007; Matsumiya et al., 2012), and these high-dose rates can produce acute toxicity in some strains (e.g., Balb/c, Yvette Ellen, pers. comm). For this reason, lower dose rates are suggested in table 5.5 as a starting point when using this agent in mice. Higher dose rates than originally suggested may also be required in rabbits (Turner et al., 2006; Leach et al., 2009; Delk et al., 2014). A slow-release preparation of meloxicam has recently become available in the United States, but no controlled trials in laboratory species have yet been published.

Naproxen Naproxen is unusual in having an exceptionally long half-life in the dog (35h) and has been used to alleviate moderate pain in this species, although, as with most analgesics, no controlled clinical trials have been undertaken. Naproxen is available as tablets and as an oral suspension.

Coxibs — Deracoxib, Eterocoxib, firocoxib, Paracoxib, Roficoxib, and Robenacoxib The coxibs are a group of NSAIDs with high selectivity for COX-2 (Hinz et al., 2007). The degree of inhibition of COX-1 and COX-2 may vary in different species, but generally, when used at therapeutic dose rates, their effect is primarily on COX-2. Initially, these agents were only available as oral preparations, but injectable formulations are now available. Since these agents have minimal effects on COX-1 in most species, there are no effects on platelet function. The coxibs still have adverse effects on the gastrointestinal system when administered for prolonged periods, but these effects are less than those produced by older NSAIDs (Fiorucci and Distrutti, 2011; Kim and Giorgi, 2013). Very limited data are available on their efficacy in controlling postoperative pain in laboratory species. Robenacoxib, for example, was relatively ineffective in mice at dose rates below those that resulted in significant side-effects (Beninson et al., 2018). However, the preclinical evaluation of these agents in rodents suggests they should be effective analgesics (Riendeau et al., 2001; Lees et al., 2022).

Opioids (narcotic analgesics)

A wide range of different opioid analgesics is available for use in animals. The different drugs vary in their analgesic potency, duration of action, and effects on other body systems. Opioids are classified by their activity at specific opioid receptors. The most clinically important of these are the mu and kappa receptors. Morphine and other opioids such as pethidine (meperidine), fentanyl, and alfentanil are mu agonists (they bind to and activate mu receptors). The analgesic action of full agonists increases with increasing dose rates. Other opioids (e.g., buprenorphine) are classed as partial mu agonists. Increasing the dose of these agents eventually reaches a plateau, with no further analgesia being produced. These effects are most relevant when considering the use of analgesics as components of balanced anaesthetic regiments, when mu agonists can prevent responses to surgical stimuli. Partial agonists may not achieve as great a degree of analgesia, although in the postoperative period, the degree of analgesia provided by both groups of agents is usually sufficient to control postsurgical pain. Butorphanol is a partial agonist at mu receptors and a full agonist at kappa receptors. Some analgesics are agonists at kappa receptors, but antagonists at mu receptors. These are generally referred to as mixed agonist/antagonist analgesics (nalbuphine, pentazocine). Both partial agonists and antagonists can be used to reverse the effects of full mu agonists such as fentanyl, used as part of balanced anaesthetic regimens.

Opioid agonists and partial agonists relieve pain without impairing other sensations. However, they can cause some undesirable side-effects. All opioid agonists can produce some degree of respiratory depression, but this is rarely of clinical significance in animals, unless high doses of pure mu agonists (e.g., fentanyl) are used. If respiratory depression occurs, it can be treated by the administration of the opioid antagonist drug naloxone. Administration of naloxone will also reverse the analgesic effects of the opioid, and it may be preferable to correct the respiratory depression by the use of doxapram. Alternatively, if a mu agonist opioid such as morphine or fentanyl has been used, the respiratory depression can be reversed using nalbuphine or butorphanol, and some analgesia maintained because of the action of these latter two agents at kappa receptors. Repeated administration of these agents may be required, and the animal should be observed carefully for several hours to ensure adequate respiratory function is maintained.

Opioids may also cause sedation or excitement, their effects varying considerably in different animal species (Le Bars et al., 2001). The effects on behaviour also depend upon the dose of the drug which has been administered (Flecknell, 1984).

When administered at dose rates appropriate for providing postoperative analgesia, opioids have minimal effect upon the cardiovascular system (Bowdle, 1998). Higher dose rates, such as those that might be administered when using opioids as part of a balanced anaesthetic regime, can cause bradycardia, (Pugsley, 2002), although this can be prevented by administering atropine. In addition, morphine, pethidine (meperidine), and some other opioids can stimulate histamine release and produce a peripheral vasodilatation in some species. Clinically significant hypotension is usually seen only after administration of high-dose rates or after rapid intravenous administration.

Opioids can cause vomiting in some animal species, notably in nonhuman primates and dogs. This side-effect is seen primarily when opioids are administered to pain-free animals (e.g., as preanaesthetic medication) and is less frequent when administered postoperatively. Apart from causing vomiting, opioids may delay gastric emptying, increase intestinal peristalsis, and cause spasm of the biliary tract. These effects may preclude the use of opioids in certain experimental procedures, but generally, the effects are of minimal clinical significance in animals. The detailed pharmacology of opioids has been extensively reviewed; general introductions to the field can be found in a number of sources (Grimm et al., 2015; Pasternak, 2012; Pasternak, 2014; Vuong et al., 2013).

Drugs available

Opioid agonists **Morphine** Morphine is obtained from opium and has been used as an analgesic in humans for many years. It has been extensively studied in a range of experimental animals and is also used in veterinary clinical practice). Its duration of action in most animals is 2–4 h, e.g., Gades et al., 2000, but slow-release oral formulations are also available. Initial trials of oral slow-release morphine in rats indicated it had a prolonged duration of action in antinociceptive tests (Leach et al., 2010a), and it may be of value for providing prolonged postoperative pain relief. Rapid intravenous injection in the dog can cause transient hypotension, because of histamine release, but this is not a problem if the drug is given by continuous intravenous infusion (see below). Although morphine remains one of the most useful and potent analgesics, it is relatively short acting in many species (<4 h), and its administration after neuroleptanalgesic anaesthetic techniques in laboratory species can, not surprisingly, result in severe respiratory depression. It is also a drug with significant abuse potential.

Pethidine (meperidine): Pethidine (meperidine) has been widely used as an analgesic in veterinary practice in the UK, but it has a relatively short duration of action in many species (<2 h). It has a spasmolytic action on smooth muscle in some species, and this has led to its recommendation for use in specific clinical situations such as colic in horses. Both oral and injectable formulations are available.

Methadone: Methadone has been used clinically as an analgesic in the horse, dog (Ingvast Larsson et al., 2010), and cat (Dobromylskyj, 1993), and dose rates for use in other species can be extrapolated from the results of experimental analgesiometry (Flecknell, 1984). Methadone does not tend to cause vomiting and has a slightly more rapid onset than does morphine. In addition to its activity at mu receptors, it is an NMDA antagonist, and this may add to its efficacy as an analgesic (Holtman and Wala, 2007). Both injectable and tablet formulations are available, and it is currently marketed for veterinary use in Europe.

Oxymorphone: Oxymorphone has actions similar to morphine and has been reported to be an effective analgesic in dogs and cats (Pypendop et al., 2014). Its pharmacokinetics and activity in antinociceptive tests has been evaluated in rats (Lemberg et al., 2006) and other species (Kelly et al., 2011). Because of its relatively short duration of action, oxymorphone offers no particular advantages in comparison with morphine; however, slow-release preparations of this analgesic have been produced and evaluated in rodents and other species (Krugner-Higby et al., 2003, 2009; Smith et al., 2013). If these slow-release preparations become available commercially, then they may be of considerable value in providing prolonged postoperative pain relief (Prommer, 2006).

Hydromorphone: Hydromorphone, like oxymorphone, is a pure mu agonist, with greater potency than morphine but a similar duration of action. It is used for analgesia in dogs and cats in veterinary practice in the USA (Bateman et al., 2008). Pharmacokinetic and antinociceptive data are available in a number of species (Robertson et al., 2009; KuKanich and Spade, 2013). Slow-release injectable formulations have been produced for research purposes (Smith et al., 2013) and shown to be effective in rats (Smith et al., 2006). Oral slow-release capsule preparations of hydromorphone are available commercially, and these may be of value for providing prolonged pain relief in larger species.

Codeine and dihydrocodeine: Codeine and dihydrocodeine are morphine derivatives of low and moderate potency, respectively. Codeine is used in combination with paracetamol for the relief of mild to moderate pain. Limited data on the efficacy of codeine to treat postoperative pain in animals are available (Martins et al., 2010). Dihydrocodeine is also available as an oral preparation and is an effective analgesic in human beings. To date, no information concerning its clinical efficacy in animals is available, however extensive information on its antinociceptive properties in laboratory rodents and other species is available (Miranda et al., 2013; Steagall et al., 2015).

Fentanyl: Fentanyl is a potent, relatively short acting synthetic opiate. Its main use in laboratory animal anaesthesia is in the neuroleptanalgesic combinations Hypnorm (fentanyl/fluanisone) and Innovar-Vet (fentanyl/droperidol). Because of its short duration of action (under 30 min in most species; Grimm et al., 2015) fentanyl is most widely used for providing analgesia during surgical procedures. If it is to be used to control postoperative pain, it should be administered as a continuous infusion or transdermally (see below).

Alfentanil: Alfentanil is a synthetic opioid related to fentanyl. It has pharmacodynamic properties similar to fentanyl but has a more rapid onset and shorter duration of action. Alfentanil can be administered by continuous infusion to provide analgesia during surgical procedures, and its short duration of action enables good moment-to-moment control of the intensity of the analgesic effect.

Sufentanil: Sufentanil is a highly potent mu opioid (approximately 60 times more potent than fentanyl in humans) used primarily for the provision of analgesia as part of balanced anaesthetic regimens (Camu and Vanlersberghe, 2002).

Remifentanil: Remifentanil is a very short acting mu agonist. Its short duration of action is primarily due to hydrolysis by nonspecific blood and tissue esterases. This has led to its use to provide analgesia as part of balanced anaesthetic regimens in humans and animals (Murrell et al., 2005; Komatsu et al., 2007). Even after very prolonged periods of administration, its effects are absent within a few minutes of ceasing intravenous infusion. Administration by other routes are unpredictable and not recommended (Alves et al., 2007).

Opioid mixed agonists/antagonists and partial agonists **Pentazocine:** Pentazocine has been reported to provide effective analgesia in a range of animal species (Taylor and Houlton, 1984; Craft and McNiel, 2003; Adetunji et al., 2009). It has been reported to produce dysphoria in humans (Zacny et al., 1998), but it is uncertain whether similar effects occur in animals. Generally, the sedative effect of pentazocine is less than that of morphine. Availability of this agent is now limited in some countries.

Butorphanol: Butorphanol has a veterinary product licence as an analgesic in several countries and is believed to provide postoperative analgesia in a variety of species (Flecknell and Liles, 1990; Waterman et al., 1991; Carroll et al., 2005). It is a partial mu agonist and can be used to reverse the action of fentanyl and is a kappa agonist (Hedenqvist et al., 2000). Its relatively short duration of action (<2 h) limits its value for postoperative pain relief. It is useful as a component of balanced anaesthetic mixtures (e.g., ketamine/medetomidine/butorphanol) in a range of species (see Chapters 1 and 5).

Buprenorphine: Buprenorphine is a potent partial mu agonist that has the advantage of having a prolonged duration of action in comparison to other opioids, in many species (Cowan et al., 1977a, b; Roughan and Flecknell, 2002; Sadar et al., 2018). The drug has been used in veterinary clinical practice in dogs and horses (Hunt et al., 2013), cats (Sramek et al., 2015) and a wide range of laboratory animal species (Roughan and Flecknell, 2002). It is available as an injectable formulation, a slow-release injectable formulation, a slow-release skin patch, and as tablets for sublingual administration in humans.

Buprenorphine has been reported to cause pica (eating of bedding) in rats (Clark et al., 1997; Bosgraaf et al., 2004) a behaviour that may reflect nausea (Mitchell et al., 1977). This uncommon but undesirable side-effect may occur with other opioids and may be preventable with methylnaltrexone (Aung et al., 2004); however, it is best managed by avoiding the use of opioids in susceptible strains of rat.

Since buprenorphine is a partial agonist that has been shown to be effective in reversing the effects of full mu agonists (Flecknell et al., 1989b), it has been suggested that mu agonists such as morphine cannot be given after buprenorphine has been administered. Paradoxically, this does not appear to be the case, and it has been demonstrated that within the analgesic dose range, a switch from buprenorphine to morphine is possible, without a loss of analgesic efficacy. There also appeared to be no refractory period between termination of buprenorphine analgesia and onset of the effects of morphine (Kögel et al., 2005).

Recently, slow-release formulations of buprenorphine have been marketed, and these have been shown to provide analgesia for up to 3 days in rodents (Carbone et al., 2012; Foley et al., 2011; Chum et al., 2014; Jirkof et al., 2014; Schreiner et al., 2020; Levinson et al., 2021). This is potentially an extremely useful means of ensuring effective pain relief following major surgery and pharmacokinetic data are now available for a range of species including marmosets (Fitz et al., 2021), macaques (Mackiewicz et al., 2019). Rabbits (Andrews et al., 2020), Guinea pig (Smith et al., 2016), sheep (Zullian et al., 2016) as well as rats and mice. However, there may be disadvantages if this agent is administered to animals after minor procedures when the duration of pain may be much shorter and its intensity mild. Further studies are needed to confirm the risk/benefit profile of these agents in rodents following a range of surgical procedures. At present, it is advisable to use the slow-release formulation only when pain assessment confirms that moderate to severe pain is likely to persist for 2–3 days.

Nalbuphine: Nalbuphine has been reported to provide effective analgesia in dogs (Flecknell et al., 1991) and rats (Flecknell and Liles, 1991). It has a duration of action of 2–4 h in most species. It rapidly and effectively antagonizes the effects of mu agonists such as fentanyl, while maintaining an analgesic effect at kappa receptors. It is therefore particularly suitable for reversal of opioid-based anaesthetic regimens.

Other agents

Tramadol: Tramadol is an opioid agonist that also has an analgesic action mediated via the inhibition of serotonin and noradrenaline reuptake in the spinal cord. Both oral and injectable formulations are available. Although it has been advocated for use in animals as an alternative to more potent opioids because of its second mode of action (Giorgi, 2008), it is rapidly metabolized in several species. The main metabolite has moderate opioid activity but no effects on serotonin and noradrenaline. It has been assessed in animal models relevant to postsurgical pain (Affaitati et al., 2002; Dürsteler et al., 2007; Guneli et al., 2007; Martins et al., 2010; McKeon et al., 2011; Rätsep et al., 2013) and its pharmacokinetics have been studied in dogs (Kukanich and Papich, 2004), rats (Garrido et al., 2003), mice (Beier et al., 2007), goats (De Sousa et al., 2008) rabbits (Souza et al., 2008), and piglets (Vullo et al., 2014). Tramadol may provide a useful alternative to opioids in a range of species, but variations in metabolism may produce considerable variations in analgesic efficacy. Initial trials in postoperative pain have produced variable results, but the high oral bioavailability of tramadol have led to its extensive use for the control of chronic pain in dogs.

    Tapentadol: Tapentadol is a relatively recently marketed analgesics, which in people has a lower incidence of adverse effects in comparison to equivalent doses of opioids such as morphine (Hartrick and Rodríguez Hernandez, 2012; Giorgi, 2012). It acts at mu opioid receptors and has noradrenaline reuptake inhibitory activity. Pharmacokinetics of tapentadol have been reported in dogs, (Giorgi et al., 2012) cats (Lee et al., 2013), and goats (Lavy et al., 2014) and its efficacy has been assessed in rodent antinociceptive models (Schiene et al., 2011). Preliminary studies indicate it may be of value for the control of postoperative pain in rabbits (Giorgi et al., 2013).

Local anaesthetics

As discussed earlier in this section, local anaesthetics can be used both as adjuncts to general anaesthesia and to provide postoperative pain relief. This is likely to be more effective if a longer lasting local anaesthetic (e.g., bupivacaine) is used. These techniques are well established in larger species (Grimm et al., 2015) but only limited data are available in rodents. This is presumably due to the practical difficulties associated with the use of the very small volumes of drug that can safely be administered. Nevertheless, this offers a potentially valuable means of providing analgesia when concerns related to drug interactions and a particular scientific protocol preclude the use of NSAIDs and opioids. The use of local anaesthetic can also be incorporated into a multimodal analgesic regimen. Mixtures of lidocaine and bupivacaine have been shown to provide effective analgesia after local infiltration at the time of surgery in mice (Leach et al., 2012) and guinea pigs (Ellen et al., 2016), and numerous studies in larger species have shown similar results. A very helpful review of use of local anaesthetics in fish, reptiles, and amphibia is available (Chatigny et al., 2017).

Timing of analgesic administration

One of the most important advances in the control of postoperative pain has been the realization that the timing of analgesic intervention may have a significant bearing on the intensity of postoperative pain. The concept was originally formulated early in the 20th century, by Crile (1913), based on clinical observations. Crile suggested using regional blocks with local anaesthetics, in conjunction with general anaesthesia, to prevent postoperative pain in humans and the 'formation of painful scars caused by alterations in the CNS as a result of the noxious stimulation caused during surgery'. The discovery that changes in the central processing of noxious stimuli occurred in response to peripheral injury (Coderre et al., 1993; Woolf and Chong, 1993) increased interest in this concept. After demonstration that the changes in the CNS were suppressed to a greater extent by administration of opioids before rather than after injury (Woolf and Wall, 1986; Kissin, 2000), the concept of 'preemptive analgesia' was developed. This advocated administration of analgesics before noxious stimulation began to prevent the adverse CNS changes that this stimulation induces. To be most effective, preemptive analgesia must prevent the noxious stimuli from reaching the CNS. It should also aim to reduce or eliminate peripheral inflammation, which increases input into the CNS and so aggravates central hypersensitivity.

The clinical application of this approach in humans has had mixed results (Grape and Tramèr, 2007), but it has been recognized that administering analgesics before the return of consciousness has significant advantages. As a result, the approach has been broadened and incorporated into a concept of 'preventive analgesia'. This approach aims to ensure that postoperative pain treatment starts before surgery and lasts long enough after surgery to avoid pain-induced sensitization of nociceptive processes (Katz et al., 2011). In animals, a positive effect of preemptive drug administration has been found experimentally (Woolf and Wall, 1986; Lascelles et al., 1995) and clinically in animals that are given opioids (Lascelles et al., 1997) and NSAIDs (Welsh et al., 1997). In addition, as in humans, ensuring pain relief has been provided before the animal recovers consciousness is clearly preferable to not administering analgesics until pain is experienced.

It is important to appreciate that a single dose of analgesic, administered prior to surgery, will not usually be all the analgesia that will be required. Additional analgesic medication will still be needed in the postoperative period, but this pain will be more easily controlled because preventive analgesia has been used. A further practical advantage of preventive analgesia is that it will often reduce the dose of anaesthetic drugs required, and by integrating analgesic therapy into a balanced anaesthetic technique, the potential adverse effects of anaesthesia can be improved, in addition to providing more effective pain relief.

Adopting preventive analgesia does not necessarily imply administration of opioids or NSAIDs before surgery. Crile's original concept, of using local anaesthetics, should also be considered. In addition, the use of anaesthetic agents with analgesic properties can be incorporated into a 'preventive' analgesia strategy. Of particular relevance to laboratory animals are the effects of ketamine. This drug has the potential to reverse central hypersensitivity because of its actions as an NMDA antagonist. Experimental studies have confirmed its efficacy, but clinical trials in humans have given mixed results (Visser and Schug, 2006). Its clinical benefit in animals is uncertain, but it is reasonable to suggest that the very high doses used in rodent anaesthesia should have beneficial effects in reducing the severity of postoperative pain.

Administration of NSAIDs preoperatively could potentially increase the risk of adverse side-effects related to renal function. However, these concerns are most relevant to clinical veterinary practice when animals may have chronic renal disease (Lascelles et al., 2007). The adverse effects are also only of concern during periods of hypotension. Preoperative administration in healthy human patients is not considered to be a significant risk and it seems likely that this will apply to healthy animals. NSAIDs with significant COX-1 activity decrease platelet function and so could increase bleeding times during surgery; however, this has not proven to be a significant problem (Moss et al., 2014; Mathiesen et al., 2014; Lewis et al., 2013). In some circumstances, it may not be possible to administer analgesics preventively; nevertheless, administering analgesics as soon as practicable is of significant benefit. The longer pain is established, the greater will be the degree of central hypersensitivity, and the more difficult pain management becomes.

'Multi-modal' pain therapy

Postoperative pain arises from the activation of a multiplicity of pathways, mechanisms, and transmitter systems. Administering a single class of analgesic often fails to suppress all these mechanisms, even when high-dose rates are used. Multi-modal pain therapy advocates the use of several different analgesics to provide more effective analgesia. In humans, this concept has been widely adopted and has the advantage that lower doses of each different analgesic can often be used, when they are given in combination (Ong et al., 2010). There are good experimental data in animals to support this concept (e.g., Martin et al., 2004; Miranda et al., 2008), and some evidence for efficacy in alleviating postoperative pain in animals is now available (Steagall and Monteiro-Steagall, 2013). It is an easy technique to use, and the balance of evidence suggests it will be of benefit. For example, the use of an opioid such as buprenorphine can be combined with an NSAID such as carprofen. The opioid acts centrally to limit the input of nociceptive information into the CNS and so reduces central hypersensitivity. In contrast, the NSAID acts centrally to limit other central changes induced by the nociceptive information that does get through. In addition, the NSAID peripheral actions decrease inflammation during and after surgery and limit the nociceptive information entering the CNS, as a result of the inflammation. By acting on different points of the pain pathways, the combination should be more effective than either drug given alone. Adding a local anaesthetic to this regimen can provide additional analgesia by blocking specific nerve pathways and so further improve the degree of pain control.

Using combinations of different classes of analgesics can also overcome some of the problems associated with differences in the speed of onset of action of the various agents. In a study comparing the degree of postoperative analgesia provided by pethidine and carprofen in cats, animals which received pethidine had good analgesia immediately following recovery from anaesthesia, compared to animals which received carprofen (Lascelles et al., 1995). In contrast, dogs receiving carprofen had better analgesia later in the postsurgical period. Clearly, combining the two analgesics would produce a more effective approach for controlling postoperative pain—immediate pain relief due to the opioid, and more prolonged analgesia provided by the NSAID.

Selection of anaesthetic and analgesic agents—Scientific and welfare considerations

Selection of a particular anaesthetic agent or anaesthetic technique will depend upon a variety of factors. Some of these will relate directly to the anaesthetic agent and its potential interactions with the research protocol, and others to its ability to produce the required depth of anaesthesia. A further series of factors relate to the practicalities of cost, the availability of equipment, and the expertise of personnel in the research unit. These various considerations are discussed in more detail below.

Whichever method is chosen, it is important to keep in mind that two primary aims of anaesthesia are to prevent pain and provide humane restraint. The anaesthetic method itself should therefore be one which causes minimum distress to the animal. For example, the use of inhalational agents may involve exposure to irritant vapour (e.g., ether, see above), and the restraint required for induction using a face mask may be stressful. Similarly, restraint for the administration of injectable agents can cause distress to the animal, as can the pain associated with injection of certain anaesthetics and the longer term consequences of myositis following intramuscular injection of irritant agents (Smiler et al., 1990; Beyers et al., 1991). Other potential problems associated with the use of chloral hydrate and tribromoethanol have been discussed earlier in this chapter. Intravenous administration usually results in smooth and rapid induction of anaesthesia, provided that the animal is restrained effectively and that the injection is carried out with the required degree of skill. Local adverse reactions can result from inadvertent perivascular administration (e.g., of thiopental). Consideration must be given to ways of minimizing any fear or distress associated with handling or physical restraint and movement of the animal from its holding room to the operating theatre or laboratory.

Selecting a method of anaesthesia that is least likely to interfere with a particular research protocol is perhaps the most difficult task. The major pharmacological and physiological effects of the various anaesthetic agents should be reviewed, and this can at least minimize the interactions between the technique and the research protocol. It is important to appreciate that a superficial consideration of the compound's effects may be insufficient. For example, if one concern is to maintain systemic blood pressure within the range found in conscious animals, then in the rat, pentobarbital might appear preferable to fentanyl/fluanisone/midazolam in some strains of the animal. However, the apparently normal blood pressure is maintained by peripheral vasoconstriction, and cardiac output is markedly depressed (Skolleborg et al., 1990). Animals anaesthetized with fentanyl/fluanisone/midazolam have lower systemic blood pressure, but elevated cardiac output. Consequently, it is important to decide which is more important to a particular study—blood pressure or cardiac output. Other anaesthetics, such as urethane, may sustain blood pressure, but only because of their stimulatory effects on the sympathetic nervous system, so animals may have elevated plasma catecholamine concentrations (Carruba et al., 1987). This information can only be gained by a careful search of the relevant literature. This then should allow evidence-based decisions to be made in relation to particular research projects (e.g., Zuurbier et al., 2014). It is important not to assume that such an assessment has been carried out by other research workers whose publications include details of the anaesthetic technique used. *Simply adopting the method of anaesthesia described in publications dealing with the particular animal model of interest will not necessarily ensure that an appropriate technique is used.*

A major consideration in this selection process is that all of the side-effects of anaesthetic agents mentioned above are dose-dependent. The more of the agent that is given, the greater the depression of body systems. Rather than trying to produce the essential components of anaesthesia with a single agent, different drugs can be combined to provide effective anaesthesia with less depression of physiological functions. This approach, of 'balanced anaesthesia' usually provides more stable anaesthesia with less likelihood of significant interactions with research protocols. Several examples of this approach have been mentioned earlier in this section, for example the use of opioids as components of anaesthetic regimens and further information is given in Chapter 4.

Having suggested that an assessment of anaesthetic–animal model interactions should be made, it is important to place such interactions in the context of the overall response to anaesthesia. There is little point in carefully selecting an anaesthetic and then allowing the animal to become hypothermic, hypoxic, and hypercapnic because of poor anaesthetic management. These common problems can have wide-ranging effects on the animal's body systems, so attention to good anaesthetic management, described in Chapter 3, is of considerable importance. A second area to consider is the animal's response to surgery. Surgical procedures produce a stress response whose magnitude is related to the severity of the operative procedure. In mammals, this response consists of a mobilization of energy reserves, such as glucose, to enable the animal to survive injury. Although this response has clear evolutionary advantages, it is considered by many to be undesirable in humans and animals which are receiving a high level of intraoperative and postoperative care (Kehlet and Dahl, 2003; Giannoudis et al., 2006). It is also often undesirable because of the potential effects on particular research protocols.

Several related endocrine responses occur, with elevation in plasma catecholamines, corticosterone or cortisone, growth hormone, vasopressin, renin, aldosterone, and prolactin, and a reduction in follicle-stimulating hormone, luteinizing hormone, and testosterone. Initially, insulin concentrations decrease and those of glucagon increase, but later, insulin concentrations rise. These hormonal responses produce an increase in glycogenolysis and lipolysis and result in hyperglycaemia. The duration of the hyperglycaemic response varies, but following major surgery, the response may persist for 4–6 h. More prolonged changes in protein metabolism occur, leading to negative nitrogen balance lasting several days (Desborough, 2000). Even minor surgical procedures can produce relatively prolonged effects. For example, blood vessel cannulation in rats produced an elevation in corticosterone for several days (Fagin and Shinsako, 1983), and more subtle disruptions of circadian rhythmicity of hormonal secretions can persist for similar periods (Desjardins, 1981). Research workers are often reluctant to refine their anaesthetic methodology because it is thought that the anaesthetics used in the new technique may affect their animal model in the postsurgical period. In some instances, there will be a sound scientific basis for this opinion, based on a critical review of the relevant literature. In other circumstances, the effects of anaesthesia may be relatively unimportant when compared with the effects of surgical stress. Similar concerns are also expressed about the use of postoperative analgesics, and once again, the side-effects of any analgesics used should be considered alongside the other effects of surgery and anaesthesia (see Chapter 5). Clearly, it is logical to consider all the factors that may interact with a particular study and to develop an anaesthetic and surgical procedure which is humane and provides minimum interference with the overall aims of the research project.

Chapter 3

Managing and monitoring anaesthesia

First steps in an anaesthetic protocol

Following induction of anaesthesia with one or more of the drugs described in Chapter 2, if surgery is to be undertaken, then the surgical site should be clipped to remove hair and the skin disinfected. These steps are essential to maintain asepsis, but they do increase the rate of heat loss, so measures to maintain body temperature should be started immediately. After preparing the surgical site, the animal should be positioned to enable the required surgical or other procedures to be carried out. A compromise must usually be made between a position considered ideal by the research worker and one that avoids compromising the function of the animal's body systems. Care must be taken to ensure that the animal's head and neck remain extended, so that the tongue or soft palate does not obstruct the larynx. The limbs should not be tied out in such a way that thoracic respiratory movements are impeded, and care must be taken during surgery that undue pressure is not placed on the chest wall or abdomen. In smaller species, the use of elastic bands or ties to position the animal can lead to excessive extension of the limbs and consequent interference with respiratory movements. Similarly, elastic bands placed around the abdomen interfere with both diaphragmatic movements and the venous return from the hindquarters and abdominal viscera. This and other techniques that aim to immobilize the animal physically are rarely needed and should be avoided. If it does become necessary to retract the limbs, these should not be pulled into full extension and the anchoring bandages should be tied loosely. This is particularly important during prolonged anaesthesia, when constricting ties around the limbs can lead to tissue damage and peripheral limb oedema, which causes considerable discomfort to the animal in the postoperative period.

If an endotracheal tube is used, it should be tied firmly to the animal's jaw. Taping the anaesthetic breathing system to the operating table helps to prevent it dragging on the endotracheal tube and dislodging it. The risk of inadvertent disconnection is reduced by using light-weight disposable breathing systems (see Chapter 1) and purpose made anchoring devices (Fig. 3.1). Particular care must be taken if an animal requires repositioning during an operative procedure.

Laboratory Animal Anaesthesia and Analgesia. https://doi.org/10.1016/B978-0-12-818268-0.00008-5
91

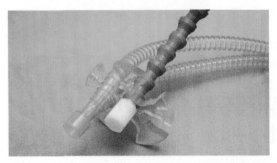

FIG. 3.1 Anchoring system for breathing circuits, infusion lines and monitoring cables (Intersurgical).

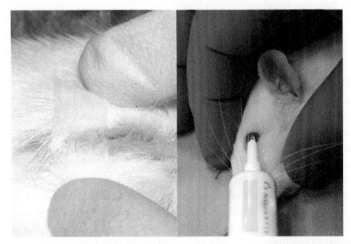

FIG. 3.2 Methods of protecting an animal's eyes during anaesthesia, by application of ophthalmic ointment or 'liquid tears' (right) or by taping the eyes shut (left)(or by using both methods, left).

Turning the animal may result in kinking of the endotracheal tube, and it is best temporarily to disconnect the animal from the breathing system while moving it.

During anaesthesia, the protective reflexes that prevent damage to the eye are usually lost, so the cornea is susceptible to drying and damage. To reduce this danger, the eyelids should be taped closed with a small piece of adhesive dressing or filled with bland ophthalmic ointment or 'liquid tears' (e.g., 'Visco-Tears', Ciba Vision or 'Lacri-lube', Allergan) (Fig. 3.2).

Monitoring anaesthesia

All general anaesthetics produce a loss of consciousness, but they also depress many other vital functions, and this can result in several undesirable effects. If these are not recognized and managed, then animals may recover poorly or may die during anaesthesia. If they do recover, the quality of scientific data obtained in subsequent studies may be compromised. If you are conducting a study in anaesthetized animals, then these changes can have an immediate impact on the quality, reliability, and reproducibility of your data.

On occasion, the degree of depression may become excessive, and the animal dies. This should be a very rare event when anaesthetizing healthy laboratory animals. The death of an animal during anaesthesia should stimulate a review of the entire process of animal selection, choice of anaesthetic, and pre- and intraoperative care. In people, anaesthetic mortality rates are approximately 34 per million (Bainbridge et al., 2012). Mortality rates in veterinary clinical practice have been reported as 1:400 (in cats) and 1:600 (in dogs) (Brodbelt et al., 2008). When anaesthetizing healthy, young adult laboratory animals, it does not seem unreasonable to expect a mortality rate of <1:1000. Anaesthetic mortality rate can usually be reduced by careful preparation, as described in Chapter 1, and by using appropriate supportive measures such as maintaining body temperature, providing oxygen or assisting ventilation, and avoiding blood loss during surgery. Although these measures should always be applied, we need to be sure that they are effective, and this requires that we monitor the animal. We can achieve this by using a combination of direct, clinical observation, and assessment and using electronic monitoring devices. The extent of our monitoring will depend upon the duration and complexity of the procedure, the requirements of our particular research goals, and the size and species of animal that is being anaesthetized.

As a routine, we should monitor depth of anaesthesia, respiratory function, cardiovascular function, and body temperature. We may also need to monitor urine output and make other more specialist observations, depending upon the potential effects on our specific study. Monitoring of an anaesthetised animal does not necessarily involve the use of complex electronic apparatus; although as will be discussed later, such equipment can prove extremely valuable. Even when using sophisticated devices, basic clinical observation, such as noting the colour of the mucous membranes, the pattern and rate of respiration and the rate and quality of the pulse are of fundamental importance. These simple clinical observations are easy to undertake and will often detect problems before they become irreversible.

Although simple clinical observation by the anaesthetist should never be neglected, when the roles of anaesthetist and surgeon or anaesthetist and theatre technician are combined, uninterrupted or even regular observation is often impossible. In addition, fatigue during prolonged procedures may lead to human error, so the use of electronic equipment to provide continuous monitoring of physiological variables can be invaluable. Certain variables can only be measured directly by using electronic equipment. When anaesthetizing animals for prolonged periods or during complex or high-risk procedures, the additional information provided by such apparatus can greatly assist in anaesthetic management. A further advantage of electronic monitoring equipment is that it usually enables acceptable limits for each monitored variable, for example, respiratory rate, to be set at the start of the period of anaesthesia. An audible or visible alert is triggered when these preset limits are exceeded. As mentioned earlier, the degree of monitoring required will depend upon the nature and duration of the surgical procedure.

Whatever monitoring is to be undertaken; it is essential to make a record of the information obtained. Problems during anaesthesia almost always develop gradually, rather than occurring as sudden catastrophes. If the observations made are recorded, preferably as simple graphs, adverse trends are easily detected, and appropriate corrective action can be taken. A second advantage of such a record is that it enables a retrospective review of a series of anaesthetics, so that techniques can be evaluated critically and improved.

As discussed earlier, it is only through practical experience that the ability to assess the significance of changes of physiological variables during the administration of a particular anaesthetic can be developed. Although the production of written records may seem unduly time-consuming, these records provide an invaluable source of reference both for the current anaesthetist and for less experienced staff who may be required to undertake the procedure in the future.

Assessment of depth of anaesthesia

Following the administration of an anaesthetic, it is essential to assess that the required depth of anaesthesia has been achieved. Depth of anaesthesia is usually assessed from a combination of measures including the presence or absence of responses to painful stimuli, changes in the pattern and depth of respiration, changes in muscle tone, and changes in heart rate and blood pressure. More sophisticated techniques for assessment of depth of anaesthesia have been developed for use in people, for example, measurement of the electroencephalogram (EEG) and of sensory or somatic evoked potentials. Although these techniques are not yet widely applied in animals (Silva et al., 2011; Otto et al., 2012; Silva and Antunes, 2012; Sandercock et al., 2014; Ruíz-López et al., 2020; Mirra et al., 2022), they may be of value in some circumstances (see 'Long-term anaesthesia', Chapter 4).

After the introduction of ether into clinical use in people, anaesthesia was divided into a series of levels and planes, (Guedel, 1920). This approach is now of very limited use although it is still referred to in some anaesthetic textbooks. The widespread variation in response to anaesthesia in different animal species and the use of several drugs in combination make such a scheme virtually unworkable in modern laboratory animal anaesthetic practice.

Although the effects of different anaesthetics vary, the initial effects are broadly similar. After administration of a volatile anaesthetic agent or the intraperitoneal injection of a drug such as pentobarbital, most animals become ataxic (wobbly), lose the ability to turn over when placed on their back (loss of righting reflex) and eventually remain immobile. At this depth of anaesthesia, they can easily be roused by painful stimuli, so anaesthesia must be allowed to deepen until these responses are lost if a surgical or other painful procedure is to be undertaken. This gradual onset of anaesthesia will not be seen if an injectable anaesthetic such as propofol is given intravenously, since loss of consciousness occurs within a minute or less.

Responses to painful stimuli

Anaesthetics are often administered to produce both unconsciousness and to block the perception of pain. Consequently, the response to painful stimuli is an essential part of the assessment of the depth of anaesthesia. In most species, this can be done by pinching the toes, tail, ears, or nose, and observing the animal's response. To assess limb withdrawal reflexes, the hindlimb should be extended and the web of skin between the toes pinched between the anaesthetist's fingernails. If the limb is withdrawn, or the animal vocalizes, it indicates that the depth of anaesthesia is insufficient to allow surgical procedures to be carried out. A slight, barely perceptible movement may remain, and in most circumstances, this indicates a sufficient depth of anaesthesia to carry out surgery. In small rodents, it may be difficult to pinch the toes; hence, pinching the tail provides a convenient alternative stimulus. In many species, the hindlimb withdrawal response is lost at lighter planes of anaesthesia than the forelimb response, but loss of hindlimb responses is normally sufficient to allow surgery to be undertaken without the animal responding. Besides using the limb withdrawal response, the reaction to pinching an ear can be observed in rabbits or guinea pigs. At light levels of anaesthesia, the animal responds to ear pinching by shaking its head and at very light levels by vocalizing. The loss of a response to painful stimuli does not occur uniformly in all body areas. On occasion, it may be possible to begin to perform a laparotomy without eliciting either any movements or any autonomic responses, such as an increase in heart rate, in an animal that still shows a limb withdrawal reflex. However, further surgical stimulation, such as cutting or clamping the abdominal muscles or handling the abdominal viscera, may produce reactions indicating an inadequate depth of anaesthesia. If this occurs, then surgery should stop, and the depth of anaesthetic increased, for example, by increasing the vapourizer setting if an inhalant anaesthetic is in use.

Although withdrawal responses provide a simple indication of depth of anaesthesia, the degree of suppression of these responses does not necessarily parallel loss of consciousness. Use of movement responses to assess depth of anaesthesia may therefore result in animals being maintained at planes of anaesthesia deeper than those required for the production of loss of consciousness and amnesia (Antognini et al., 2005). Withdrawal responses are mediated primarily by spinal mechanisms, and the depth of anaesthesia required to suppress these responses is greater than that needed for loss of consciousness. In people, neuromuscular blocking (NMB) drugs are frequently used to prevent movement, as this enables the use of lower doses of anaesthetics. Although this approach is generally effective, it can result in awareness during anaesthesia (Pandit and Cook, 2013).

In animals, NMB drugs are used much less frequently, so anaesthetics need to be relied upon not only to produce unconsciousness, but also to suppress movement. It is therefore usually impracticable to maintain only light planes of anaesthesia since surgery cannot be carried out safely or reliably. Consequently, it is recommended that absence or very marked suppression of withdrawal responses be used as an indication of the onset of surgical anaesthesia.

Alterations in eye reflexes

In larger species, such as the dog, cat, pig, sheep, and primates, the palpebral reflex (blinking when the edge of the eyelid is lightly touched) is lost during the onset of light surgical anaesthesia with barbiturates, volatile anaesthetics, and some other drugs. Use of ketamine causes the loss of this reflex at lighter levels of anaesthesia, and the use of neuroleptanalgesic combinations has unpredictable effects on the reflex. The palpebral reflex is difficult to assess in small rodents, and in rabbits it may not be lost until dangerously deep levels of anaesthesia have been attained. In larger species, as anaesthesia deepens the corneal reflex is lost (blinking in response to brushing the cornea with a damp swab). In small mammals, loss of this reflex is very variable, but loss usually indicates a very deep plane of anaesthesia. The position of the eyeball can also be of use once experience has been gained with the species of animal and the particular anaesthetic technique that is to be used. For example, in dogs anaesthetized with a volatile anaesthetic such as isoflurane, or with propofol, the eye rotates downward as a surgical plane of anaesthesia is attained. At very deep planes of anaesthesia, the eye rotates back to a central position, but the palpebral reflex is absent, which enables this stage to be distinguished from very light anaesthesia. Since the position of the eyeball, and other changes such as the degree of pupillary dilatation and the occurrence of side-to-side movement of the eye (nystagmus) vary both between species and with different anaesthetics, they cannot be relied upon as indicators of the depth of anaesthesia and should always be combined with observation of other clinical signs.

Alterations in cardiovascular and respiratory functions

Most anaesthetics cause a dose-dependent depression of the cardiovascular and respiratory systems. The way in which this depression is manifested can vary considerably with different anaesthetics. Both the rate and depth of breathing may change, and so may the pattern of breaths. Cardiovascular system depression usually results in a fall in arterial blood pressure, but this may be associated with either a fall or a rise in heart rate.

Given these wide variations in response, it is dangerous to generalize about the effects of different depths of anaesthesia. However, once experience has been gained with a particular anaesthetic technique in a particular animal species then these changes can be used to help assess the depth of anaesthesia. Methods of monitoring the cardiovascular and respiratory system are discussed as follows.

Monitoring body temperature

Body temperature is one of the easiest physiological variables to monitor during anaesthesia. Rectal temperature can be monitored simply by using a glass clinical thermometer, but this requires repeated adjustment and replacement of the instrument in the rectum to record the changes in body temperature that may occur during anaesthesia. A second disadvantage is that the lowest temperature measurable by many instruments designed for clinical use, including some electronic thermometers, is 35°C. The body temperature of small animals can rapidly fall below this value, and the onset of hypothermia may be overlooked. It is much more satisfactory to purchase an electronic thermometer that can provide continuous display of a wide range of body temperatures. The rectum is often the most convenient site for placing a temperature probe, but deep body or core temperature will often be underestimated. If the probe is positioned in the middle of a mass of faeces, its response time to the changes in temperature will be slow. For these reasons, it may be preferable to use a probe placed in the oesophagus, but it must be located in the lower part of the oesophagus to avoid the cooling effects of respiratory gases in the upper airway. Probe sizes of thermometers are usually suitable for placement in the rectum of all commonly used species, but smaller probe sizes need to be used in mice (Fig. 3.3).

Measurement of skin surface temperature is also valuable, and this can conveniently be carried out by taping a temperature probe between the animal's digits. In a healthy anaesthetized animal, the temperature differences between the core and the periphery rarely exceed 2–3°C. An increase in this temperature gradient indicates that peripheral vasoconstriction is occurring and the various possible causes of this should be investigated. It is also useful to place a temperature probe between the animal and any heating devices that are being used

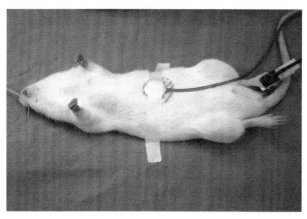

FIG. 3.3 Respiratory monitor using a pressure sensor. The device shown is designed for use during MRI procedures.

to maintain body temperature. This will detect any over-heating problems that might occur and enable measures to be taken to correct these and prevent superficial burns.

If routine temperature monitoring of a range of different species is to be undertaken, it is worth purchasing a more sophisticated electronic thermometer that allows the simultaneous use of temperature probes of different designs. Suitable-sized probes for rectal or oesophageal placement in mice, rats, rabbits, and larger animals are available, together with skin surface temperature probes, needle probes, and other special-purpose probes. Thermometers for measuring temperature at the tympanic membrane in people have an extremely rapid response time, and these may be used in larger animals (Hanneman et al., 2004) but their accuracy and reliability varies considerably when used in different species (Sousa et al., 2011; Brunell, 2012). If use of one of these devices is contemplated, it should be carefully validated using a conventional electronic probe before reliance is placed on the data obtained.

Hypothermia is one of the commonest problems to occur during anaesthesia, and its prevention and management are discussed in detail later in this section.

Respiratory system

Many anaesthetics depress respiratory function, and this can result in hypoxia, hypercapnia, and a consequent respiratory acidosis. The development of hypoxia can be prevented by administration of oxygen, something that is often done when using inhalant anaesthetics. It is equally important to provide oxygen supplementation when using injectable anaesthetics, since animals often develop marked hypoxia when breathing room air and this can have serious consequences (Blevins et al., 2021).

The routine use of 100% oxygen is, however, controversial. Administering 100% oxygen to animals (or people) for prolonged periods can cause 'oxygen toxicity' – but exposure for more than 6–12 h is needed before significant problems begin to occur (Stogner and Payne, 1992; Horncastle and Lumb, 2019). Giving 100% oxygen for shorter periods (e.g., 1 h) can cause some alveoli in the lungs to collapse (Wilding et al., 2017). These areas of atelectasis reinflate at the end of anaesthesia and animals remain well oxygenated during anaesthesia. Other lung functions remain within the normal range. If animals breathe room air (21% oxygen) then most become hypoxic during anaesthesia. In small rodents, with injectable anaesthetics, oxygen saturations of less than 60% are not uncommon unless oxygen supplementation is provided. These degrees of hypoxia have numerous detrimental effects. Ideally, we would administer 30%–40% oxygen, but this may not be easy to achieve unless you have both an oxygen and an air supply. On balance, it is advisable to administer oxygen (100%) and to consider reducing the concentration (to 30%–40%) for longer procedures

(>4 h). Susceptibility to the adverse effects of oxygen toxicity differs between species and in different ages of animals. Neonatal rodents are much less susceptible than adults ((Stogner and Payne, 1992).

Although providing supplementation with oxygen will prevent hypoxia, anaesthetized animals often become hypercapnic and acidotic (e.g., Svorc et al., 2018; Gaarde et al., 2021) and assisted ventilation is required to correct this (see Chapter 4).

Monitoring respiratory function

Clinical observations

Simple clinical observations of the animal's pattern, depth, and rate of breathing must always be made. These observations will assist in detecting any deterioration in respiratory function. In larger animals, movement of the anaesthetic breathing system's reservoir bag can be monitored if one is present. In addition, an oesophageal stethoscope can be used to monitor breath as well as heart sounds, or a conventional stethoscope placed on the chest wall.

Respiratory monitors

The respiratory rate can be conveniently monitored with electronic devices. The most inexpensive of these use a thermistor, mounted either in the anaesthetic breathing system close to the endotracheal tube or face-mask connector, or placed near the animal's nostrils. Some of these devices are sufficiently sensitive to monitor breathing in animals weighing as little as 300 g. An alternative technique for monitoring respiratory rate relies upon movements of the chest wall to trigger a pressure sensor (Fig. 3.4). These devices can be used with animals weighing as little as 30 g and are supplied with a number of imaging systems. When buying a respiratory monitor, check that it will function reliably with the range of species that you plan to anaesthetize and that an alarm can be set to detect respiratory arrest (apnoea). If buying a more sophisticated instrument that allows upper and lower limits for respiratory rate to be set, make sure the range is wide enough to be appropriate for the species that will be monitored.

Assessment of lung gas exchange

Although measurements of the mechanical aspects of breathing usually provide a reasonable indication of respiratory function, some attempt must also be made to assess the adequacy of lung gas exchange. This can be judged clinically simply by observing the colour of the visible mucous membranes and the colour of any blood which is shed at the surgical site. Although such simple clinical monitoring will show the onset of severe hypoxia, a more sensitive measure of blood oxygen saturation can be obtained using a pulse oximeter. Neither clinical observation nor use of a pulse oximeter will allow detection of a build-up of

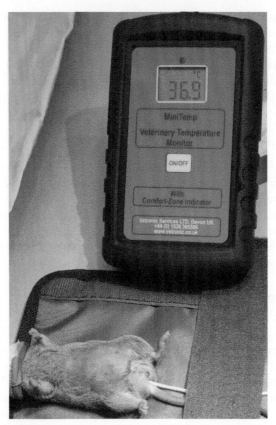

FIG. 3.4 Electronic thermometer with a rectal probe suitable for use in mice and other small rodents (Vetronics, UK).

carbon dioxide (hypercapnia), and this requires either use of a capnograph or measurement of arterial blood gases.

Pulse oximetry

Pulse oximeters measure the percentage oxygen saturation of arterial blood by detecting changes in the absorption of light across tissues, for example, across the tongue or a digit. A variety of probes of different shapes and sizes are available, the majority are designed for use in people. Both reusable and disposable probes can be obtained. Besides measuring the saturation of the haemoglobin with oxygen (SpO_2), the instrument measures the variation of this signal with each heart beat and uses this to calculate the heart rate (Chan et al., 2013). Although the absorption spectra of haemoglobins vary between species, they are sufficiently similar to allow instruments designed for use in people to be used successfully in most mammals (Gibney et al., 2011; Thawley and Waddell, 2013).

Attaching a pulse oximeter to an animal gives three useful pieces of information:

- The percentage saturation of haemoglobin allows detection of hypoxaemia (low blood oxygen concentration) due, for example, to respiratory depression, airway obstruction, or anaesthetic equipment failure.
- The heart rate reading is useful in detecting changes in rate associated with cardiovascular system depression, or tachycardia caused, for example, by carrying out surgical procedures at an inadequate anaesthetic depth.
- The strength of the pulsatile signal, usually displayed as a bar graph or as a waveform, provides some indication of the flow of blood through the tissues. This is often more informative than a simple indication of heart rate since it reflects the mechanical action of the heart. A fall or loss of signal can be due to a fall in blood pressure or to onset of vasoconstriction.

Pulse oximeters have been shown to be reasonably accurate at normal oxygen saturation levels (80%–99%) but become increasingly inaccurate as saturation falls. They therefore only provide a general indication of the adequacy of tissue oxygenation and cannot be relied upon to record low saturations accurately. Nevertheless, they are considerably more reliable than simple clinical assessment, and since development of low saturation requires immediate corrective action, their relative inaccuracy in this range is rarely of clinical importance.

Pulse oximeters are sensitive to movement artefacts, and this can cause difficulty if they are used in the later stages of recovery from anaesthesia. They will fail to provide a signal if the pulsatile blood flows through the tissues falls, as occurs during shock. In very small animals, the low volume of tissue available for monitoring limits the reliability of many currently available instruments. Several manufacturers' instruments can be used successfully in animals weighing more than 200 g, although the upper heart rates displayed, and the corresponding high heart rate alarm, may be limited to 250 beats per minute. Instruments specifically designed for veterinary use are now widely available (Appendix 4), but only a few have upper rate limits above 250 beats per minute. Pulse oximeters sufficiently sensitive for use in mice have also become available (Fig. 3.5). One such model provides heart rate, oxygen saturation, respiratory rate, and an indication of depth of respiration and respiratory effort (Fig. 3.6).

Suitable sites for probe placement include the tongue, ears, tail, nail bed, and across the footpad in rats and guinea pigs (Figs. 3.7 and 3.8). If a poor signal is obtained, then try shaving the fur or hair, or reposition the probe to different area. If the anaesthetic agent used produces marked vasoconstriction (e.g., ketamine and dexmedetomidine) then this can cause some instruments to fail. If the probe is on the tongue, remove the probe, moisten the tongue, and replace it. Some sensors function less well in bright light, so try shielding the probe with a drape or swab.

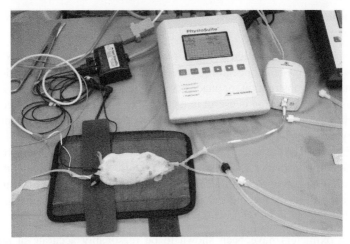

FIG. 3.5 Pulse oximeter suitable for use in mice (Mouse Physiosuite, Kent Scientific) (model shown includes capnography, temperature maintenance and monitoring and a ventilator).

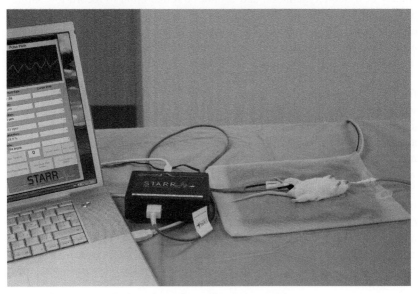

FIG. 3.6 The 'Mouseox' pulse oximeter in use (Starr Instruments).

End-tidal carbon dioxide

An indication of carbon dioxide exchange can be obtained by monitoring the concentration of carbon dioxide present in the exhaled gas using a capnograph. The maximum concentration detected at the end of exhalation, the end-tidal concentration, reflects the concentration of carbon dioxide present in alveolar gas. Considerable additional information can be obtained from the waveform

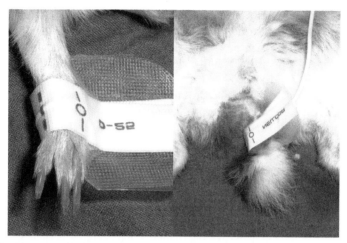

FIG. 3.7   Placement of pulse oximeter probes on a guinea pig and a rabbit.

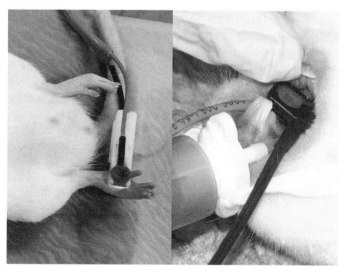

FIG. 3.8   Placement of pulse oximeter probes on a rat and a rabbit. The angled probe (right) is placed into the mouth across the surface of the tongue.

that shows the changing concentration of carbon dioxide during the respiratory cycle (O'Flaherty, 1994). A capnograph can alert the anaesthetist to an abnormal build-up of carbon dioxide caused by respiratory failure and to rebreathing of exhaled gas caused by inadequate fresh gas flows in the anaesthetic breathing system. It also indicates changes in respiratory rate and pattern. Sudden reductions in end-tidal carbon dioxide may indicate a fall in cardiac output.

When used with larger species, a capnograph allows the fresh gas flow in a breathing system to be adjusted to prevent rebreathing in an individual animal.

The flow required varies from that calculated, as described in Chapter 1, and is often lower. This can result in very significant savings in anaesthetic gases and volatile anaesthetic. When used with closed breathing systems, a capnograph also monitors the effectiveness of the absorption of carbon dioxide.

Capnographs are designed to either sample expired gases from a tube placed close to the endotracheal tube (side-stream systems) or have the carbon dioxide sensor placed directly in the anaesthetic breathing system, at the point of connection of the endotracheal tube (main-stream sampler) (Bednarski and Muir, 2011). Main-stream sampling gives a more rapid response and may be slightly more sensitive, but they introduce additional dead space in the breathing system (see Chapter 1, Anaesthetic Breathing Systems). Most instruments were originally designed for use in adult humans, and this dead space can be significant when using the equipment in small animals. The dead space can be reduced by using a paediatric adaptor and by modifying the anaesthetic breathing system connectors. Alternatively, the sensor can be placed in the expiratory limb of the breathing system but mixing of gases during breathing can reduce the accuracy of measurement.

Side-stream samplers are generally satisfactory for most species, but low dead space adapters should be used for small animals (Fig. 3.9). Their suitability in small animals also depends on the instrument's gas sampling rate. Most capnographs sample 150–200 mL of gas per minute, but many have a paediatric setting of around 50 mL/min. Since the minute volume of a 200 g rat will be approximately 120–200 mL/min, even sampling at a rate of 50 mL/min can lead to dilution of the gas that has been breathed out by the animal with fresh gas from the anaesthetic breathing system. This will result in an underestimation of the end-tidal carbon dioxide concentration. However, provided the gas flow in the breathing system is not altered, capnograph readings will indicate trends during anaesthesia in these small animals, and so are useful, particularly in animals maintained using a mechanical ventilator. If blood gas analysis is carried out at the start and end of the procedure then the capnograph readings can be related to arterial PCO_2 values, and the constant readout from

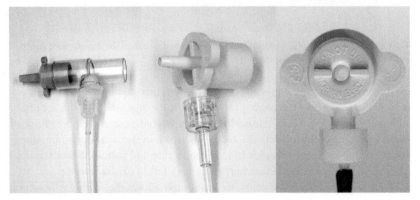

FIG. 3.9 Side-stream capnograph adaptors.

the capnograph provides reassurance that the carbon dioxide tension remained constant. An alternative is to purchase an instrument specifically designed for use in laboratory rodents that operates at very low gas sampling rates. These instruments sample at 5–20 mL/min, and so can provide accurate readings in mice and rats (Beck et al., 2013).

Blood gas analysis

The most accurate method for measuring the adequacy of lung gas exchange is to obtain arterial blood samples and carry out blood gas analysis. Blood gas analysers will measure the partial pressure of oxygen, carbon dioxide and pH of the blood and, in addition, will calculate the blood bicarbonate concentration and the base excess. Analysers designed for use in children and infants require sample volumes as low as 0.1 mL, so their use in monitoring blood gases in small animals becomes practicable. Handheld analysers are now available (Fig. 3.10). Although costs of each sample are high in comparison to conventional bench top instruments, their overall running costs can be much lower. A major problem with both types of analysers is the difficulty in obtaining arterial blood samples, particularly in smaller animals. When using either type of instrument the temperature of the animal must be recorded, since the instrument applies a correction to its measurements based on this. Since hypothermia is relatively common in anaesthetized small animals, this can be a significant source of error. Instruments designed for use in people carry out their calculations based on data from human haemoglobin. Results are generally applicable to animals, but for greater accuracy, instruments are available which allow data on animal haemoglobin to be used. Interpretation of blood gas data can be complex, but simply establishing that PCO_2, PO_2 and pH are within acceptable limits is often of significant benefit. A full and easy-to-follow account of interpretation of blood gas data can be found in Martin (1999).

A reasonably close approximation of arterial carbon dioxide and oxygen concentration may be obtained noninvasively and continuously by using transcutaneous oxygen and carbon dioxide monitors (Rodriguez et al., 2006).

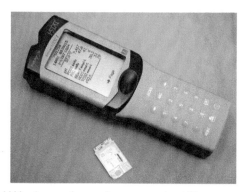

FIG. 3.10 Handheld blood gas analyser and measurement cartridge.

These instruments have been less used in animal anaesthesia, but there have been reports of their use and their accuracy in small rodents (Ramos-Cabrer et al., 2005; Barter and Hopper, 2011; Sahbaie et al., 2006).

Measurement of tidal and minute volume

In some circumstances, it is also useful to assess the depth of respiration by measuring tidal volume. Both tidal and minute volumes (the volume of gas breathed in 1 min) can be measured using a Wright's respirometer. The standard model of this instrument can measure tidal volumes down to 200 mL. A paediatric version is also available which has a range of 10–250 mL and is appropriate for use in animals ranging in size from large guinea pigs to medium-sized dogs. Respirometers are used primarily to perform intermittent measurements of tidal and minute volume and are most widely used to assess that mechanical ventilators are delivering an appropriate volume of gas. The relatively large dead space of the instrument makes its permanent placement impracticable in the breathing system of a small animal, and in patients of all sizes, build-up of water vapour can cause the failure of the instrument.

Cardiovascular system

Clinical observations

The rate, rhythm and quality of the peripheral pulse can be assessed in rabbits, cats and larger animal species. The femoral artery is easily palpable, but if the animal is covered with sterile surgical drapes, both this and other pulse points may be inaccessible. In the dog and pig, the sublingual artery and the digital artery can be palpated, but some practice is needed before these pulse points can be used with confidence. The assessment of the quality of the pulse will give a rough indication of the adequacy of systemic arterial pressure. Some indication of the adequacy of tissue perfusion can be gained by observing the capillary refill time in the visible mucous membranes. The gums are usually the most accessible site, and the refill of the capillaries following blanching by digital pressure can be observed in larger species. In normal animals, following blanching by pressing with a finger, the mucous membranes regain their normal colour in less than a second. If refill is significantly delayed (>1 s), it indicates poor peripheral tissue perfusion and possible circulatory failure.

The heart sounds and heart rate can be assessed using a stethoscope positioned on the chest wall or, in dogs and larger animals, by means of an oesophageal stethoscope. In small rodents, the heartbeat can be palpated across the thorax, but the heart rate will be too rapid to count (>250 bpm) in most animals.

Blood pressure

Systemic arterial pressure

Direct or indirect recording of systemic arterial blood pressure can be carried out in most animal species (Van Vliet et al., 2000; Kurtz et al., 2005; Bass et al., 2009;

Thal and Plesnila, 2007; Yeung et al., 2014). Direct measurements are invasive, requiring arterial cannulation, but this is relatively straightforward in most larger species. Cannulation can be carried out either following surgical exposure of a suitable artery or by puncture through the skin using a catheter and introducer. The femoral artery can be cannulated in this way in dogs, pigs, sheep, and larger primates. Percutaneous cannulation of the femoral artery in the cat and rabbit requires considerable technical skill. In rabbits and sheep, the central ear artery provides a convenient vessel for percutaneous catheterization (Fig. 3.11).

Direct blood pressure monitoring has the advantage of providing a rapid indication of changes in pressure and of recording accurately over a wide range of blood pressures. Blood pressure can also be monitored indirectly and noninvasively using a sphygmomanometer. Instruments designed specifically for use in animals are now available, and these are preferable to those used in people since an appropriate-sized cuff for occlusion of the artery must be used for accurate measurement (Kittleson, 1983) (Appendix 4). The use of a Doppler probe to detect arterial blood flow, coupled with an inflatable cuff and a pressure sensor, can be used to measure arterial blood pressure in a range of animal species. These instruments are available commercially and can be used to measure arterial pressure in the caudal artery of rats (Harvard Apparatus Ltd.,

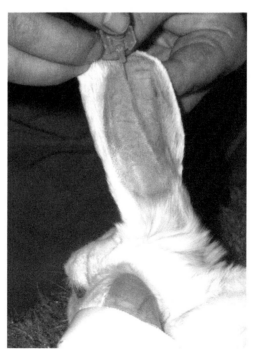

FIG. 3.11 Arterial catheter placed in the central ear artery of a rabbit.

Appendix 4). Comparisons of direct and indirect blood pressure measurements have been made in a number of species including dogs (Bosiack et al., 2010), cats (Acierno et al., 2010), pigs (Knaevelsrud and Framstad, 1992) primates (Mitchell et al., 2010), rabbits (Ypsilantis et al., 2005), guinea pigs (Kuwahara et al., 1996) and rats (Ikeda et al., 1991). In mice, a modified commercial non-invasive blood pressure device correlated well with direct measurements (Thal and Plesnila, 2007).

The main disadvantage of indirect monitoring is the intermittent nature of the information obtained. The most widely used automated instruments, which use an oscillometric technique to detect the arterial pressure changes, take readings at a minimum interval of a minute. During periods of cardiovascular instability, this interval may be too long to allow effective emergency treatment. A second problem is that when blood pressure falls, the instrument may fail to detect the reduced amplitude signals.

Pulse oximetry, which is described above, provides a measure of heart rate and gives a crude but effective indication of the pulsatile flow in the tissues.

Central venous pressure

Central venous pressure can be measured by inserting a catheter into the jugular vein and advancing it so that its tip lies in the cranial vena cava. The catheter can be introduced through the skin or following surgical exposure of the vein. The simplest method of recording central venous pressure is to connect the cannula to a water manometer that has had its baseline (zero) reading set at the estimated level of the animal's right atrium. Water manometer systems are generally unsatisfactory in smaller animals such as rodents and rabbits; and in most species it is preferable to use an electronic pressure transducer.

Pressure transducers for arterial and venous pressure are relatively expensive items of equipment, but a range of disposable transducers is available for use in people (Gould Medical Ltd., Appendix 4). The initial purchase cost of these transducers is considerably less than that of nondisposable transducers, and provided absolute asepsis is not required, they can be reused successfully on numerous occasions.

Electrocardiography

The electrical activity of the heart can be monitored by an electrocardiogram (ECG). Instruments designed for use in people are normally acceptable for monitoring larger animals, but the maximum heart rate that can be displayed is usually 200 or 250 bpm. Small rodents and rabbits frequently have heart rates greater than 250 bpm, and this may limit the usefulness of some of these monitors. Purpose-designed instruments for animal use are now available (Appendix 4), which enable low-voltage ECG signals and rapid heart rates to be detected (Farraj et al., 2011). ECG electrodes designed to stick on the skin can be used successfully in larger animals, provided any hair in the area of electrode placement is carefully removed. Electrodes supplied for use in infants and children are suitable for cats, rabbits, and small primates, but needle electrodes are usually required for small rodents. Electrode placement on the left and right forelimb and right hindlimb will provide a standard ECG trace, but the signal amplitude from small animals may be insufficient to produce an adequate display on some monitors. Whenever possible, it is preferable to have a demonstration of an ECG on the species concerned before purchasing the instrument.

Some monitors simply extract and display the heart rate from the ECG waveform, but this is of limited value. Both the heart rate and the ECG trace should be displayed and constantly updated. Upper and lower rate limits can usually be set, although the restricted range of these settings in some instruments may limit their use in smaller animal species. It is important to appreciate that the ECG indicates only the electrical activity of the heart and not adequate circulatory function. It is possible to have a cardiac output of zero and a normal ECG!

The heart rate can also be obtained using a pulse oximeter (see above) or a Doppler flow probe positioned over a suitable artery. An ECG monitor is of most importance during procedures where cardiac arrhythmias or other disturbances in cardiac function may be anticipated, for example, during thoracic surgery. It is also particularly useful during long-term anaesthesia, when disturbances in acid–base and electrolyte balance can lead to arrhythmias.

Anaesthetic equipment function

Before administering an anaesthetic, it is important to check that all the equipment to be used is functioning properly (see Chapter 1). Even if the equipment is functioning correctly at the start of the anaesthetic, it is important to monitor its continued normal function.

Anaesthetic breathing system disconnection

The risk of inadvertent disconnection of the animal, the anaesthetic breathing system and the anaesthetic machine can be reduced by using safe-lock type connectors. The most frequent point of disconnection is at the junction of the breathing system and the endotracheal tube. It is possible to position a thermistor-type apnoea alarm in the breathing system and this can provide an alert if disconnection occurs. When anaesthetizing larger animals, pressure monitoring can be used in the breathing system that will detect both low pressure due to disconnection and high pressure caused, for example, by a malfunctioning expiratory valve. An oxygen analyser, positioned within the fresh gas flow of the breathing system, will detect disconnection of the breathing system from the anaesthetic machine and any failure of the oxygen supply. Some machines are fitted with an audible alarm that is activated if the oxygen pressure falls below a lower limit.

Infusion pumps

If anaesthesia is being administered by continuous intravenous infusion, it is useful to have a warning system that will detect if the pump fails, or the infusion reservoir or syringe is emptied. This is particularly important if NMB agents are being administered, as these will prevent any spontaneous movements of the animal that might occur as anaesthesia becomes lighter. Older style infusion pumps generally have no warning devices, so it remains the anaesthetist's responsibility continuously to monitor their function. The more recently available microprocessor-controlled infusion pumps may be fitted with a variety of devices to alert the anaesthetist to a malfunction, but even these should be regularly inspected throughout the operative period. The main features to consider when purchasing such devices are listed in this chapter.

Anaesthetic problems and emergencies

Monitoring of the state of the animal during anaesthesia will enable early warning to be obtained of impending problems and emergencies, so that corrective action can be taken. There is little purpose in using the monitoring procedures described above unless the information obtained is of value and influences the course of action taken should problems arise. In clinical anaesthesia, the successful resuscitation of the patient is of paramount importance, but in a research setting, additional factors must be considered. An animal that has developed problems during anaesthesia, for example, severe respiratory depression, may no longer be a suitable animal model for some studies. A second consideration is that extensive emergency therapy may result in some additional pain and distress to the animal concerned. These factors must be considered, preferably *before* starting a procedure, so that an appropriate course of action in the event of emergencies can be planned. It may also be necessary to include these plans in your study protocol, for both regulatory and practical reasons.

As mentioned earlier, emergencies rarely happen without warning—keeping an anaesthetic record will allow trends to be identified and corrective measures taken before serious problems occur. The following section outlines the major indications of impending problems and suggests appropriate corrective measures.

Hypothermia

Hypothermia is a frequent cause of anaesthetic deaths. Hypothermia prolongs recovery time from anaesthesia (Pottie et al., 2007) and increases the potency of volatile anaesthetics (Regan and Eger, 1967). The MAC of isoflurane, for example, decreases by 5% for each 1°C fall in temperature (reviewed by Franks and Leib, 1996). It is a particularly common problem in small rodents and birds, but also occurs in larger species, especially during prolonged anaesthesia. Small mammals and birds lose heat rapidly because of their high surface area to body weight ratio. The homeostatic mechanisms that control body temperature are depressed during anaesthesia and severe hypothermia can result. Hypothermia can develop rapidly in small animals; the author has recorded reductions in body temperature of 5–10°C in as little as 15–20 min in anaesthetized mice (Caro et al., 2013, in-house data, Newcastle).

Although supplying oxygen to anaesthetized animals is beneficial, the cold, dry gases from an anaesthetic machine will cool the animal. Shaving the animal before surgery will remove insulating hair and the use of cold skin disinfectants will cause further heat loss. During surgical procedures, exposure of the viscera and use of swabs soaked in cold saline, or the administration of cold intravenous fluids, will also cool the animal.

Hypothermia prolongs recovery from anaesthesia and, if severe, can result in death of the animal. It can also have direct and indirect effects on research data, by its effects on a range of biological processes (Sheffield et al., 1994; Kumar et al., 2005; Scott and Buckland, 2006; Riley and Andrzejowski, 2018). For example, it has been shown to influence implantation rates after embryo transfer (Bagis et al., 2004) and to affect outcomes in orthopaedic studies (Constant et al., 2022). It is therefore essential to take effective measures to prevent even mild hypothermia from developing.

Preventive measures

Careful pre- and intraoperative management can reduce any fall in body temperature. Most animals will require some additional heating and insulation to minimize heat loss. Effective insulation can be provided either by wrapping the animal in cotton wool, followed by an outer wrapping of aluminium foil, or by using the bubble packing which frequently forms part of the packaging of laboratory equipment, or other insulating materials. After wrapping the animal in an insulating layer of material, a window can be cut to expose the operative field (Fig. 3.12). When insulating small rodents, ensure that the tail is included in the wrapping, since heat loss from this part can be considerable. Use of a surgical drape, which is good practice as part of measures to maintain asepsis, is also beneficial in maintaining body temperature in small rodents (Celeste et al., 2021). These simple measures will help reduce heat loss, but supplemental heating is essential for small animals, even for brief periods of anaesthesia (Fig. 3.13).

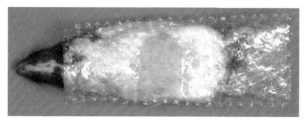

FIG. 3.12   Maintaining body temperature in a rat using bubble packing.

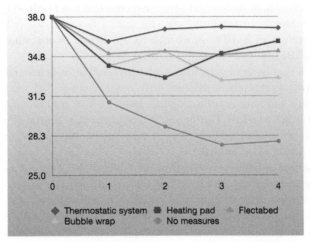

FIG. 3.13 Body temperature in anaesthetized rats when using different methods to maintain body temperature (in house data, Newcastle university).

Ideally, active warming should be started as soon as possible, since the animal will lose heat as soon as it becomes anaesthetized (Rufiange et al., 2020).

Supplemental heating can be provided by heat lamps and heating blankets, but care must be taken not to burn the animal. A thermometer placed next to the animal, or between the animal and a heating pad, will show whether excessive heat is being applied. The probe temperature should not exceed 40°C. It is possible to cause hyperthermia by over-enthusiastic or uncontrolled heating, and this can result in superficial burns or even the death of the animal. To avoid such problems, and provide effective, well-controlled warming, it is preferable to use a thermostatically controlled heating blanket, regulated by the animal's body temperature using a rectal probe (Kent Scientific, VetTech Solutions, Appendix 4) (Fig. 3.14). Even when using these types of units, some can develop 'hot spots' so monitoring the temperature of the pad beneath the animal is still advisable (Zhang et al., 2017). If such a unit is not available, a simple heating pad or lamp can be used which, provided the animal's rectal temperature is monitored, can be switched on and off manually as required. It is important to switch on heating pads and lamps before they are required, to allow their temperature to stabilize and to prevent a period of inadequate heating when the pad or lamp is warming up. Thermostatically controlled pads should be set up with the probe in contact with the blanket, so that they reach body temperature before the animal is anaesthetized.

Heating blankets may use electrical elements, have circulating warm water, or employ warm air. Warm water heating systems may not provide sufficient warmth for small animals because of the fall in water temperature between the water reservoir and the blanket, but are effective in larger species (Sikoski et al., 2007). Forced air warming systems (Fig. 3.15), such as the Bair Hugger

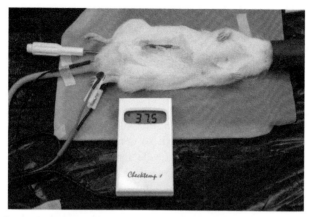

FIG. 3.14   Rat on thermostatically controlled heat pad, with temperature sensor in rectum and a second temperature probe placed between the heat pad and the rat.

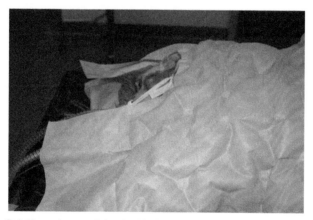

FIG. 3.15   'Bair Hugger' warm air heating blanket.

(Appendix 4), provide excellent maintenance of body temperature (Rembert et al., 2004), but the design of the blankets makes them best suited for use in larger (>3–4 kg) animals.

Respiratory system

Signs of impending failure

Respiratory rate

Respiratory rate should be recorded before anaesthesia, so that any subsequent depression in rate can be assessed. If the animal is calm and relaxed then the assessment will be reasonably accurate, but many rodents and rabbits will have a marked increased respiratory rate in the immediate preanaesthetic period, caused by fear and apprehension. In these circumstances, all that can be done is to estimate the normal respiratory rate based on published data (Appendix 1). As a general guide, in rodents and rabbits, during anaesthesia, a fall in the respiratory rate to less than 50% of the estimated normal respiratory rate indicates impending respiratory failure. The pattern and depth of respiration may also change, and animals may show a gasping pattern of respiration, or respiratory movements may become very shallow.

Changes in respiratory pattern and rate with varying depths of anaesthesia differ depending upon the agent used; so considerable experience is needed to assess their significance across a wide range of techniques and species. Nevertheless, when using a single anaesthetic in one species, it is relatively easy to develop an appreciation of the effects of increased or decreased depth of anaesthesia. This learning process can be speeded by always taking the opportunity to observe animals which have been killed humanely with an overdose of anaesthetic. If possible, undertake euthanasia using an overdose of the specific anaesthetic or anaesthetic mixture intended for later use in your research protocol.

Aside from a falling respiratory rate causing concern, a rise in rate may occur due to a lightening of the depth of anaesthesia, and this also requires corrective action. The animal should be carefully assessed for other signs of a reduced depth of anaesthesia (see 'Assessment of depth of anaesthesia' section, above), since an increased respiratory rate and depth may also occur if carbon dioxide accumulates in the breathing system. This can occur during closed system anaesthesia if the soda-lime carbon dioxide absorber has become depleted, or if there is a failure of the fresh gas supply in any breathing system.

Tidal volume

A progressive fall in tidal volume (the volume of each breath) frequently indicates impending respiratory failure. As with most other monitored variables, it is important to record the trends that occur during the period of anaesthesia. An apparent sudden failure of respiration is nearly always preceded by a progressive deterioration in tidal and minute volumes.

Lung gas exchange

Mucous membrane colour: Any noticeable blue colouration of the visible mucous membranes indicates the onset of severe hypoxia. In most species, oxygen saturation must fall below 50% before any evidence of cyanosis is detected. Development of cyanosis must therefore be considered an emergency requiring immediate corrective action. Assessment of the colour of the mucous membranes indicates only a lack of oxygen, and the mucous membranes may remain a normal pink colour despite an animal having greatly elevated blood carbon dioxide content. This can occur when an animal is receiving oxygen but has depressed respiratory function.

Pulse oximetry: A more accurate assessment of the degree of oxygenation of the arterial blood can be obtained using a pulse oximeter. Oxygen saturation is normally 95%–98% in animals that are breathing room air. Animals breathing oxygen will have a saturation of 100%. Falls of more than 5% indicate the onset of mild hypoxia, and a reduction of more than 10% requires immediate corrective action. Readings below 50% indicate severe, life-threatening hypoxia. It is important to note that one of the most common causes of an apparent sudden change in oxygen saturation is the pulse oximeter probe becoming displaced. Probe position should always be checked, and repositioned, while preparing to take action to correct hypoxia (see 'Corrective action' section below). Pulse oximeters can also show reduced oxygen saturation due to a fall in tissue perfusion due to cardiovascular failure, hypothermia, and vasoconstriction caused by anaesthetic agents. If respiratory function appears normal, always consider other possible causes of a fall in oxygen saturation. If the animal is breathing 100% oxygen, if respiration stops it will take 1–2 min for oxygen saturation to fall. If breathing room air, saturation will fall within 30 s or so. It is therefore important to continue to monitor breathing pattern even when using a pulse oximeter.

End-tidal carbon dioxide: Animals that are breathing spontaneously should have an end-tidal carbon dioxide concentration in the range of 4%–6%. During positive pressure ventilation, a concentration of 4%–5% should be maintained, so that arterial carbon dioxide tensions are maintained within the normal physiological range. A gradual rise in end-tidal carbon dioxide concentration indicates progressive hypercapnia and corrective action should be taken. Increased concentrations can also occur because of failure of the fresh gas supply, exhaustion of the soda lime during closed system anaesthesia or problems with the anaesthetic breathing system. If the capnograph trace fails to return to zero, this usually indicates that rebreathing of exhaled gas is occurring, and this can be prevented by increasing the fresh gas flow or reducing the breathing system dead space. A gradual fall in carbon dioxide concentration can indicate increased ventilation but may also occur during hypotension and decreased cardiac output. Sudden reductions in end-tidal carbon dioxide concentrations can indicate airway obstruction, disconnection of the animal from the breathing system or cardiac arrest. Assessment of the respiratory rate and tidal volume will help distinguish the likely cause. As experience is gained, considerable information can be obtained from the capnograph waveform (Marshall, 2004) (www.capnography.com).

Blood gases: It is important to establish a baseline measurement of blood gas values as soon as possible following the induction of anaesthesia. This may be compared with normal values for the particular species, but these are broadly similar for most animals (Table 3.1). A progressive fall in blood oxygen concentration, or a rise in carbon dioxide concentration, usually accompanied by a fall in pH, indicates inadequate gas exchange. Animals breathing room air (20% oxygen) will normally have an arterial PO_2 of 11–12.5 kPa (82–95 mmHg); a fall below 10.5 kPa (80 mmHg) requires corrective action. It is important to note

TABLE 3.1 Blood gas values for animals breathing air.

	Arterial blood		Venous blood	
PCO$_2$	3.8–5.3 kPa	28–40 mmHg	3.8–5.6 kPa	28–42 mmHg
PO$_2$	11–12.5 kPa	82–94 mmHg	5.3–8 kPa	40–60 mmHg
pH	7.35–7.45 (units)		7.3–7.39 (units)	

For species specific data see Brun-Pascaud et al., 1982 (rat); Lee et al., 2009 and Iversen et al., 2012 (mouse); Bar-Ilan and Marder, 1980, Eatwell et al., 2013 (rabbit), Lee et al., 2012 (Rhesus macaque).

that animals receiving oxygen will normally have much higher arterial partial pressures of oxygen. Values in the range of 40–53 kPa (300–400 mmHg) can be anticipated. In these circumstances, a fall in PO$_2$ below 90–112 mmHg (12–15 kPa) in an animal breathing 40%–60% oxygen should be considered serious. A rise in PCO$_2$, from a typical baseline of 5 kPa (37.5 mmHg) to above 6.5 kPa (50 mmHg) indicates mild to moderate hypercapnia. Increases greater than 8 kPa (60 mmHg) indicate severe hypercapnia and consequent respiratory acidosis. Detailed interpretation of blood gases data is complex, but not difficult to master. An excellent source of reference is provided by Martin (1999).

Corrective action

Impending respiratory failure requires immediate corrective action. The following list provides a quick guide to dealing with the most frequently encountered problems:

- If an anaesthetic breathing system and a source of oxygen are in use, quickly check that oxygen is still being supplied.
- Check that the breathing system is correctly assembled and still connected to the animal and to the anaesthetic machine.
- If inhalational agents are in use, reduce the concentration to zero and remember to switch off any nitrous oxide and to increase the oxygen flow to compensate for the reduced total gas flow.
- If injectable agents are being administered, stop any continuous infusions and consider whether a reversal agent should be administered. For example, if a neuroleptanalgesic anaesthetic combination has been used, respiratory depression can be reversed using a specific antagonist such as naloxone or diprenorphine (Revivon: C-Vet) (Tables 6.1 and 6.2). Since this will reverse the anaesthetic and analgesic actions of the combination, it must not be administered if surgical procedures are still in progress.
- Fill the breathing system with oxygen using the emergency oxygen switch on the anaesthetic machine and assist ventilation for a few respiratory cycles. This can be done by squeezing the reservoir bag, or temporarily occluding

the end of the reservoir limb of the system. If the chest inflates easily, listen to both sides of the chest (in larger, $\geqslant 1$ kg, animals) to assess whether they are being ventilated. If the endotracheal tube has moved down so that its tip is in one bronchus, this causes only one lung to be ventilated, and the tube must be repositioned.

- Observe the movement of the chest to ensure that gas is moving in and out of the lungs. If it is not, check the endotracheal tube—this may have become kinked, pushed too far down the airway or become blocked with secretions.
- If excessive secretions are present (indicated by bubbling noises during ventilation), disconnect the breathing system and clear the tube using gentle suction. Although a vacuum suction device is very useful, a simple technique is to use an appropriate-sized catheter attached to a 10–50 mL syringe.
- If an endotracheal tube is in place, but the chest cannot be inflated, and suction and repositioning the tube do not resolve the problem, then it may have become kinked or blocked. To replace a tube, pass an introducer down the tube, remove the tube and thread a new tube down over the introducer. If this is not possible then a laryngoscope will be needed to replace the tube.
- If the animal has not been intubated, check that the head and neck are extended, open the animal's mouth and pull its tongue forward to ensure that this is not obstructing the larynx.
- If oxygen is not being administered, but an oxygen supply is available, try to administer 100% oxygen as soon as possible. If an anaesthetic breathing system is in use, continue assisting ventilation. If a breathing system is not connected, assist ventilation by manual compression of the thorax. This can be carried out successfully even in small rodents, when compression with the thumb and forefinger can be used to produce some respiratory gas movements.
- Ventilation can also be assisted using a face mask in some species (dog, cat, and primate), but in others (e.g., rabbit), this approach often only inflates the stomach. In small rodents, ventilation can be assisted by extending the head and neck, placing a syringe barrel over the nose and mouth, and gently blowing down the nozzle (Fig. 3.16).
- Consider other possible causes of depressed respiration. Check on the activities of the surgeon, for example, whether movements of the animal's chest are being restricted, either by using the thorax as a support or by inappropriate positioning of retractors or packs.
- Respiration can be stimulated by the administration of an analeptic such as doxapram. This agent can be used in all species (Table 6.3) but as its action is of relatively short duration repeated doses may be required every 15–20 min.
- If assisted respiration and administration of oxygen have improved respiratory function, observe the animal carefully to check whether any deterioration occurs when these measures are stopped. If respiration appears

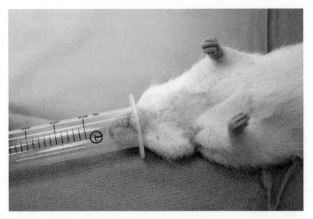

FIG. 3.16 Assisting ventilation with a syringe barrel placed over the mouth and nose of a rat.

stable, recommence administering the anaesthetic drugs if these have been stopped and continue to observe the animal carefully. If respiratory function deteriorates, recommence assisted ventilation and preferably connect the animal to a mechanical ventilator. Try to reduce the depth of anaesthesia, but this may be limited by the continuance of any surgical procedures.

Cardiovascular system

Most anaesthetic drugs have a depressant effect on cardiovascular function, and overdosage of anaesthetic is probably the most common cause of cardiac failure. Both the heart rate and the force of contraction can be depressed, and in addition, cardiac arrhythmias may occur. These may also be caused by hypoxia and hypercapnia due to respiratory failure. If the circulation is severely depressed and insufficient oxygen is delivered to the body tissues, peripheral circulatory changes may occur which lead to the development of shock. Besides the adverse effects of anaesthesia or respiratory system failure, loss of blood and body fluids may result in a reduction in the circulating blood volume. If blood volume falls excessively, cardiovascular failure and cardiac arrest will occur. Severe hypothermia (body temperature approximately 25 °C) will also result in cardiac arrest.

Clinical signs of cardiac failure

Appearance of the mucous membranes

Progressive circulatory failure may be detected in larger species by deterioration in capillary refill time, assessed by blanching the peripheral mucous membranes by pressing with a finger. Any noticeable delay in refill indicates a reduction in tissue perfusion, which may also produce moderate cyanosis (bluish tinge) of the mucous membranes. Cyanosis is more frequently associated with respiratory failure and, if it is due to cardiovascular failure alone, it indicates severe circulatory disturbance. Severe circulatory failure due to hypovolaemia will produce a blanching of the visible mucous membranes.

Peripheral temperature

Severe circulatory failure is also associated with a fall in peripheral temperature, and the animal's limbs will become noticeably cool to the touch. This can be detected more readily by using a temperature probe taped between the animal's digits and comparing the peripheral temperature with rectal temperature. This temperature change develops slowly, so it will not be of immediate value if rapid haemorrhage has occurred.

Blood pressure

Systematic arterial pressure will fall during the development of cardiac failure. Usually, the reduction is gradual and regular monitoring of blood pressure will allow corrective action to be taken before severe changes have occurred. If a pulse oximeter is in use, a fall in signal strength or complete loss of the signal may occur because of hypotension. As mentioned above, a fall in end-tidal carbon dioxide tensions can indicate hypotension. It is advisable to maintain mean arterial blood pressure above 60–70 mmHg, to avoid problems caused by poor tissue perfusion. A fall in mean arterial pressure below 45 mmHg can result in a failure of renal blood flow, severe metabolic disturbances and death.

Changes in heart rate or rhythm

Circulatory disturbances may also be associated with changes in heart rate or rhythm. An increased heart rate that is not associated with increased surgical stimulation can be due to blood loss. Severe slowing of the heart can be caused by vagal stimulation, for example, when traction is applied to the viscera, or when the vagus nerve is handled during surgical procedures in the neck. This can be sufficiently severe to cause marked hypotension and can even result in cardiac arrest.

Corrective action

When attempting to correct signs of cardiovascular failure, it is helpful if there is some indication of the likely cause. However, whatever the causative factor, the following measures should be undertaken:

- An immediate priority must be to ensure an unobstructed airway, preferably by endotracheal intubation. If intubation is possible, the animal's lungs should be ventilated with 100% oxygen, or at least this should be administered via a face mask. If assisted ventilation cannot be provided using an anaesthetic breathing system, intermittent compression of the chest wall should be commenced. In large animals, the air movements produced by this technique can be readily appreciated, but even in small rodents, gentle, and rapid compression of the thorax between thumb and forefinger can result in effective ventilation.

- If complete cardiac arrest has occurred, external cardiac massage should be undertaken. In larger species, this is best achieved by placing the animal on its side and firmly compressing the chest over the region of the heart (just behind the point of the elbow). The compression should be applied smoothly and maintained for about half a second and at a rate of 60–70 compressions/min. With smaller animals, the chest should be held between thumb and forefinger and the area over the heart compressed regularly and rapidly, about 90 times/min. Even in small rodents, some circulatory support can be maintained whilst other corrective measures are being carried out. Combining assisted ventilation and external cardiac massage in small rodents requires practice and it is usually easier to compress all areas of the thorax simultaneously.
- After adequate ventilation has been established and cardiac massage attempted if it is necessary, an intravenous line should be inserted for drug and fluid therapy. To avoid the need to carry out emergency venepuncture, it is good practice to tape a suitable catheter in a superficial vein, either during or shortly after induction of anaesthesia, in all except the smallest animals. If anaesthetic overdose is suspected, a specific antagonist should be administered if available. The use of drugs to restore stable cardiac rhythm and output requires considerable care and presupposes that arterial pressure and the ECG are being monitored. However, as an emergency measure, adrenaline (epinephrine) 0.1–0.2 mg/kg should be given if asystole is suspected, or lidocaine (2 mg/kg) administered if the heart is fibrillating. Arrhythmias will often respond to lidocaine or to other antiarrhythmic agents such as bretylium (5–10 mg/kg). Complete heart block or low cardiac output can be treated by atropine injection (0.02 mg/kg). If cardiac arrest has occurred, all drugs need to be administered by intracardiac injection. If no intravenous access is available, but an endotracheal tube has been placed, both adrenaline (epinephrine) and lidocaine can be instilled down the tube, at 2–2.5 times the i/v or intracardiac dose rate.
- After treatment of cardiac failure, sodium bicarbonate may be administered to correct the acidosis that is usually present. Although elaborate formulae are available for calculation of the dose required (see, e.g., Grimm et al., 2015), a useful guide for emergency use is 1 mmol/kg of body weight. If cardiovascular failure has arisen primarily from hypovolaemia, maintenance of adequate ventilation and effective fluid therapy will usually rapidly restore a normal acid–base balance without the administration of sodium bicarbonate.

The use of drugs to treat cardiac failure poses considerable problems for the inexperienced anaesthetist. Detailed descriptions of the techniques available are provided by Costello (2004). All of the more sophisticated means of correcting and treating cardiac failure, including measures such as defibrillation, which are used in people, can be applied in animals, and if high-risk procedures such as cardiac surgery are planned then expert advice from a veterinary anaesthetist should be sought. A summary of emergency measures is given in Table 3.2.

TABLE 3.2 Basic guide for coping with cardiovascular emergencies, and infusion rates of some drugs commonly used for cardiovascular support.

For all cardiovascular problems

1. Administer 100% oxygen and ventilate and turn off anaesthetic vapourizer or anaesthetic infusion

2. If blood loss, transfuse (in order of preference)

a. Whole blood

b. Haemaccel or hespan (or equivalent products)

c. Lactated Ringer's solution

If rapid blood loss has occurred replace estimated blood loss as quickly as possible, otherwise 10–15 mL/kg/h

1. If low arterial pressure, administer:

a. Dopamine infused at 5–10 µg/kg/min, then 1–5 µg/kg/min after volume replacement or

b. Adrenaline 1 µg/kg (0.2 mL per 20 mg of 1:10,000), then infuse 0.05–0.5 µg/kg/min

2 Cardiac arrest: start external cardiac massage

a. Fibrillating

i. Lidocaine 2 mg/kg iv (4 mL of 1% per 20 kg), if no response administer 5 mg/kg iv (10 mL of 1% per 20 kg) plus use defibrillation
and/or

ii. Bretylium 5–10 mg/kg plus use defibrillation

iii. Adrenaline 30 µg /kg (6 mL per 20 kg of 1:10,000)

iv. Sodium bicarbonate 1 mmol/kg initially, reassess after blood gas analysis

b. Asystole

i. Adrenaline as above, repeat in 2 min if no response

c. Heart block or severe bradycardia

i. Atropine 0.02 mg/kg (0.6 mL per 20 kg)

ii. If continued treatment required: isoprenaline 5–20 µg/kg/min

Drugs for cardiac support

Bretylium	5–10 mg/kg	To prevent dysrhythmias
Dobutamine	2.5–10 µg/kg/min	To increase cardiac output
Dopamine	1–5 µg/kg/min	To increase heart rate and cardiac output, decrease renal blood flow and increase peripheral vascular resistance at higher doses
	5–20 µg/kg/min	To increase renal and mesenteric blood flow
Lignocaine	30–70 µg/kg/min	To prevent dysrhythmias

For detailed information, see Thomas and Lerche (2022) and Dugdale et al. (2020).

Fluid balance

It is of vital importance to support the circulation by correcting any fluid imbalances, and hypovolaemia should always be considered a possible primary cause of cardiovascular failure. Blood loss during surgery can be very gradual, and assessment of the volume lost is frequently highly inaccurate. One simple measure is to weigh the swabs used during surgery. This should always be done, as it is rapid, simple and can be applied in all species. Weigh a dry swab, and then weigh any swab used to control haemorrhage or clean the surgical site. It is sufficiently accurate to assume that 1 g is the equivalent of 1 mL of blood. This will provide a reasonable estimate of blood loss, but additional blood will have been lost by seepage into surgical wounds, body cavities and surgical drapes. Additional losses of plasma occur by exudation both into traumatized tissues and into the peritoneal cavity during prolonged abdominal surgery [approximately 100–200 mL/h] in people (Wiklund and Thoren, 1985). A further depletion of the extracellular fluid (ECF) occurs due to water loss by evaporation from the respiratory tract and from any surgical wounds and exposed viscera. As a routine, fluid should be replaced at a rate of 10 mL/kg of body weight per hour using either Hartmann's solution or 0.9% saline. It is common practice to warm fluids to body temperature before administration (Dix et al., 2006); however, infusing fluids at 20°C rather than 38°C will have minimal effects on the animal's body temperature compared with other sources of heat loss. The effect of infusing fluids at 40°C would be greater, especially if administered rapidly, so it is recommended that fluids are warmed if practicable, but this should not delay or prevent their administration.

A healthy, unanaesthetized animal can withstand the rapid loss of 10% of its circulating volume. Once the loss exceeds 15%–20% of circulating volume, signs of hypovolaemia and shock may develop. In an anaesthetized animal, many of the physiological mechanisms that act to maintain cardiovascular stability are depressed and hence less severe losses can still have serious effects. If blood loss exceeds 20%–25% of the circulating volume, replacement with whole blood may be necessary. Smaller losses can be replaced by the infusion of crystalloid solutions or plasma volume expanders. Blood volume is approximately 70 mL/kg of body mass, so a 30 g mouse has a total blood volume of about 2.1 mL. It is easy to appreciate that any blood loss in these small species can rapidly become significant. A key measure in preventing problems is therefore to ensure careful surgical technique, with rapid and effective control of any haemorrhage.

Blood for transfusion can be obtained from a donor animal of the same species and collected in acid citrate dextrose solution (1 part ACD to 3.5 parts blood, using ACD from a blood collection pack manufactured for storing human blood). It is preferable to use the blood within 4–6 h as platelet function and red cell viability is likely to be well maintained during this period. More prolonged storage at 4°C is possible, but the storage characteristics of blood from many animal species have not been properly evaluated. Although cross matching will rarely be possible when dealing with laboratory animals, in the author's experience the incidence of adverse reaction to an initial transfusion appears to be low. Selection of donors of the same breed or strain as the recipient may help reduce the likelihood of transfusion reactions. Use of blood from a single individual, rather than pooled from several donors, will also help to reduce the risk of an adverse reaction. When using an inbred strain of rodents, there are obviously no problems of this nature.

Blood should be replaced at a rate of 10% of the calculated blood volume every 30–60 min. If severe and rapid haemorrhage has occurred, the estimated volume of blood lost should be transfused as rapidly as possible. If whole blood is unavailable, either previously stored plasma or a plasma volume expander such as Haemaccel (Hoechst) or Hespan (Du Pont) should be administered. Administration of dextrans can cause hypersensitivity reactions in some strains of rat (Cotran et al., 1968), so it is preferable to use colloidal products such as 'Haemaccel' in this species. If stored plasma is to be used, it should be warmed to body temperature before infusion. If these fluids are unavailable, or if blood loss has been less severe, then Hartmann's solution or 0.9% saline should be administered, at the rate described for whole blood and at a volume of three to five times the estimated blood loss. Considerably greater volumes are needed because these crystalloids are distributed throughout the ECF, unlike blood, plasma, and plasma volume expanders that remain in the circulatory system. Some controversy exists concerning the merits of crystalloids and plasma volume expanders for restoring the circulating volume following severe haemorrhage. Such controversy should not be a deterrent to the use of fluid therapy, and it should be remembered that it is almost always better to give than to withhold fluids.

In small animals in which intravenous therapy is difficult, 0.9% sodium chloride or Hartmann's solution can be administered intraperitoneally to correct intraoperative fluid loss. It is often particularly convenient to replace intraoperative water losses and anticipated postoperative deficits by the administration of 0.18% sodium chloride with 4% dextrose by subcutaneous injection at a rate of 10–15 mL/kg. These routes of administration result in slow absorption and will be of no immediate value in treating cardiovascular failure but will help maintain fluid balance in the postoperative period.

Vomiting and regurgitation

Vomiting or regurgitation of stomach contents may occur either during induction of anaesthesia or during the recovery period. It is a potentially serious problem and requires prompt treatment. Inhalation of gastric contents can produce immediate respiratory obstruction, asphyxiation and death, or lead to the development of aspiration pneumonia.

If vomiting occurs, the animal should immediately be placed in a head-down position and the vomit aspirated from the mouth and pharynx. If an effective suction apparatus is not available, one can be improvised from a large-diameter catheter and a 50 mL syringe. Since speed of reaction is of paramount importance, such apparatus should be available as standard equipment in the anaesthetic preparation room and recovery area.

If aspiration of vomit has occurred, oxygen should be administered, and ventilation supported if respiratory distress develops. A broad-spectrum antibiotic should be administered, and corticosteroids given immediately by the intravenous route (30 mg/kg methylprednisolone). If administration is delayed, steroids may be of little benefit.

It is obviously preferable to reduce the incidence of vomiting and its associated problems by withholding food preoperatively when appropriate (see Chapter 1) and by rapid endotracheal intubation of all animals whenever this is practicable.

Chapter 4

Specialized techniques

Use of neuromuscular blocking agents

Neuromuscular blocking (NMB) drugs or 'muscle relaxants' produce paralysis of the skeletal muscles. They may be used either to aid stable mechanical ventilation by blocking spontaneous respiratory movements or, more frequently, to provide more suitable conditions for surgery. If skeletal muscle tone is eliminated by using a NMB agent, exposure of the surgical site can be achieved more easily and with less trauma to the surrounding tissues. NMB drugs are also used in neurophysiological and other studies, to enable very light planes of anaesthesia to be maintained. Under these conditions, if an NMB had not been administered, spontaneous muscle movements could occur which would interfere with data collection.

The NMB drugs in common clinical use are classified as either depolarizing or nondepolarizing agents (Bowman, 2006). Depolarizing agents, such as suxamethonium, act similarly to the normal transmitter at the neuromuscular junction, acetylcholine. They bind to muscle receptors and trigger a muscle contraction but then produce a persistent depolarization, so preventing further muscle contractions. When drugs that act in this way are administered to an animal, generalized disorganized muscle twitches (fasciculations) are produced before complete skeletal muscle paralysis.

Nondepolarizing or competitive blocking agents do not cause a muscle contraction before producing paralysis. Drugs in this group include pancuronium, vecuronium, and rocuronium (Table 4.1). Since these agents act by competing with acetylcholine for receptor sites at the neuromuscular junction, their action can be reversed by increasing the local concentration of acetylcholine. This can be achieved by administering drugs such as neostigmine that block the activity of the enzymes which normally break down acetylcholine. As an alternative, steroid NMB agents (e.g. rocuronium and vecuronium) can be reversed using sugammadex, an agent that selectively binds to the NMB drug and prevents it acting on the neuromuscular junction (de Boer et al., 2006; Booij et al., 2009). NMB agents must be used with great care since their administration prevents all movements in response to pain. It would be possible, but obviously inhumane, to carry out a surgical procedure on an animal which had been paralysed but was still fully conscious. This is a recognized clinical problem in people (Tasbihgou et al., 2018), and it is for this reason that the use of NMB

Laboratory Animal Anaesthesia and Analgesia. https://doi.org/10.1016/B978-0-12-818268-0.00005-X

TABLE 4.1 Dose rates for neuromuscular blocking agents (mg/kg, by intravenous injection).

Muscle relaxant	Mouse	Rat	Guinea pig	Rabbit	Cat	Dog	Sheep	Goat	Pig	Nonhuman primate
Alcuronium	–	–	–	0.1–0.2	0.1	0.1	–	–	0.25	–
Atracurium	–	–	–	–	0.2	0.5	0.5	–	–	0.3–0.6
Gallamine	–	1	0.1–0.2	1	1	1	1	4	2	–
Pancuronium	–	2	0.06	0.1	0.06	0.06	0.06	0.06	0.06	0.08–0.1
Rocuronium	–	1.2	0.9	1.0	0.6	0.4–1.0	0.5	–	0.5-1.2	0.1–0.5
Suxamethonium	–	–	–	0.5	0.2	0.4	0.02	–	2	–
Tubocurarine	1	0.4	0.1–0.2	0.4	0.4	0.4	0.4	0.3	–	–
Vecuronium	–	1	–	–	0.1	0.1	0.05	0.15	0.15	0.04–0.06

drugs in experimental animals is subjected to careful control in many countries, for example special permission is required to use these agents in the United Kingdom, and Institutional Animal Care and Use Committee review is required in the United States. NMB agents are nevertheless extremely useful adjuncts to anaesthesia and enable, for example the use of balanced anaesthetic regimens such as an opioid, an hypnotic, and a muscle relaxant to provide stable surgical anaesthesia. Dose rates of several different NMB agents are given in Table 3.1.

If NMB drugs are used, other methods of assessing the depth of anaesthesia must be adopted. As a preliminary step, the proposed anaesthetic technique, excluding the NMB drug, should be administered to an animal of the same species and the proposed surgical procedure carried out. This will establish that the degree of analgesia and unconsciousness will be sufficient to allow surgery to be carried out humanely. Since considerable individual variation in response to anaesthesia occurs and some inadvertent alteration in the technique can arise, for example due to equipment malfunction, it is also necessary to provide an independent assessment of the depth of anaesthesia. Several indicators of anaesthetic depth are of use. Despite muscle paralysis, twitching of muscles may occur in response to a major surgical stimulus and this indicates that the depth of anaesthesia is inadequate. In humans, pupillary size may alter in response to surgical stimulation, but this sign is of little value in most animals, particularly if atropine has been included in the preanaesthetic medication.

Changes in blood pressure and heart rate are the most widely used indicators of adequacy of the depth of anaesthesia. Dramatic changes in heart rate or blood pressure are believed to indicate a depth of anaesthesia insufficient for the surgical procedures that are being undertaken. It has been suggested that increases in heart rate and blood pressure by 10%–20% indicate the need for additional anaesthesia. However, many anaesthetics do not block these autonomic responses and 10%–20% increases in heart rate can be seen in animals that have not received NMB drugs, and yet these animals show no movement in association with the stimulus. If inadequately anaesthetized, most animals respond to surgical stimuli with a rise in blood pressure, but some animals may show a fall in pressure. So despite their widespread acceptance, these parameters may not always be reliable indicators of adequate anaesthesia (Whelan and Flecknell, 1992).

An alternative method of monitoring the depth of anaesthesia is to use the EEG. Although this requires specialist equipment and expert interpretation, these may be available, especially if neurosurgical or neurophysiological studies are being carried out. Simple changes in the unprocessed EEG, such as onset of burst suppression, can be useful when using some anaesthetic agents, for example halothane. Various derived measures, for example total power and spectral edge frequency have also been used to assess depth of anaesthesia (Silva and Antunes, 2012); however, these measures generally cannot be used easily with balanced anaesthetic techniques which involve simultaneous use of hypnotics and analgesics. These same difficulties occur in human subjects, and great efforts have been made to develop monitoring devices that can measure loss of consciousness. The most recently developed have been bispectral index (BIS) monitors (Appadu and Vaidya, 2008), and these are now widely used in human patients, particularly in North America. Studies suggest that these and similar indices may also be of value in some species (Antognini et al., 2005; Lamont et al., 2004; Martín-Cancho et al., 2006; Otto et al., 2012; Velasco Gallego et al., 2021) but results may vary (Romanov et al., 2014). The attraction of the BIS monitor is that it provides a single number as an index of conscious-ness, or depth of anaesthesia. The disadvantage is that, like the EEG from which it is derived, it is primarily intended to assess the degree of loss of consciousness and is most predictive when a single anaesthetic agent is used. It is less reliable when using balanced anaesthesia. A further drawback is that it is designed for use in human beings, and the mathematical processing used to create the 'index' has been derived from measures made in large numbers of human subjects. Despite these problems, BIS monitors may be of use, particularly for long-term anaesthetic procedures with neuromuscular blockade, but extensive validation for each specific protocol will be needed before these monitors can be relied upon. It is also apparent that BIS values may vary between species at equivalent anaesthetic depths (Lamont et al., 2004). Given the difficulties of monitoring the level of consciousness in paralysed animals, a simpler approach is to allow the action of the muscle relaxant to subside periodically. The animal will then be capable of responding to painful stimuli with voluntary movements.

Allowing the actions of the muscle relaxant to subside will not always be practicable, especially during prolonged neurophysiological studies, however, it is almost always feasible to delay administration of the relaxant until after the start of the surgical procedure. This allows an initial assessment of the adequacy of the depth of anaesthesia to be obtained. It also avoids difficulties in interpret-ing changes in heart rate and blood pressure that can occur as a side-effect of ad-ministration of some muscle relaxants (Appadu and Vaidya, 2008). Decisions as to what constitutes an appropriate depth of anaesthesia, especially in paralysed animals, remains controversial. It has been suggested that very much lighter planes of anaesthesia should be used routinely (Antognini et al., 2005); but this approach does not take account of our current poor knowledge of indicators of consciousness in animals. A more conservative approach (Drummond et al., 1996) is recommended by most regulatory authorities, scientific journals and is adopted at the author's own institution. Before using NMB agents, it is always advisable to consult an experienced veterinary anaesthetist.

The degree of neuromuscular blockade can be monitored using a peripheral nerve stimulator. This device delivers a small electrical stimulus, either using skin electrodes or needle electrodes, to a peripheral nerve supplying muscle. In a nonparalysed animal, the stimulation causes a muscle twitch. In larger species, the medial aspect of the elbow can be used, or the medial carpal region. Full details of these techniques can be found in a number of veterinary anaesthesia texts (Dugdale et al., 2020).

Controlled ventilation

Many anaesthetic agents depress respiration, and this can lead to the production of hypercapnia, hypoxia, and acidosis. To maintain blood carbon dioxide and oxygen concentrations within normal levels, it is often necessary to assist ventilation. If the thoracic cavity is opened, the normal mechanisms of lung inflation are disrupted, and it is usually necessary to ventilate the animal's lungs artificially. It is not necessary to use a mechanical ventilator provided a suitable anaesthetic breathing system is in use (see Chapter 1) but using a ventilator will often be more convenient than manually assisting ventilation. A mechanical ventilator will often allow the precise control of the duration of inspiration and expiration, the volume of gas delivered to the lungs and the pressure reached in the airway during inspiration. It is not necessary to administer a NMB agent to carry out artificial ventilation but, unless the animal is deeply anaesthetized or is hyperventilated to produce hypocapnia, spontaneous respiratory movements may occur, and these may interfere with ventilation and surgery.

Mechanical ventilators

Ventilators for use with animals may have either been specifically designed for these species or may be adapted from their original use as ventilators for human subjects (Table 3.2). Ventilators are designed to achieve controlled ventilation of the animal's lungs by means of the application of intermittent positive pressure to the airway. This may be achieved either by delivering gas directly to the anaesthetic breathing system or, indirectly, by compressing a rebreathing bag or bellows, which in turn delivers gas to the animal.

A variety of techniques have been devised to control the delivery of gas to the patient and to determine the patterns of gas flow and gas pressure that occur during ventilation. It might be thought that all that was required of a ventilator was to deliver the required volume of gas to the lungs at a predetermined rate. However, since the characteristics of the patient's lungs, changes in airway resistance and leaks in the anaesthetic breathing system can all influence the volume of gas delivered, different techniques for terminating inspiration have been devised.

There are basically only two ways in which gas can be delivered during inspiration. The ventilator may deliver gas at a set pressure pattern: the pressure is determined by the machine, but the patient's airway characteristics will influence the volume of gas which is delivered; this is because the pressure reached in the airway depends upon the resistance to flow provided by the patient's lungs. If the ventilator is set to achieve a predetermined pressure, it will be reached earlier, and less gas will be delivered, if the patient's lungs provide a higher resistance to flow.

In contrast, a ventilator may be set to produce a fixed flow pattern, which will be uninfluenced by the patient's lung characteristics. Under these circumstances, the flow of gas will be constant but the pressure that develops in the airway will vary depending upon the patient's lung characteristics.

It is important to understand how these two types of ventilators, termed 'pressure generators' and 'flow generators' respectively, are switched or cycled from inspiration to expiration. This can be achieved in several different ways, but the most frequently used method in animal ventilators is time cycling. Here, the change to expiration occurs after a preset time and is uninfluenced by changes in the patient's lungs. If a time-cycled ventilator is used, the pressure developed in the lungs, the gas flow and the volume delivered can all vary. The actual values of these variables will depend both upon the characteristics of the patient and upon whether the ventilator is a pressure or flow generator. If the power of the ventilator is very great relative to the resistance of the patient's lungs, then although time-cycled, the ventilator may in fact deliver a preset volume during inspiration.

An alternative to time cycling is to determine the volume of gas that should be delivered during inspiration based on the animal's estimated tidal volume and change from inspiration to expiration when this volume has been delivered. In contrast, the changeover may be triggered not when a fixed volume of gas has been delivered, but when a predetermined airway pressure has been reached.

Once the lungs have been inflated and expiration begins, some mechanism must be used to trigger inspiration. In practice, only two techniques are used: either the changeover can occur after a fixed time or after airway pressure falls to a preset level.

The apparent complications introduced by the mechanics of ventilator design do have real effects on the patient. For example, if a fixed tidal volume is delivered, there will be no compensation for leaks in the anaesthetic breathing system so, if any leaks are present, there will be a fall in the volume of gas delivered to the lungs. A ventilator set to deliver gas until a preset pressure is achieved will compensate for leaks in the anaesthetic breathing system, but an increase in the animal's airway resistance will result in a fall in the tidal volume delivered to the lungs. Ventilators that deliver gas at a fixed flow with a high generating pressure and that are either time or volume cycled, are unaffected by changes in the patient's lungs, but they may produce excessive airway pressures.

In selecting a ventilator for use in laboratory animals, the most important factor to be considered is the ability to ventilate a wide range of animal species. It should be emphasized that the successful delivery of small tidal volumes (e.g., less than 50 mL) often requires a leak-proof anaesthetic breathing system and minimal compliance of breathing system components such as connecting tubing. Additional features that may be needed are the ability to apply PEEP (positive end expiratory pressure) and a facility for humidification of gases. It is also important to select a machine that is simple to use and is reliable and easy to maintain. The author's personal preference for a suitable multipurpose ventilator is the Merlin ventilator (Vetronic Services, Appendix 4) (Fig. 4.1)

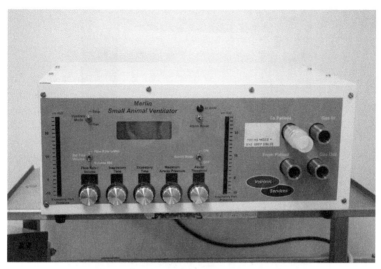

FIG. 4.1 Merlin ventilator suitable for use with animals above 1 kg body weight (Vetronics).

which can deliver a wide range of tidal volumes ranging from 50 to 800 mL. For small rodents, the ventilators produced by Kent Scientific (see Appendix 4) are versatile and can ventilate animals from 10 to 500 g (Fig. 4.2).

An important practical consideration is that some ventilators require a source of compressed gas to provide the driving power for the ventilator. If a piped gas supply is available, then this does not represent a particular problem. If small gas cylinders are used to drive the ventilator, then large numbers of cylinders may be required during a prolonged anaesthetic, even when used on a relatively small animal. Since the driving gas does not reach the animal's lungs, a compressor delivering medical air is one possible solution. Alternatively, a large cylinder of compressed air can be provided as the driving gas. If none of these solutions are thought practicable, then a mechanically driven ventilator is required. Most of these ventilators are designed to ventilate the animal either with room air or with gas provided from an anaesthetic machine. If gas is supplied from an anaesthetic machine, then it is important that a pressure relief valve is incorporated into the breathing system between the fresh gas inflow and the ventilator to prevent over-inflation of the animal's lungs. Most ventilators designed for clinical use incorporate this highly desirable feature.

Practical considerations

Controlled ventilation usually requires placement of an endotracheal tube, or if the animal is not intended to recover, a tracheostomy can be performed, and the trachea cannulated. Ventilating using a face mask is not usually successful, because of the difficulty of providing a suitable fitting mask, and the risk of inflating the stomach, which can interfere with respiratory movements. This approach

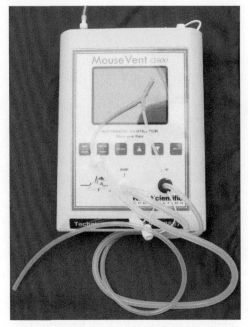

FIG. 4.2 'Mouse vent' small rodent ventilator (Kent Scientific).

has been described in rats (Rindfield and McBrian, 2012) however (Fig. 4.3) and shown to provide comparable control respiratory function (Krutrök et al., 2022). Although ventilation can be assisted after placement of a laryngeal mask, this is not recommended for anything other than short term respiratory support.

The ventilator needs connecting to the animal using a suitable breathing system. In larger species, the systems described in Chapter 1 can be used, but often

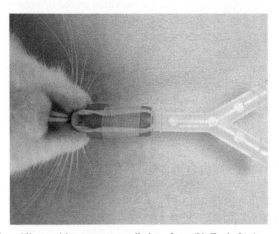

FIG. 4.3 Mask enabling positive pressure ventilation of rats (VetEquip Inc.).

a circle system will be preferred because of the much lower gas flows needed. Small animals (less than 500 g) are often connected to ventilators using a simple 'Y' connector and plastic tubing connected to the inspiratory and expiratory ports of the ventilator. The ventilator is supplied with fresh gas either simply from room air or, preferably, is supplied with a gas mixture from an anaesthetic machine. When using ventilators designed for small rodents, check the manufacturer's instructions regarding the methods of connecting the fresh gas supply. It is possible to over-pressurize some ventilators unless a separate pressure relief valve is placed between the anaesthetic gas supply and the ventilator. One easy way of achieving this is to place a standard pop-off valve and rebreathing bag on the anaesthetic machine gas outlet and connect this to the 'gas-in' port of the ventilator. The flow rate of gas from the anaesthetic machine needs only be equal to the animal's minute volume (see Chapter 1, Tidal and minute volume), but it is often difficult to set this accurately so slightly more gas than needed is supplied. This will result in gradual inflation of the reservoir bag. This can be prevented from over-filling by minor adjustments to the flow rate, or by partly opening the pop-off valve.

Remember that if an inhalant anaesthetic is being used, changing the vaporizer setting will not produce an immediate change in the concentration of anaesthetic delivered to the animal, because of mixing with gas in the rebreathing bag. To speed this process, fully open the pop-off valve, empty the bag by squeezing it, and then close the valve again. This same technique should be used with larger animals and circle breathing systems.

To ventilate an animal, first calculate the required tidal volume (approximately 7–10 mL/kg body weight) and select a suitable respiratory rate. Generally, a rate slightly lower than the normal resting rate, when conscious, is adequate. Suggested initial ventilation rates are given in Table 4.2. This process may be more complex since some ventilators do not provide direct settings for these variables. If a setting for tidal volume is not provided, then the ventilator should have a setting for inspiratory time and inspiratory flow rate. Since

$$\text{Tidal volume} = \text{inspiratory time} \times \text{inspiratory flow rate}$$

The tidal volume needed can be calculated. Setting these variables may also change the breathing rate, since

$$\text{Breathing rate}\left(\text{breaths per minute}\right) = \frac{60}{\text{inspiratory time} + \text{expiratory time}}$$

Separate controls for inspiratory and expiratory time may not be provided; some ventilators have only a control for the inspiratory time, and one for the inspiratory: expiratory (I:E) ratio. During IPPV, the heart and large veins in the thorax are compressed during inspiration, in contrast to the negative pressure that develops in the thorax during inspiration with spontaneous ventilation. The positive pressure produced during IPPV can reduce cardiac performance and cause a fall in blood pressure. To reduce this effect, inspiration should be

TABLE 4.2 Suggested ventilation rates for laboratory animals.

Species	Breaths/min
Pig, dog (<20 kg)	15–25
Pig (>20 kg), sheep (>20 kg), dog (>20 kg)	10–15
Primates (>5 kg)	20–30
Marmosets	40–50
Cat and rabbit (1–5 kg)	25–50
Guinea pig	50–80
Rat	60–100
Other small rodents	80–100

Tidal volumes of 10 mL/kg are normally required. Whenever possible the adequacy of ventilation should be assessed by monitoring the end-tidal carbon dioxide concentration or by arterial blood gas analysis.

completed in as short a period as possible but must not be too rapid as this could result in high airway pressure. Conventionally, I:E ratios are set to be 1:2, but ratios of 1:3 and 1:4 will often cause less cardiac depression, while maintaining inflation pressures below 20 cmH$_2$O.

After setting the rate and tidal volumes, and I:E ratio (if possible), set the maximum inspiratory pressure—this should be less than 15 cmH$_2$O for small animals and should not exceed 25 cmH$_2$O in most circumstances.

To monitor inflation pressures, if the ventilator is not equipped with a pressure monitor, place a needle in the inspiratory side of the anaesthetic breathing system and attach it to a pressure transducer. Besides checking that excessive pressures do not develop, by setting appropriate limits on the pressure monitor, it can act as an alert should the animal become disconnected from the breathing system or the ventilator malfunction.

When the chest is open, the lungs collapse completely, and to prevent this many ventilators allow a positive pressure to be maintained at the end of expiration (PEEP). Only very low pressures, ranging.

from 1 to 5 cmH$_2$O, are normally required for small animals. PEEP can be applied either via a specific feature on some ventilators, or by attaching a PEEP valve onto the ventilator. In some models of rodent ventilator (e.g., the Harvard volume cycled model), PEEP can be achieved simply by immersing the end of the tubing from the expiratory gas port into a few centimetres of water.

If a muscle relaxant is not being used to prevent spontaneous respiratory movements, then these can occur and interfere with the breathing cycles produced by the ventilator. One technique that can often reduce or eliminate these spontaneous movements is to increase the respiratory rate by approximately

50%, and slightly over-ventilate the animal for a few minutes. The respiratory rate can then be reduced slowly, and in many animals any spontaneous movements will remain suppressed or will be occurring in synchrony with the ventilator.

Setting up and managing IPPV can seem daunting, but it is particularly useful in long anaesthetics ($\geqslant 1$ h). Many veterinary or medically qualified anaesthetists should be able to provide expert advice. Once some simple protocols have been established, IPPV should be a relatively easy technique to master. A recommended article that provides a straightforward account of IPPV for veterinary practice are Dugdale (2007).

Long-term anaesthesia

When animals are anaesthetized for only a short period, their ability to withstand numerous disruptions to their normal physiology will often enable them to survive even very poor anaesthetic techniques. As the period of anaesthesia is extended, the adverse effects caused by poor technique become increasingly important. Similarly, the undesirable side-effects of many anaesthetic drugs become more apparent, and a considerably higher standard of intraoperative care becomes necessary. Long-term anaesthesia is of course an arbitrary term, but here it is used to describe anaesthesia lasting longer than 60 min.

There is little practical difference between anaesthesia from which the animal will be allowed to recover and that in which the animal will be killed at the end of the procedure. Prolonged, nonrecovery anaesthesia, often undertaken to enable the study of physiological mechanisms or drug metabolism, usually requires stable anaesthesia with minimal depression of the various body systems. However, since recovery is not required, cumulative effects of drugs become less important, provided physiological stability can be maintained.

Choice of anaesthetic agent

Injectable agents—Shorter acting anaesthetics

It might be thought that the simplest method of prolonging anaesthesia would be to give repeated doses of an injectable anaesthetic. Two problems arise if this approach is adopted. Giving intermittent doses of the drug will cause the depth of anaesthesia to vary considerably, although this can be overcome by administering it as a continuous infusion so that steady plasma concentrations of the anaesthetic are maintained. A second problem arises because of the pharmacokinetics of the anaesthetic. Following an initial injection of, for example a barbiturate, the blood concentration of the drug rises rapidly and the concentration in tissues with high relative blood flows, such as the brain, also increases rapidly. Redistribution of the drug to other body tissues then follows, with equilibration with body fat occurring most slowly. As this redistribution occurs, the concentration of drug in the brain falls. Recovery from the anaesthetic effects of the drug is primarily due to this redistribution, rather than to drug metabolism or excretion. If a second dose of anaesthetic is given, redistribution occurs more slowly, since the body tissues already contain some of the drug, and the duration of anaesthesia is prolonged. Repeated doses will have progressively greater effects. In addition to extending the duration of surgical anaesthesia, the sleeping time following anaesthesia is also very prolonged. If the animal does eventually wake up, the residual effects of the drug may persist for 24–48 h. For this reason, repeated incremental doses of drugs such as the barbiturates are not an ideal way of prolonging anaesthesia. The cumulative effects of different types of anaesthetic do vary considerably and some, such as alphaxalone and propofol, are rapidly metabolized following their administration. These drugs can be used to produce prolonged periods of anaesthesia without causing greatly extended recovery times (Chambers, 2019). The change in recovery rate following different durations of infusion is characterized by the 'context-sensitive half-life' of different anaesthetic agents (Hughes et al., 1992).

Whichever injectable anaesthetic is used, it is preferable to administer incremental doses of the drug by the intravenous route, so that its effects on the depth of anaesthesia will be seen rapidly and be readily adjusted. Administration by other routes is possible with some drugs, but the depth of anaesthesia will vary less predictably.

Drugs available

Barbiturates

Recovery following repeated doses of barbiturates is very prolonged, so the use of these drugs for procedures from which the animal is expected to recover consciousness is not recommended. Incremental doses of barbiturates can be used for nonrecovery experiments, but the hypotension and respiratory depression that may result can cause serious problems. In addition, the depth of anaesthesia will vary considerably and may be insufficient to allow surgical procedures to be undertaken in rodents and rabbits. In larger species, continuous infusion of pentobarbital or repeated administration can be used successfully for long-term anaesthesia, but recovery is very prolonged and often associated with long periods of involuntary excitement and ataxia. The drug is therefore best reserved for use in nonrecovery procedures.

Alphaxalone

Evaluation of the effects of long-term infusions of alphaxalone relies largely on extrapolation from data on the previous formulation which was a mixture of alphaxalone and alphadolone. It is likely that similar effects will be seen when the newer, currently available, product is used for prolonged anaesthesia (Ferre et al., 2006; Ndawana et al., 2015). Even after several hours of continuous infusion of alphaxalone/alphadolone, recovery was rapid (Cookson and Mills, 1983) and it was shown to be useful for producing long-term anaesthesia in primates, cats, sheep, pigs, rats, mice and guinea pigs (Gumbleton et al., 1990; Green et al., 1978; Whelan et al., 1999; Vijn and Sneyd, 1998; Schwenke and Cragg, 2004; Moll et al., 2013; Ruane-O'Hora et al., 2009). In rabbits, the poor degree of analgesia and the respiratory depression that is produced at high dose rates limits the usefulness of this drug unless ventilation is assisted, or additional analgesia provided by the addition of a potent opioid such as alfentanil. This approach is of value in all species, since the infusion rates of alphaxalone can be reduced, while still maintaining a surgical plane of anaesthesia if this is required.

Initially, an induction dose of the drug should be given, followed by a continuous infusion at the rate quoted in Table 3.3. The animal should be monitored to ensure the depth of anaesthesia is appropriate and the infusion rate increased or decreased as required. Stable anaesthesia is usually achieved within 30–60 min and will be established more rapidly as experience is gained with a particular species and strain of animal.

Propofol

Propofol has been shown to have little cumulative effect, and this drug has been used to provide prolonged anaesthesia in a number of species (Hall and Chambers, 1987; Brammer et al., 1993; Robertson et al., 1992; Aeschbacher and Webb, 1993; Fanton et al., 2000; Murayama et al., 2005; Tzabazis et al., 2004). Maintenance of full surgical anaesthesia with propofol alone requires relatively high infusion rates, and this may result in more prolonged recovery times in some species. It is often preferable to supplement propofol anaesthesia with a potent opioid such as alfentanil. This allows lower infusion rates of propofol to be used, and since the opioid can be reversed using a partial agonist such as butorphanol, recovery is generally rapid (Flecknell et al., 1990a). When using higher doses of opioids with propofol, respiration may be depressed, and it is preferable to connect the animal to a ventilator. This also has the advantage of improving respiratory function during prolonged anaesthesia.

Infusion with propofol will result in marked lipaemia since the commercial preparation of the drug formulated as an emulsion in soya bean oil. This seems to have little clinical significance, but potentially could interfere with some experiments. Various water-soluble pro-drugs of propofol are under development for medical clinical use and these may offer alternatives for animal use (Zhang et al., 2020; Zhou et al., 2013).

Ketamine

Ketamine is metabolized moderately rapidly, and incremental doses can be given to extend the period of anaesthesia. The recovery rate is prolonged after repeated administration and severe respiratory depression can occur. If repeated doses or a continuous intravenous infusion are to be used, it is usually necessary to monitor respiration and to have facilities for mechanical ventilation available.

It is a poor anaesthetic and analgesic in most rodents (see Chapters 2 and 5) so is almost always administered in combination with medetomidine or xylazine or a sedative such as diazepam to eliminate the muscle rigidity, which occurs when ketamine is used alone (see Chapter 2).

Ketamine can be used in combination with propofol to provide stable, long-term anaesthesia in rats (Welch, personal communication; Kiefer et al., 2022). After induction of anaesthesia with isoflurane, an intravenous catheter is placed in the tail vein and a loading dose of ketamine (50 mg/kg) and propofol (3 mg/kg) is administered. This is followed with an infusion of ketamine (50 mg/kg/h) and propofol (50 mg/kg/h) commenced. The infusion rates can then be varied to produce the required depth of anaesthesia.

Etomidate and metomidate

Etomidate and metomidate are potentially useful drugs to produce long-term anaesthesia. Rapid metabolism of these agents occurs and continuous infusion results in only a mild cumulative effect on recovery time. The drugs suppress adrenal cortical activity when used in this way (Fellows et al., 1983; Ge et al., 2013) and this side-effect must be considered if they are to be administered to experimental animals. Neither drug produces sufficient analgesia to allow surgical procedures to be carried out and an opioid such as fentanyl should be administered to produce full surgical anaesthesia. Metomidate and etomidate have relatively little depressant effect on the cardiovascular system (Valk and Struys, 2021) and when used with an opioid they produce good surgical anaesthesia and maintain stable cardiac function. Analogues of etomidate that have no suppressive effect on adrenal cortical activity are being developed for clinical use in man (Valk and Struys, 2021).

Neuroleptanalgesic combinations

These combinations, when administered with a benzodiazepine, produce excellent surgical anaesthesia in rodents and rabbits (Chapters 2 and 5), but several problems arise when they are used to produce long-term anaesthesia. Neuroleptanalgesic preparations consist of a mixture of an opiate analgesic and a potent tranquillizer. If repeated doses of a fixed-dose preparation are given, relative overdosage with the tranquillizer may occur since it usually has a longer duration of action than the analgesic component. In practice, this seems to have only a minor effect in prolonging recovery times when fentanyl/fluanisone (Hypnorm, VetaPharma) is administered to rats, mice and rabbits. The problem can be avoided by inducing anaesthesia with the neuroleptanalgesic combination and a benzodiazepine and then maintaining anaesthesia with an infusion of an analgesic alone (e.g., fentanyl). Repeated doses of the benzodiazepine are usually required only every 4–6 h.

A more serious side-effect can be the respiratory depression that is frequently seen following the administration of neuroleptanalgesics. This is not usually so severe as to necessitate assisted ventilation, but a moderate hypercapnia and respiratory acidosis will develop. During prolonged anaesthesia it is preferable to assist ventilation by using a mechanical ventilator.

The neuroleptanalgesic combination that has been used most extensively in rodents and rabbits is fentanyl/fluanisone (Hypnorm), together with diazepam or midazolam. The combination of fentanyl and dropiderol (Innovar-vet) differs in its effects and is generally less suitable when used in this way (Marini et al., 1993). Repeated doses of Hypnorm can be given every 20–30 min to maintain anaesthesia in rats, mice, rabbits and guinea pigs, following an initial dose of Hypnorm together with a benzodiazepine, although the depth of anaesthesia will fluctuate markedly. It is preferable to administer a 1:10 dilution of the drug by intravenous infusion. In other species, such as the dog and pig, a combination of fentanyl or alfentanil and midazolam can be used to provide long-lasting surgical anaesthesia (Flecknell et al., 1989a) (Table 3.3). If marketed more widely, the novel and less cumulative benzodiazepine remimidazolam may prove useful as a component of long term anaesthetics in animals (Kilpatrick, 2021).

Injectable agents—Use of longer acting anaesthetics

An alternative to administering repeated doses or a continuous infusion of short-acting agents is to select an anaesthetic with a very prolonged duration of action.

Urethane

Urethane has been widely used for the production of long periods of anaesthesia in a range of laboratory species, although its mechanism of action remains uncertain (Hara and Harris, 2002). It is reported to cause minimal depression of the cardiovascular and respiratory systems (Buelke-Sam et al., 1978; Princi et al., 2000; Janssen, 2004). It should be noted, however, that this cardiovascular stability is in part due to sustained sympathetic nervous system activity, associated with high circulating levels of adrenaline (epinephrine) and noradrenaline (norepinephrine) (Carruba et al., 1987). Although respiratory function is usually stable, problems of airway patency can arise, especially in small mammals and intubation and ventilation may be required (Moldestad et al., 2009). The properties and effects of urethane have been extensively reviewed elsewhere (Maggi and Meli, 1986a, b, c). Urethane has been reported to be both mutagenic and carcinogenic (Field and Lang, 1988) and although the experimental studies on its potency are somewhat limited, it is now widely regarded as a potential hazard to staff. Before using urethane, it is suggested that other anaesthetics are assessed, and an alternative regime is used whenever possible. If it can be shown that the use of other anaesthetics would frustrate the purpose of the experiment and a decision is taken to use urethane, it is recommended that it be treated as a moderate carcinogen. In most institutes there will be guidelines for the safe handling of such materials, and these will usually include the use of gloves and face masks when handling the substance and use of fume cupboards or similar cabinets for preparing solutions from the dry powdered drug.

If such precautions are adopted, urethane can be used in a reasonably safe manner and is a valuable anaesthetic for providing long-lasting, stable surgical anaesthesia (see review in Abdelkhalek et al., 2021). In view of its carcinogenic action in rodents, and irritant properties after intraperitoneal injection, urethane should only be used for nonrecovery procedures.

Although classed as a long-acting anaesthetic, urethane's duration of action can vary considerably, and it also causes peritoneal effusions when administered intraperitoneally. An alternative approach is to lightly anaesthetize the animal with a volatile anaesthetic, place an intravenous catheter and administer urethane by this route (Millar et al., 1989; Pagliardini et al., 2014).

Chloralose

When prolonged anaesthesia is required and surgical interference is to be kept to a minimum, chloralose may be used. This drug is an hypnotic and has little analgesic action, although this varies considerably between different species and strains of animal and in some individuals surgical anaesthesia is produced (Luckl et al., 2008). It is usually necessary to administer a short-acting anaesthetic, such as propofol while carrying out any surgical procedures, following which chloralose can be administered to produce long-lasting, light anaesthesia. This drug is believed to be particularly valuable for studies of the cardiovascular system, since the various autonomic reflexes are well maintained (Holzgrefe et al., 1987).

Chloralose is prepared by heating the powdered drug in water at 60°C to form a 1% solution. Care must be taken to avoid boiling the drug and the solution must be cooled to 40°C before administration. Administration in propylene glycol improves solubility and is claimed to reduce problems of acidosis associated with administration of chloralose (Shukla and Shukla, 1983). A more stable solution can also be produced using cyclodextrin (Storer et al., 1997). The onset of action following intravenous administration is about 15 min, so even if surgical procedures are not to be undertaken, it is preferable to administer a short-acting drug to induce anaesthesia, followed by the chloralose. The drug produces 8–10 h of light anaesthesia in most species (see Tables 6.3–6.25 for dose rates). Chloralose is normally used only for nonrecovery procedures, because of the prolonged recovery time. However, it has been used successfully for recovery procedures (Luckl et al., 2008).

In addition to the use of chloralose as the sole anaesthetic, various combinations with urethane have been described, which aim to reduce the quantity of urethane required, and provide improved analgesia in comparison to chloralose alone (Korner et al., 1968; Sharp and Hammel, 1974; Hughes et al., 1982). These combinations do not, of course, circumvent one of the main difficulties of using urethane, its classification as a carcinogen. An alternative approach is to provide additional analgesia using opioids in combination with chloralose (Rubal and Buchanan, 1986).

Inactin (thiobutobarbital)

Inactin, a thiobarbiturate, has been widely used as a long-acting anaesthetic in rats. In this species it produces surgical anaesthesia in some strains of animal, with well-maintained systemic arterial pressure (Buelke-Sam et al., 1978). Despite near-normal arterial pressure, blood flow to specific organs may be significantly reduced, due to depressed cardiac output (Holstein-Rathlou et al., 1982; Walker and Buscemi-Bergin, 1983; Rieg et al., 2004), and it should not be assumed that cardiovascular function is normal. Nevertheless, this agent can be extremely useful for producing 3–4 h of general anaesthesia in some strains of rodents (Ailiani et al., 2014).

Inhalational agents

All of the modern anaesthetic agents can be used to provide prolonged anaesthesia, and when used for extended periods many of the factors related to their use for shorter procedures are similarly relevant (see Chapter 2). There is very little practical difference between administering an inhalational agent for half an hour, and for 8 h. Once the animal has been anaesthetized, it will remain anaesthetized if supplied with an appropriate maintenance concentration of anaesthetic.

Recovery times after prolonged periods of anaesthesia using inhalational agents are longer than after shorter periods of anaesthesia, and the differences between agents becomes of greater practical importance (Eger and Johnson, 1987; Bailey, 1997; De Wolf et al., 2012). The other advantages of sevoflurane and desflurane, of being able to rapidly alter the depth of anaesthesia more rapidly than when using isoflurane can also be a significant advantage during prolonged anaesthesia.

When using volatile anaesthetics for prolonged periods it is essential to select an anaesthetic breathing system with minimal dead space and resistance. It is also important to ensure that adequate supplies of compressed gas cylinders and anaesthetic agent are available (Appendix 2). It is not uncommon to exhaust four or five gas cylinders during a prolonged period of anaesthesia, particularly if the compressed gas source is also used to drive a mechanical ventilator.

Nitrous oxide/relaxant anaesthesia

An alternative technique that has been claimed to produce prolonged, stable anaesthesia is the use of NMB agents in combination with nitrous oxide. This type of regime is totally unacceptable for use in animals, since it will not provide sufficient depth of anaesthesia to allow surgical procedures to be carried out humanely, or even produce loss of consciousness reliably.

Confusion appears to have arisen because of the widespread use of relaxant/nitrous oxide techniques in people considered at high risk of anaesthetic complications. The potency of inhalational anaesthetics is commonly expressed as the MAC (see Chapter 2). In humans, the MAC value of nitrous oxide is 95% and when used alone it can produce loss of consciousness and moderate analgesia. In animals, the MAC value ranges from 150% to 220% (Steffey et al., 1974; Weiskopf and Bogetz, 1984; Tranquilli et al., 1985; Mahmoudi et al., 1989; Gonsowski and Eger, 1994) (Table 2.4). When used alone, it cannot produce sufficient analgesia for even the most superficial surgical procedure and does not even appear to produce loss of consciousness in most species. The occurrence of awareness during relaxant/nitrous oxide anaesthesia is a recognized problem in human beings (Hardman and Aitkenhead, 2005). In animals, the low potency of nitrous oxide will almost invariably result in awareness in animals paralysed by NMB agents. Even if surgical procedures are not carried out, this is likely to cause considerable distress to the animal.

There have been suggestions that following completion of surgery using conventional anaesthetic techniques involving NMB agents, the surgical wounds can be infiltrated with local anaesthetic, and anaesthesia continued using nitrous oxide alone. Besides the problem of awareness discussed above, the local anaesthetic agents used (lidocaine) have a short duration of action and movements at the sites of surgical incision could result in pain once the drug's effects had disappeared. For these reasons the technique is considered unacceptable by the author.

Management of long-term anaesthesia

Selecting an anaesthetic regimen

Although the use of a single, long-acting agent has the attraction of simplicity, the two most widely used agents, urethane and chloralose, are suitable only for nonrecovery procedures. As discussed above, both have significant disadvantages when used as the sole anaesthetic agent, but their particular pharmacological profiles may make them suitable for specific research studies (Table 4.3).

Although it is possible to use a volatile anaesthetic or shorter-acting injectable drug as the sole agent for prolonged anaesthesia, in many circumstances the use of a balanced anaesthetic regimen has significant advantages. As discussed in Chapter 2, when a single anaesthetic agent is used, significant depression of body systems occurs, particularly when surgical planes of anaesthesia are produced, and these effects are often of even greater importance during prolonged anaesthesia.

A widely used approach in medical and veterinary anaesthesia is to include an infusion of a potent opioid, such as fentanyl or alfentanil, to an anaesthetic regimen. This greatly reduces the dose of injectable agent, or the concentration

TABLE 4.3 Suggested regimens for total intravenous anaesthesia for long-term anaesthesia.

Species	Regimen
Cat	Propofol 7.5 mg/kg i.v., then 0.2–0.5 mg/kg/min
	Alphaxalone 5 mg/kg i.v., then 0.1–0.2 mg/kg/min i.v.
Dog	Propofol 5–7.5 mg/kg i.v., then 0.2–0.4 mg/kg/min; addition of alfentanil (2–3 µg/kg/min) enables propofol rate to be reduced to 0.14–0.18 mg/kg/min
	Midazolam 50–100 µg/kg i.v. and alfentanil 10–20 µg/kg, then midazolam 5 µg/kg/min and alfentanil 4–5 µg/kg/min
	Alphaxalone, 2 mg/kg then 0.1–0.2 mg/kg/min i.v.
Mouse	Propofol 26 mg/kg i.v. then 2–2.5 mg/kg/min i.v.
Nonhuman primate	Propofol 7–8 mg/kg i.v. (after ketamine (10 mg/kg i.m.) then 0.2–0.5 mg/kg/min i.v.; addition of alfentanil (1–10 µg/kg/min) enables propofol rate to be reduced to 0.1–0.2 mg/kg/min
Pig	Propofol 2–2.5 mg/kg i.v. after ketamine (10 mg/kg i.m.), then 0.1–0.2 mg/kg/min, addition of alfentanil (20–30 µg/kg i.v.), then 2–5 µg/kg/min enables the dose of propofol to be reduced to 0.05–0.1 mg/kg/min
Rabbit	Fentanyl/fluanisone 0.3 mL/kg i.m. and midazolam (1–2 mg/kg i.v.), then fentanyl 2–5 µg/kg/min
Rat	Propofol 10 mg/kg i.v., then 0.5–1.0 mg/kg/min i.v.
Sheep	Propofol 4–6 mg/kg i.v., then 0.3–0.5 mg/kg/min i.v.

Note that regimens using opioids often require IPPV to maintain adequate ventilation.

of volatile anaesthetic needed to maintain anaesthesia. For example, reductions of 30%–50% in the concentration of inhaled anaesthetics needed to maintain anaesthesia can easily be achieved (Criado et al., 2003). Fentanyl and alfentanil have been widely used for this purpose, but remifentanil is even more suitable for prolonged anaesthesia, as it is rapidly eliminated (within a few minutes) even after several hours of continuous infusion. This characteristic makes it easy to both vary the depth of anaesthesia and produce rapid recovery. As with all opioids, some respiratory depression is produced, so the availability of assisted ventilation is recommended.

Delivery techniques for shorter acting injectable agents

Several different methods can be used, varying in cost and reliability.

Burette infusion sets and drip-rate controllers

Anaesthetic can be administered using a paediatric burette (Fig. 4.4), although often the drug will need to be diluted to allow better control of the infusion rate. Paediatric burettes deliver 60 drops per millilitres so allowing greater control over the infusion rate than the standard adult type apparatus. It is important to remember that this method of delivery will be very sensitive to partial occlusion of the catheter caused, for example by changing the position of the animal or by the formation of thrombi in the catheter tip. In addition, gradual movements of the drip control device will result in changes in the infusion rate. For these reasons, if simple drip sets are used for infusion of anaesthetics they must be monitored carefully and frequently. The degree of control over the infusion rate can be improved by use of a drip-rate controller, which varies the infusion rate by changing the diameter of the drip tubing. The simplest and least expensive of these are disposable devices, but greater accuracy can be achieved using electronically controlled devices that measure the flow by counting the fluid drip rate. Electronic controllers also incorporate an alarm to alert the anaesthetist to cessation of flow caused for example, by occlusion of the catheter or exhaustion of the fluid reservoir. All of these devices will fail should occlusion of the catheter occur.

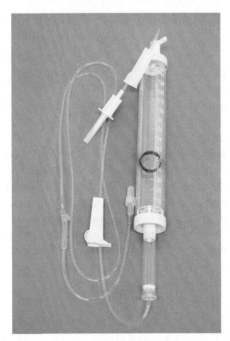

FIG. 4.4   Paediatric burette.

Infusion pumps

Catheter occlusion is less likely to occur when using an infusion pump, since the driving pressure generated by the pump tends to maintain catheter patency. Infusion pumps are available from several different manufacturers and vary considerably in their suitability for laboratory animal anaesthesia. When selecting a pump, the most important considerations are as follows:

1. Can the pump deliver a wide range of different infusion rates? Ideally, the range should extend from microlitres per hour to millilitres per minute and be capable of being varied in small increments.
2. Can the pump accept syringes of different sizes, from a variety of different manufacturers?
3. Is the pump fitted with an occlusion alarm, a 'syringe empty' alarm, a 'bubble' detector and a power failure or low-battery alarm?
4. Is a battery backup provided in case of failure of the electrical supply or inadvertent disconnection?
5. Is the pump small, light, portable, easily cleanable and robust?
6. Is it easy to set and vary the infusion rate and are any necessary calculations carried out by the pump's own microprocessor?
7. Is an interface provided for microcomputer control of pump operation and is appropriate software provided to simplify this control process?

Pumps can broadly be divided into those designed for clinical use in people or animals and those designed for laboratory or research use. Pumps designed for clinical use normally have a full range of alarms and alerts but may require purchase of specific disposable items for each use of the apparatus. They may also be designed to operate with a limited range of drug and fluid reservoirs that are most suited for use with larger (>3–5 kg) subjects. Laboratory-style pumps are often general-purpose devices that may lack many of the features found on pumps designed for clinical use but may be very versatile in the range of infusion rates and syringe types. Several pumps specifically designed for drug infusion are now available, and these often combine many of the desirable features listed above. Designs suitable for both small and larger species are available (Figs. 4.5 and 4.6).

As with other anaesthetic apparatus, it is helpful to obtain potentially suitable infusion pumps on a trial basis, to ensure that they have all the features required and prove reliable during routine operation.

Setting up an infusion

Whichever method of infusion is used, initial adjustments to the infusion rate will be required after induction of anaesthesia, but once experience has been gained with a particular anaesthetic technique, stable infusion rates and depth of anaesthesia can be established relatively rapidly. Initially the infusion rate should be based on the pharmacokinetics of the anaesthetics used, although it must be appreciated that even when full details of these have been published

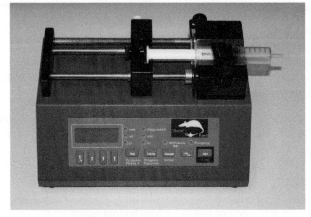

FIG. 4.5 Laboratory-style infusion pump.

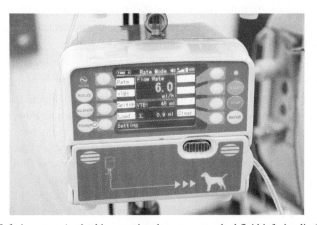

FIG. 4.6 Infusion pump (peristaltic operation that uses a standard fluid infusion line) (Burton's Veterinary UK).

for a particular species, considerable between-animal variability will occur. Nevertheless, if the drug has been well-characterized, then the required infusion rate can be estimated from its volume of distribution (the theoretical space in the body available to contain the drug) and its rate constants (Mather, 1983).

A simple analogy may be helpful to those unfamiliar with pharmacokinetics. If a particular concentration of dye is needed in a sink filled with water, the concentration of dye needed to be added is equal to the volume of water in the sink multiplied by the target concentration. If the sink's taps are turned on, and the plug is pulled out, then the situation becomes more complicated. In these circumstances, dye must be added continuously to maintain the desired concentration. If dye is added at a constant rate, then eventually a situation will be reached where the rate at which it is removed is equal to the rate at which it is added, a situation known as 'the steady state'. These same considerations apply to continuous intravenous infusion of anaesthetics. If anaesthetic is infused at a constant rate, eventually the rate of removal from the plasma will equal the rate of infusion. Under these circumstances:

$$\text{Maintenance infusion rate} = \text{Clearance} \times \text{Plasma concentration}$$

Unfortunately, this is an oversimplification for many anaesthetics, as their kinetics are better described by more complex models than a single sink, or single compartment. Many intravenous anaesthetics are characterized by one compartment with rapid distribution and elimination, and one or more compartments with slower equilibration and elimination times. The rapid distribution compartment is often thought to represent the blood and other well-perfused tissues. Drugs with these characteristics will have a single rapid half-life, and one or more slower half-lives. These are calculated from the rate of fall of the plasma concentration after administration of a single intravenous dose of the compound. The half-life of a compound is the time taken for its plasma concentration to fall by 50%.

If the anaesthetic is infused at a constant rate, it will require 4–5 half-lives to achieve a steady state. The more usual alternative is to administer an initial loading dose to induce anaesthesia, followed by a constant infusion. The problem with this latter technique is that if the drug's pharmacokinetics are best represented by a multicompartment system, then the plasma concentration will fall rapidly as redistribution to other compartments occurs. If additional anaesthetic is given rapidly to compensate, then dangerously high plasma levels can be attained. One method of estimating the loading dose required to achieve a steady plasma concentration rapidly has been described by Norwich (1977) as:

$$\text{Loading dose} = \text{Maintenance infusion rate} \times \frac{\text{Half-life}}{0.693}$$

The slow half-life is used with anaesthetics modelled using multicompartment systems. This method can result in high plasma concentrations, so if the required loading dose exceeds the recommended safe induction concentration, a safer approach is to multiply the maintenance rate by the half-life of the anaesthetic. This would prolong the time taken to reach a steady state but would reduce the chance of overdose. An alternative approach is to use two infusions, an initial rapid rate followed by a slow maintenance rate, with the rates determined by the drug clearance and the half-life (Wagner, 1974; Musk et al., 2005). More sophisticated modelling of drug pharmacodynamics and pharmacokinetics has led to the use of computer controlled infusion systems (Sneyd and Rigby-Jones, 2010). These approaches required knowledge of the pharmacological characteristics of the anaesthetic agent in the particular species. Although most data and clinical applications are in people, research data is available and this can be used to develop similar approaches in animals (Tzabazis et al., 2004; Hacker et al., 2005).

If the half-life of the drug is not known, but practical experience has been gained by giving intermittent injections of the anaesthetic to maintain anaesthesia, then the total quantity of drug given in a specific period can be used to estimate an infusion rate. It may also be possible to extrapolate half-lives of anaesthetics between species, as has been suggested for antibiotics, using the relationship of body weight$^{0.75}$ (Morris, 1995; Riviere et al., 1997; Huang and Riviere, 2014).

After establishing an infusion rate, it may be necessary to dilute the anaesthetic to provide a volume that can more easily be controlled using an infusion pump. In theory, many pumps can deliver very low volumes, but the actual rates, especially when using plastic syringes, may vary, as the plunger in the syringe may not move smoothly and continuously in response to the pump. Increasing the volumes that are being infused may help provide more stable infusion rates. However, care must be taken not to infuse too much fluid, especially in smaller animals. As a general guide, infusion rates should not exceed 10%–15% of the animal's blood volume each hour (i.e., <7–10 mL/kg/h).

As mentioned earlier, all the potential problems and adverse effects of anaesthesia assume greater importance during a prolonged period of unconsciousness. All the factors discussed in Chapter 3 should be considered, but some additional care will also be required.

Respiratory and cardiovascular function

Since all anaesthetics depress respiration to some extent, it is advisable to administer oxygen to all animals that are anaesthetized for prolonged periods. It is also preferable to intubate the animal's trachea and provide facilities for mechanical ventilation. Mechanical ventilation is essential if an attempt is to be made to provide stable blood gas levels during anaesthesia.

In a spontaneously breathing animal, the depression in respiration caused by anaesthesia produces a rise in PCO_2. The rebreathing that occurs because of equipment dead space will also contribute to this rise. In most animals, this will have little clinical consequence for an hour or so, but after this period problems associated with hypercapnia and respiratory acidosis may become apparent.

One approach to control this problem is periodically to assist ventilation by manual compression of a reservoir bag or by intermittent occlusion of a T-piece. Since, during anaesthesia, respiratory drive is influenced strongly by blood oxygen tension, temporarily increasing oxygen tension by ventilating with 100% oxygen can produce a short period of apnoea. In addition, an elevation in blood carbon dioxide tension increases the release of catecholamines and these have a stimulating effect on the cardiovascular system. If carbon dioxide tensions are reduced by a short period of assisted ventilation, this can produce a fall in cardiac output. The previously elevated carbon dioxide tensions will also have produced a peripheral vasodilatation, and this will persist during the period of assisted ventilation. The fall in cardiac output, coupled with the persistent vasodilatation may produce a period of hypotension. These problems are best avoided by ensuring that the animal's initial ventilation is adequate and if a minute volume is low, mechanical ventilation should be started early during the anaesthetic and maintained throughout its duration. Ventilation with 100% oxygen is safe for short and medium duration periods of anaesthesia, but during prolonged anaesthesia (e.g. for >12 h) it is important to provide oxygen at an inspired concentration of 30%–40% to avoid the risk of oxygen toxicity (Clutton et al., 2011; Kallet and Matthay, 2013).

A second problem occurring during long-term anaesthesia is caused by a build-up of bronchial secretions, which can block small airways (Moldestad et al., 2009). Use of atropine or glycopyrrolate can help to reduce the quantity of these secretions, but partial airway obstruction may still occur. A free flow of bronchial mucus can be produced by humidifying the inspired gas mixture. Although purpose-made nebulizers are to be preferred, simply bubbling gases through a temperature-controlled water bath appears satisfactory during controlled ventilation of rats. An alternative approach using a disposable nebulizer has been used successfully when anaesthetizing rats (Martenson et al., 2005). When anaesthetizing larger species, disposable humidifiers can be incorporated into the anaesthetic breathing system, however, these have a relatively large volume, and the increase equipment dead space precludes their use in smaller (≤5 kg) animals.

During prolonged periods of anaesthesia, metabolic acidosis may gradually develop. This can only be detected by monitoring arterial blood gases and pH and may be corrected by administration of sodium bicarbonate. Gradual fluid loss from surgical wounds, the respiratory tract and by urine formation should be replaced by continuous infusion of balanced electrolyte solutions (Hartmann's solution). During prolonged anaesthesia it is useful to monitor urine production, by catheterizing the bladder, to check on continued renal function. Urine production is normally approximately 1–1.5 mL/kg/h.

Hypothermia and fluid balance

In addition to the problems of providing adequate ventilation, all the monitoring and management techniques described in Chapter 3 assume much greater importance. Particular attention should be given to the prevention of hypothermia, and fluid balance should be carefully monitored. Although fluid deficit is the major concern during prolonged surgery and anaesthesia, it is important to avoid fluid overload, caused by a combination of enthusiastic intravenous therapy and the infusion of large volumes of anaesthetic drugs. As a general guide, total fluid infusions of up to 10% of circulating volume per hour (7 mL/kg/h) are well tolerated by most animals for the first hour of anaesthesia, followed by approximately 5 mL/kg/h.

Posture

A problem which is of considerable importance in human anaesthetic practice, but which receives little attention in laboratory animal anaesthesia is the damage that can be caused to muscles and nerves by the imposition of abnormal positions during anaesthesia. To avoid unnecessary postoperative discomfort, try to ensure that the animal is placed in as normal a posture as possible. Avoid 'tying out' the limbs and instead use positioning pads. Try to protect pressure points such as the elbow, hock and the wings of the pelvic bones. If possible, change the animal's position and massage these pressure points every 1–2 h. The eyes should be protected, preferably by taping them shut, to avoid corneal desiccation. The addition of a bland ophthalmic ointment or 'liquid tears' (e.g., 'Visco-Tears', Ciba Vision or 'Lacri-lube', Allergan) is also of use and this has the advantage of providing some protection during postoperative recovery. The mouth, nose and pharynx can become blocked with viscous secretions, and these should be removed using gentle suction before the animal is allowed to recover.

Staff fatigue

It is widely recognized that the likelihood of technical errors increases when personnel are fatigued, and this general effect is of particular relevance to staff conducting anaesthesia (Gregory and Edsell, 2014). When undertaking very prolonged procedures, it is essential to have sufficient staff available to provide time for regular rest periods and for adequate sleep periods. Although use of caffeine by the anaesthetist may transiently improve performance (at doses between 200 and 600 mg—equivalent to 2–6 shots of espresso coffee) (Philip et al., 2006), this is not a solution for prolonged (24–48 h) procedures and can also result in side-effects including sleep disturbance, palpitations and addiction.

Anaesthesia of pregnant animals

Pregnant animals require special care when anaesthetized. Consideration must be given both to the adverse effects of anaesthesia on the mother and also its effects on the foetus(es) (Thaete et al., 2013). The increasing size of the foetus in the last third of pregnancy leads to an increase in abdominal pressure and consequent interference with respiratory movements. This may be of minimal importance under normal circumstances but may be of considerable significance when the mother is placed in an abnormal posture during anaesthesia. The pressure of the uterine contents on the abdominal blood vessels may also interfere with venous return.

To minimize these problems, care should be taken to avoid maintaining the animal in dorsal recumbency. Wherever possible, position the animal so that it is lying on one side. It may be advisable to carry out endotracheal intubation and assist ventilation, particularly during the last third of pregnancy (Davis and Musk, 2014). Good anaesthetic practice, such as providing oxygen by face mask to the animal before induction assumes greater importance, but care must also be taken to reduce stress. Pregnant animals should not be fasted before inducing anaesthesia, as this can have adverse metabolic effects both on mother and foetus. The foetus is extremely sensitive to changes in maternal acid–base balance caused, for example by hypercapnia. Maternal hypotension can seriously reduce placental blood flow and cause the foetus to become hypoxic. The foetus in many species is very susceptible to hypothermia, and special care must be taken both to maintain maternal body temperature, and to keep the foetus warm if it is exteriorized.

Placental transfer of anaesthetics

Most commonly used anaesthetics cross the placenta. This may be advantageous in providing some degree of anaesthesia in the foetus to allow surgical procedures to be undertaken. Conversely, the drug may have serious acute or long-term effects on the foetus. If the foetus is to be delivered by Caesarean operation, residual effects of the anaesthetic drug may cause sedation, respiratory depression and cardiovascular system depression.

General recommendations

The choice of a particular anaesthetic will depend upon the type of experimental procedures which are to be undertaken, but the following advice can be offered as a general strategy for anaesthetizing pregnant animals:

1. Use a balanced anaesthetic technique to reduce adverse effects such as hypotension in the mother and so minimize hazards to the foetus.
2. Use local and regional anaesthesia if possible, but this must be balanced against welfare considerations (see Chapter 3).
3. Carry out surgical and other techniques as rapidly as possible to reduce the duration of anaesthesia.
4. Whatever the anaesthetic technique, maintain good oxygenation of the mother and limit hypercapnia by assisting ventilation.
5. Maintain blood pressure with intravenous fluids and plasma volume expanders when necessary.
6. Monitor maternal blood glucose and correct any hypoglycaemia that may develop.
7. If the foetus is being delivered by Caesarean operation and opioid analgesics have been administered to the mother, administer naloxone to the neonate to reverse any respiratory depression caused by these agents. Irrespective of the anaesthetic used, administration of doxapram to stimulate respiration can be helpful.

Foetal surgery

If surgical procedures are to be undertaken on the foetus, care must be taken to ensure that it is adequately anaesthetized. The stage of gestation at which the CNS is sufficiently well developed to respond to painful stimuli varies in different species and expert advice should be sought before commencing work as to the likely stage of development of the foetus.

If the foetus is sufficiently developed to respond to noxious stimuli, then these responses should be prevented by means of an appropriate anaesthetic. There has been extensive debate concerning the capacity of the foetus to experience pain (White and Wolf, 2004), and in medical anaesthetic practice much of the debate has focused on the effects of noxious stimulation of the development of the CNS, and the effects of this after birth. These considerations will often apply to foetal surgery in animal subjects. It has been suggested that awareness occurs only after the start of parturition (Mellor et al., 2005; Mellor and Diesch, 2006), but this view has been challenged (see Bellieni, 2021 for a review). Irrespective of whether this applies to all species, preventing movement responses to noxious stimuli makes surgical procedures simpler to undertake. It may also be important to reduce nociceptor activation and the foetal stress response in order to minimize the longer-term effects of such interventions (Smith et al., 2000).

The simplest approach is to anaesthetize the mother to a sufficiently deep level so that the foetus is also anaesthetized. This is most readily achieved by using a volatile general anaesthetic such as isoflurane. However, maintenance of this depth of anaesthesia may be undesirable because of possible adverse effects, such as cardiovascular system depression, on mother and foetus or adverse effects on foetal development (Bellieni, 2022). A single dose of an anaesthetic administered by the intravenous route, although sufficient to produce anaesthesia in the mother, is very unlikely to produce anaesthesia in the foetus.

The most widely used alternative to deep general anaesthesia is to infiltrate the surgical site on the foetus with local anaesthetic. If carried out carefully, this technique appears suitable for procedures such as cannulation of superficial blood vessels. It is unlikely to be sufficiently effective for more major surgery such as laparotomy or thoracotomy.

If the mother and foetus are to recover from surgery, then postoperative analgesia should be provided for the mother. Providing effective pain relief can be essential in encouraging rapid return of food and water consumption and minimizing the endocrine stress response to surgery, all of which can have effects on the foetus. However, the positive effects of analgesia need to be balanced against the potential adverse effects of the analgesics on foetal development. Since many surgical procedures involving the foetus are undertaken to study normal or abnormal development, interactions with analgesics could compromise some studies. It is important to note that most studies of the interactions of analgesics (e.g., opioids or nonsteroidal anti-inflammatory drugs, NSAIDs) have been undertaken to assess the likely effect of these agents in pregnant human subjects. To try to model these effects, analgesic agents are almost invariably administered at high dose rates for relatively prolonged periods (e.g. Shavit et al., 1998; Ragbetli et al., 2007; Cappon et al., 2003; Slamberová et al., 2005). As with other uses of analgesics, the potential interactions of pain, surgical stress, anaesthesia and analgesic drug administration must all be considered (see Chapter 5). In most circumstances, administration of analgesics for a limited period (12–36 h) at normal therapeutic dose rates should have positive effects on studies on pregnant animals (Schlapp et al., 2015). This approach has been adopted by the author and colleagues with success.

If opioid analgesics are to be used, their preoperative administration, as part of a balanced anaesthetic technique, enables reduction of the dose of anaesthetic agents. This can limit the acute adverse effects of anaesthesia, such as hypotension.

Anaesthesia of neonates

Neonatal animals have an increased susceptibility to hypothermia and may also have poor pulmonary and circulatory function. They frequently have low energy reserves, which can lead to problems during the recovery period. In addition, any period of fasting, because of removal from their mother for the period of anaesthesia and recovery, can lead to rapid depletion of hepatic glycogen stores and result in hypoglycaemia. Depending on species, neonates have a reduced capacity to detoxify a wide range of drugs and hence their response to anaesthetics can differ considerably from adult animals.

When anaesthetizing neonates, it is essential to maintain body temperature using the techniques described in Chapter 3. Care must be taken to maintain good ventilation and to maintain fluid balance. In large species (dog, cat, sheep, and pig) the umbilical vessels provide a convenient route for intravenous infusion.

It is preferable to use inhalational anaesthetics so that recovery is rapid and normal feeding is resumed as soon as possible. Methoxyflurane is particularly safe and effective in neonates, however, this agent is now difficult to obtain, and isoflurane has been reported to be safe and effective (Danneman and Mandrell, 1997). Neonatal animals usually require higher concentrations of anaesthetic, for example young adult rats require a concentration of approximately 2% halothane for maintenance of surgical anaesthesia, whereas neonates require 2%–3%. Delivery of inhalational anaesthetics requires construction of an appropriately sized face mask, but this is relatively easy to achieve using a plastic syringe barrel (Fig. 4.7). Alternatively, a 3D printer can be used to construct a suitable sized mask (Ho et al., 2020; Steffens et al., 2022).

Several anaesthetic agents have been shown to be neurotoxic in neonates, and to produce detectable neurological deficits in later life (Sanders et al., 2013). Isoflurane anaesthesia also caused hypoglycaemia in neonatal mice (Loepke et al., 2006). Mice subjected to hypothermic anaesthesia showed only minor behavioural changes in later life (Richter et al., 2014), but rats showed small cognitive deficits (Kolb and Cioe, 2001). However, the relevance of these studies to the use of anaesthesia for relatively short surgical procedures is neonatal rodents remains unclear.

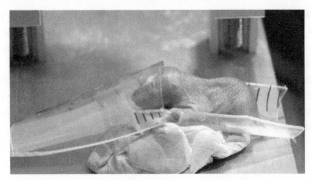

FIG. 4.7 Face-mask for delivery of volatile anaesthetics to a neonatal mouse. The mask and cradle are made from a 2 mL syringe, and stabilized with 'Blu-Tack'. Body temperature is maintained using radiant warming or a warm air blower.

Anaesthesia using hypothermia

Deliberate production of hypothermia has been used as a means of immobilizing neonatal rats and mice to enable surgical procedures to be undertaken. It is not clear whether the technique produces anaesthesia or simply immobility although it seems likely that during the period of hypothermia the degree of depression of peripheral nervous system and CNS is sufficient to prevent the animal experiencing pain. There is considerable debate concerning the capacity of neonates to experience pain – both human and animal. In case of rodents, significant postnatal brain development occurs, and the pathways responsible for nociception and pain in adults are not fully developed (White and Wolf, 2004; Fitzgerald, 2005). Although there is disagreement about the nature of pain perception, both nociception and pain can be considered undesirable because of the effects on later development. It has been suggested that recovery from hypothermia and the return of sensation to the body may be associated with nociceptor activation and pain, based on analogy with human experiences. Studies in our laboratory have shown that hypothermia in neonatal rats is associated with cfos activation, which is presumably triggered by cooling or rewarming (Rhodes, 2009). It is uncertain whether the CNS is sufficiently well developed for pain perception, but since safe and effective alternatives are available, for example isoflurane (Danneman and Mandrell, 1997), halothane, fentanyl/droperidol (Park et al., 1992), fentanyl/fluanisone (Clowry and Flecknell, 2000), or medetomidine, midazolam and fentanyl (Tang et al., 2020) it seems advisable to avoid the use of hypothermia whenever possible until its efficacy has been established.

Anaesthesia for imaging

The increased use of medical imaging (functional magnetic resonance imaging, fMRI, MRI; positron emission tomography, and PET) as research tools has introduced new requirements for anaesthesia. Animals need to be immobilized for image acquisition; however, the anaesthetic methodology should not influence the data obtained. A further requirement is that imaging may need to be repeated at relatively frequent intervals, so that progression of physiological or pathophysiological processes can be monitored. This requires standardized anaesthetic protocols that will result in reproducible effects on the animal. An added complication is that often the animal is not easily observed during the process, access for monitoring devices may be limited and some imaging studies may require several hours of data collection from an individual animal. For some imaging modalities (e.g. MRI and fMRI), specialized monitoring equipment is required. It may also be necessary to synchronize data capture with respiratory movements, or at the very least, produce stable cardiorespiratory parameters. Finally, changes in body temperature can differentially affect brain temperature and it has been suggested that this could influence results of fMRI (Zhu et al., 2004).

Anaesthetic techniques

A review of the literature indicates that a wide range of different agents is currently used to anaesthetize animals for imaging. In many instances these have probably not been selected as the most appropriate for specific purposes, so it is important to review the main requirements of each study, and develop a protocol that is compatible with these (Austin et al., 2005; Steward et al., 2005; Van der Linden et al., 2007; Hildebrandt et al., 2008; Tremoleda et al., 2012; Alstrup and Smith, 2013; Jonckers et al., 2014; Paasonen et al., 2018). Since most agents can have significant effects on brain functions, the general approach to minimizing these, by developing appropriate balanced anaesthetic regimens, has been proposed (Reimann and Niendorf, 2020). These authors also provide a comprehensive review of the effects of anaesthesia on brain function.

Although mixtures of injectable agents can be used (see Chapter 6), the depth of anaesthesia produced will vary between individuals, and within individuals at successive anaesthetics. Use of continuous intravenous infusion (e.g. with propofol) or use of inhalant anaesthetics allows anaesthetic depth to be adjusted more precisely.

Intravenous agents can be delivered via an over-the-needle catheter securely fixed in a convenient vein. It may also be advisable to splint (using a plastic splint) the catheter site to avoid inadvertent kinking due to repositioning of the limbs, or the tail in rodents. Catheter extensions can be used to connect to an infusion pump, positioned a safe distance from the scanner. Note that when using long extension lines to deliver injectable anaesthetics, two practical problems may be encountered. If using an infusion pump, the increased resistance to flow associated with long (several metres) of tubing, can result in erroneous 'catheter occlusion' alarms. This can be overcome by using a lab-style pump that lacks this safety feature. It is also important to note that because of the significant volume of anaesthetic in the infusion line, administering emergency or adjunctive agents can require infusion of dangerous additional volumes of anaesthetic agent. If other agents need to be given intravenously during imaging, a second intravenous line needs to be established.

In some circumstances, only deep sedation may be required, and drugs such as medetomidine can be used to provide sufficient immobility for imaging (Weber et al., 2006). Medetomidine may have disadvantages, however, since it produces marked respiratory depression and has a range of metabolic effects. Its major advantage is that it is reversible with atipamezole (see Chapter 2).

Inhalational anaesthetics can be delivered either via an endotracheal tube, a nasal catheter or a specially designed face mask (Steward et al., 2005). Anaesthetic breathing systems can be extended to an anaesthetic trolley positioned a safe distance from the scanner. We have found oxygen bubble tubing ideal for providing fresh gas, and disposable paediatric ventilator tubing for the expiratory limbs of breathing systems for small animals (Fig. 4.8). When an open mask system or nasal catheter is used, gas scavenging may be necessary, but in small rodents the relatively low fresh gas flows used may be rapidly diluted and extracted by normal room ventilation. When intubated, mechanical ventilation can be carried out either using an MRI compatible ventilator positioned close to the scanner (Hedlund et al., 2000), or by extending the breathing system. It is not necessary to use NMB drugs to ventilate animals (see above), but they may be required to prevent small movements that could interfere with imaging. As with any use of NMBs, they should always be used in conjunction with adequate anaesthesia e.g. (Keilholz et al., 2004), and never used to immobilize conscious animals (van Camp et al., 2003).

Monitoring equipment and management

Standard monitoring apparatus can be used for certain imaging modalities (e.g. PET), although there may be problems of access. Significant problems arise when undertaking MRI or fMRI. All sensors used must be compatible with high magnetic fields, and the instruments need to be positioned at a safe distance from the scanner. Respiratory rate can be monitored in large and small animals using pneumatic sensor systems, but these give no indication of the adequacy of respiratory gas exchange. Pulse oximetry sensors suitable for use in high magnetic fields can be purchased (e.g. Nonin Medical, Inc., Appendix 4), and these function reliably during image acquisition. Other devices, such as some ECG leads, may be safe to use, but the signal quality degrades markedly during imaging. Extension lines to allow invasive blood pressure monitoring and side-stream capnography can be used, but when long lines are used the signal may be damped or altered. For example, capnograms may fail to show a normal plateau if several metres of sample tubing are required. Nevertheless, the trends obtained from this monitoring remains of considerable value. An alternative approach when monitoring arterial pressure is to position a compatible transducer close to the animal, although this then makes it difficult to

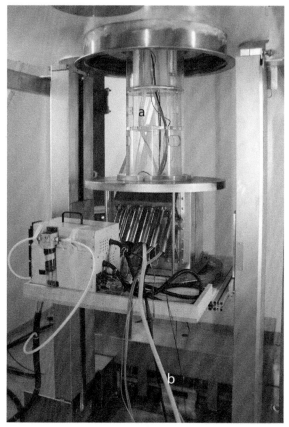

FIG. 4.8 Breathing system extended during MRI imaging, using lightweight tubing (b) on the expiratory limb of the system and oxygen bubble tubing (a) to extend the fresh gas supply.

obtain repeated arterial blood gas samples for blood gas analysis, to ensure stable conditions are being maintained. Transcutaneous gas monitoring may also be used to assess pulmonary function. This can be used to indicate trends in $PaCO_2$ (Stout et al., 2001; Ramos-Cabrer et al., 2005), and in some circumstances can correlate well with direct measures (Sahbaie et al., 2006). If the animal is not being ventilated, and capnography is not used, then respiratory movements can be monitored using simple pneumatic sensors that are compatible with the magnet.

Some specialized imaging procedures may require the animal to be placed in specific postures, for example sitting upright, which may increase the anaesthetic risk. In these circumstances careful monitoring becomes even more important.

Body temperature must be controlled, and most studies have used circulating warm water systems, although forced air warming is also suitable. MRI compatible temperature probes are available, and these should be used to monitor both the animal's core temperature, and the skin temperature that is in contact with the heat source.

At the time of writing of this edition, the considerable increase in imaging, especially of rodents, is leading to the development of purpose-made, commercially available monitoring systems (e.g., SA Instruments Appendix 4).

Chapter 5

Analgesia and postoperative care

Preoperative preparations for postoperative care

Postoperative care must be considered a natural and essential extension of good anaesthetic practice. Failure to attend to the animal's needs during this critical period will inevitably complicate recovery from anaesthesia and is in any case inhumane. Poor postoperative care will exacerbate and prolong the metabolic disturbances caused by surgery and, if seriously neglected, the animal may die. The results of a survey of anaesthetic-related mortality in small animal veterinary practice has shown that the majority of deaths (>50%) occurred in the postoperative period (Brodbelt et al., 2008). Although some risk factors in veterinary practice will differ from those in a laboratory animal facility, these results highlight the critical importance of good postoperative care.

Providing high standards of postoperative care requires careful planning and preparation. It is important to:

- Check what equipment and other resources will be needed and that these are available.
- Ensure that you and your colleagues have sufficient time to provide the required care and attention that your animal or animals will need.
- Check that any specialized housing or equipment that may be needed during the postoperative period is available.

This should be done as part of the planning of the procedure *before* you anaesthetize your animals. Preparing a protocol sheet with all the details of the procedure and what aftercare may be needed is good practice and is a mandatory requirement in many facilities. You should also include a check that the regulatory approval of the procedure includes all the proposed techniques and enables modification of analgesic regimens if this becomes necessary.

Immediately before you start the procedure, check that the recovery area has everything you might need and that warming devices are switched on and will have reached the required temperature by the time that they are needed.

All animals will require some degree of additional attention in the postoperative period, and this is often best achieved by providing a special recovery area. This will simplify the provision of the most appropriate environmental

Laboratory Animal Anaesthesia and Analgesia. https://doi.org/10.1016/B978-0-12-818268-0.00017-6

conditions, which will frequently differ from those present in a standard animal holding room. It will also highlight the special needs of animals placed in the recovery area and encourage extra attention from animal husbandry and nursing staff.

As part of your preanaesthetic preparations, you should have:

- Made sure the animals have been acclimatized for a sufficient time.
- Considered implementing positive reinforcement training so that animals co-operate with procedures such as drug administration following recovery from anaesthesia.
- Weighed the animals regularly—these data are needed both for the immediate and the longer-term assessment of the animals.
- Assessed and recorded the preprocedure behaviour, appearance, and response to handling of your animals. For example, are they active and inquisitive, like the rats shown in Fig. 5.1, or do they normally huddle under the food hopper during the light phase of their photoperiod?

Recovery from anaesthesia

Recovery from anaesthesia should be smooth, with a minimal period of involuntary excitement (a stage when the animal has not fully recovered consciousness but makes spontaneous movements). If a surgical or other painful procedure has been undertaken, analgesics should have been administered so that the animal remains pain-free (see below).

Recovery from anaesthesia follows a similar pattern in most species: reflex responses (pedal withdrawal, tail pinch etc.) return, respiratory and cardiovascular depression reverses, the animal regains its righting reflex, co-ordinated movements return, and the animal becomes fully conscious.

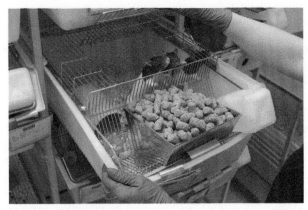

FIG. 5.1 The normal appearance and behaviour of animals should be assessed before carrying out any research procedures.

If the animal is intubated, the endotracheal tube should be removed when the laryngeal and pharyngeal reflexes return. Return of these reflexes is associated with the animal making slight swallowing movements. It may also cough, especially in response to small movements of the endotracheal tube. If the endotracheal tube was tied in place during the procedure, remove any ties so that it can be withdrawn quickly when reflex responses return.

The speed of recovery will be influenced by the anaesthetic agents used, whether the action of some components of the anaesthetic regimen have been reversed using specific antagonists (e.g. reversal of medetomidine with atipamezole), and on the effectiveness of intraoperative care, especially the maintenance of normal body temperature.

Recovery from anaesthesia can still be smooth and uneventful even when prolonged, but during the recovery period the animal's body systems will still be depressed by the anaesthetic agent. Animals that recover rapidly from anaesthesia:

- Have a more rapid reversal of cardiovascular and respiratory depression.
- Rapidly regain the ability to maintain their normal body temperature.
- Begin to eat, drink, groom, and interact with cage mates more rapidly.
- Require a shorter duration of close attention and monitoring of vital signs—although they must still be assessed regularly to ensure recovery continues uneventfully.

Full recovery from anaesthesia, with the return of normal activity and food and water consumption, may take 24–48 h or longer. The metabolic consequences of surgery and anaesthesia may persist for several days.

The recovery room environment

The recovery area for most laboratory mammals should be warm and quiet. Lighting should be subdued but adequate to allow easy observation of the animal. Higher intensity lighting must be readily available to enable more detailed examination and to allow procedures such as intravenous injection. In the immediate postoperative period, when the animal may be semiconscious and immobile, incubators for small rodents should be maintained at 35–37°C. For larger species which may be placed in a larger recovery pen, the animal's temperature can be maintained by using blankets or other insulating materials. The cage or pen temperature can also be raised by using a warm air blower. Placing warming blankets directly in the pen or cage can help maintain temperature, but they need to be removed when the animal begins to recover consciousness, to avoid the blanket being damaged. As the animal recovers consciousness, the normal physiological mechanisms that maintain body temperature will remain depressed, but the ambient temperature can gradually be reduced to 27–30°C for adult animals and 35–37°C for neonates. Once the animal has recovered from the major depressant effects of the anaesthetic, the temperature can be reduced to 25°C for adults but should be maintained at 35°C for neonates.

This gradation in temperature can be achieved by maintaining a general room temperature of 21–25°C and providing supplemental heating using warming lamps or heating pads. Ideally, an animal incubator should be used: this will allow careful control of the ambient temperature and enable easy administration of oxygen. Unfortunately, many commercially available incubators do not maintain stable temperatures. This is less of a problem with larger animals (⩾2 kg) but can result in transient hypothermia in small rodents. If available, paediatric incubators designed for use with human neonates provide excellent conditions for small rodents. These incubators are often available when being replaced by hospitals with new models. One practical point to note is that most of these infant incubators have a gap around the inner tray to allow air circulation, so small rodents need to be confined in an inner cage.

Heating pads and lamps

If an incubator is not available, heat pads that have been used to maintain temperature during anaesthesia can continue to be used in the recovery period, but the same care needs to be taken to ensure the temperature is appropriate. It should be high enough to maintain body temperature but not too high. As animals recover, temperature probes will need to be removed to avoid them being chewed and damaged.

Heating pads can also be placed beneath the cage used for recovery but need to be put in position and switched on at least 1 hour before they are needed. The temperature can then be measured before the animal is placed into the cage.

Warming lamps can be used to raise the temperature in a recovery cage or pen and are particularly useful when working with larger species (e.g. adult pigs and sheep), since heat pads placed in the pen or cage may be damaged by the animal. Heat lamps should be positioned and switched on an hour or so before they will be needed. The temperature below them should then be monitored at a position that corresponds to the anticipated height of the animal's back or sides. With a large animal, its upper body surface could be 30–50 cm closer to the lamp and reach a higher temperature than the floor of the pen.

If it is practicable to use a warm air blower, for example if the animal is in a solid-sided pen or cage, then these often allow better control of the environmental temperature. The warming units from forced-air warming blanket systems can be used as the source of warm air. These systems can also be used to warm smaller cages used to house rodents (Rembert et al., 2004).

Maintaining normothermia

Although hypothermia is a potentially serious problem in the postoperative period, care must be taken not to overheat the animal, and both the animal's rectal temperature and the temperature of its immediate environment should be carefully monitored. Surface temperatures of animals, heating pads and their surroundings can be checked quickly and easily using remote measurement thermometers, or thermal imaging cameras. Although skin temperatures measured noninvasively are usually lower than core temperatures, they are correlated and provide useful information when monitoring animals (Kawakami et al., 2018).

In small experimental units, it may be impracticable to allocate space permanently for use as a recovery room. In this situation a temporary area can be set aside for this purpose. This be achieved by equipping a suitably sized trolley with an animal incubator and other necessary equipment. This can then be moved around the unit to wherever it is required. In some instances, when performing surgery on many rodents, use of a portable incubator to provide a suitable recovery area is the most practicable solution. It has the added advantage of allowing the theatre assistant to regularly observe animals that are recovering from anaesthesia and surgery, while continuing to provide technical support to the surgeon and anaesthetist.

Following major surgical procedures, an alternative to a separate recovery room for small rodents is the use of a specialized warming rack (Fig. 5.2).

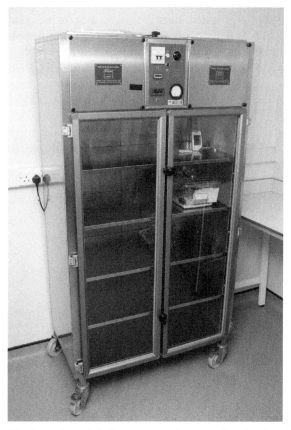

FIG. 5.2 Specialised warming rack for longer term maintenance of small rodents (Techniplast).

This can maintain animals at warmer temperatures (e.g. 25–26°C) for several days following surgery and can be of considerable benefit in reducing mortality and morbidity after major surgery.

Caging and bedding

In most instances, small rodents can be allowed to recover in their normal cages, placed either in a recovery room or inside an incubator, but sawdust or wood shavings must not be used as bedding. This type of bedding will often stick to the animal's eyes, nose, and mouth and so should be replaced by more suitable materials. A synthetic bedding with a texture like sheepskin (fleece) has proven particularly useful for all animal species and can be obtained from several different suppliers ('Vet-Bed', 'Dry-Bed'). It is washable, autoclavable, and extremely durable and appears to provide a comfortable surface for the animal. If such material is unavailable, towelling or a blanket should be used. Tissue paper is relatively ineffective as animals usually push it aside during recovery from anaesthesia and end up lying on the bottom of a plastic cage, soiled with urine and faeces. Shredded paper of a type that will not stick to the animals' orifices or wounds should also be provided, since it provides a warm and comfortable nesting material (Fig. 5.3) (e.g. 'paper shavings', RS Biotech, Appendix 4). Good quality hay can be provided for rabbits and Guinea pigs, as this will provide both insulation and a readily available source of high fibre food. Animals should not be placed in grid-bottomed cages to recover from anaesthesia but should be placed either directly in an incubator or in a temporary plastic or cardboard holding box.

Once the animal has recovered its righting reflex and is able to move in a co-ordinated way, it can be returned to its home pen or cage. Rodents that were group housed can be returned to their social group. Almost all small rodents, including those with exteriorized implants or catheters, can be housed in groups following

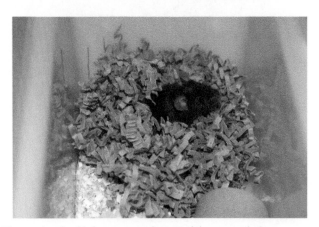

FIG. 5.3 Mouse using shredded paper as nesting material postoperatively.

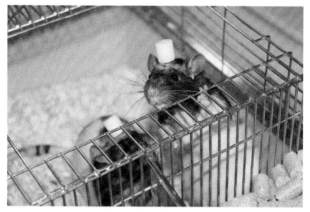

FIG. 5.4   Rats returned to their stable social groups following surgery.

surgery (Fig. 5.4). In rare circumstances, implants can be particularly delicate, and, in these cases, animals will require single housing. If single housing is required, then animals should be acclimatized to this additional stress preoperatively.

It is common practice to change the cage of rodents immediately upon recovery from anaesthesia. However, this removes existing scent markings and places animals that are already experiencing stress associated with the procedure into an unfamiliar environment. Consider replacing the bedding material and wiping the cage clean but retaining any nest that the rodent has made and any environmental enrichment items. A routine cage change can then be conducted a few days later, when the animal has largely recovered from the procedure. This is particularly important in mice, since disrupting their olfactory environment can trigger aggression towards cage mates.

Larger species will require a recovery cage or pen. Synthetic sheepskin (see above) can be used with most species for the immediate postoperative period, but deep straw beds are also suitable for small ruminants and pigs.

Nursing care

The response to human contact varies considerably among different animal species and is influenced by previous experiences. Excessive contact may have adverse, stressful effects in some small rodents and rabbits, but other species will benefit from some degree of nursing care carried out in a calm and reassuring manner. The degree of alarm caused to the animal can be reduced if it has been gradually familiarized to regular handling in the preoperative period. This process forms an important part of preoperative acclimatization in all species (see Chapter 1) and should be considered essential when planning any series of experiments.

Most cats, dogs, and many pigs will respond positively to stroking or scratching and to a reassuring, familiar voice. If the recovery period is prolonged and normal grooming activity not resumed, some animals, particularly dogs and cats, may respond favourably to regular grooming by nursing staff. Time should be provided to encourage any dogs and cats that are reluctant to eat following surgery. Most can be tempted by hand feeding. Warming the food will often make it more appetizing. Very often, the presence of a familiar staff member to encourage eating will greatly affect the animal's appetite. Similar techniques can also be useful in pigs and nonhuman primates, provided they have been properly familiarized to human contact in the preoperative period.

All species, including rodents and rabbits, should be checked regularly during recovery from anaesthesia. In the immediate postoperative period, constant attention may be needed, followed by observation every 1–4 h for the first 8–12 h. If recovery is progressing well, assessments should be continued several times a day especially following surgery when the effectiveness of pain control is needed. Particular attention should be given to cleaning the eyes, nose and mouth, which can become clogged with dried mucus or other debris. Monitoring of body weight and checking of wounds and surgical implants are also an important part of postoperative care. Rodents may be offered food pellets softened with warm water in bowls placed on the cage bottom, as many may be reluctant to reach up to food hoppers at this time (Fig. 5.5). Commercially produced nutrient gels can also be given to provide additional fluid and food (Fig. 5.6) but these may need to be offered to the animal for 2–3 days preoperatively as rodents may need to be familiarized to their taste and odour.

It is important that a daily routine is followed as far as possible. It will be an advantage if some staff are assigned specifically to the care of postsurgical animals throughout the perioperative period, as they are more likely to notice subtle changes that may take place on a day-to-day basis. Careful record keeping is essential, so that other staff attending the animal, for example, during weekends and out-of-hours, will be aware of all treatments given and the animal's progress. It is important to record not only all active interventions, but also that the

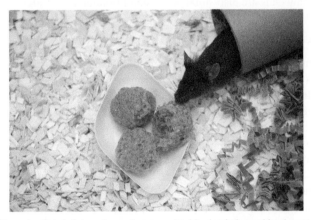

FIG. 5.5 Normal pelleted diet can be made more palatable simply by soaking in water.

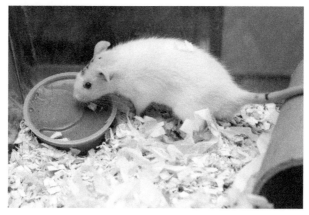

FIG. 5.6   Commercially produced nutrient gels can be given to provide additional fluid and nutrition.

animal has been examined and found to be progressing satisfactorily. Records of clinical observations and treatments must be readily available, and use of electronic record systems can be of great assistance in providing legible, easily accessible, and up-to-date information.

Fluid therapy

Additional fluid may be needed following anaesthesia, both because of fluid loss during surgery and anaesthesia and because fluid intake may be reduced postprocedure. Supplemental fluids can be provided in a variety of ways. If animals are fully conscious, then supplemental fluid can be provided by the oral route. This can be achieved either by encouraging voluntary consumption of standard diet pellets soaked in water or by using palatable gels or liquids, depending upon the species. Animals can be hand-fed food and fluids, particularly if they have been trained to accept this in the preanaesthetic period.

The voluntary water intake of all animals should be recorded postoperatively, even if this consists simply of making a rough estimate based on the level in a water bottle. If dehydration develops, it can seriously compromise the recovery of the animal. Fluid requirements of most species are approximately 40–80 mL/kg/24 h, but the presence of vomiting or diarrhoea or other abnormal losses will increase this requirement.

If the animal is fully conscious, supplemental fluid is best given by the oral route. If the animal is unable or unwilling to accept oral administration, then dextrose–saline (4% Dextrose, 0.18% Saline) or saline (0.9%) can be given quickly and easily by the subcutaneous or intraperitoneal routes (Fig. 5.7, Table 5.1). Severe dehydration causes loss of skin tone that causes it to tent and tend to remain elevated when a fold is twisted between the fingers. In

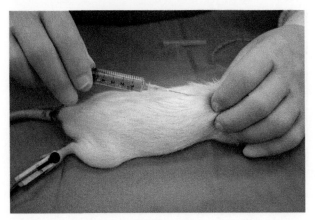

FIG. 5.7 Administration of subcutaneous fluids to a rat.

TABLE 5.1 Approximate volumes for fluid replacement therapy by intraperitoneal or subcutaneous administration.

Species	Subcutaneous (mL)	Intraperitoneal (mL)
Cat (3 kg)	50	50–100
Gerbil (60 g)	1–2	2–3
Guinea pig (1 kg)	10–20	20
Hamster (100 g)	3	3
Marmoset (500 g)	5–10	10–15
Mouse (30 g)	1–2	2
Rabbit (3 kg)	30–50	50
Rat (200 g)	5	5

larger animals, dehydration will result in the mucous membranes becoming dry to the touch. If this degree of dehydration has inadvertently been allowed to develop, fluids must be administered intravenously. If the animal is severely depressed, then it may not interfere with the intravenous line; however, as the beneficial effects of rehydration occur, it will become more active. Various bandaging and splinting techniques can be used (Fig. 5.8), and Elizabethan collars (Fig. 5.9) can be used in rats, rabbits, dogs, and cats to prevent interference with catheter sites. These bandages and collars may interfere with the animals' normal activities and may delay resumption of voluntary food and water intake. They also prevent coprophagy in rats, Guinea pigs, rabbits, and other species and may cause significant distress to some

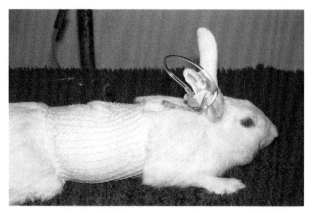

FIG. 5.8   Stockinette bandage used to secure an intravenous line.

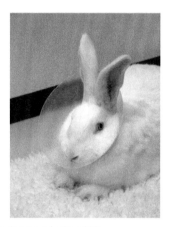

FIG. 5.9   Elizabethan collar placement in the rabbit.

individuals. It is therefore important to monitor the animals closely, to ensure the benefits outweigh possible problems.

If peripheral vessels are too constricted to catheterize, the intraosseous route can be used in small mammals. A hypodermic needle can be inserted into the proximal end of the femur or tibia, in the same manner as when taking a bone marrow biopsy or performing a marrow transplant (Zehnder, 2008). If the animal is severely depressed, this can be performed under local anaesthesia; otherwise, a light general anaesthetic using an agent such as isoflurane is required.

The monitoring of body weight in the pre- and postoperative periods can provide a good indication of the adequacy of fluid intake. Although a small fall in body weight (<1%–3% reduction) will be recorded because of the almost inevitable reduction in food intake that occurs postoperatively, most weight loss usually represents a fluid deficit.

Besides assessing food and water intake, the urinary and faecal output of the animal should be recorded, and any abnormalities investigated. As with most of these variables, a meaningful judgement can only be made if the animal has been observed in the preoperative period. A reduction in urine output may be the result of dehydration, urinary tract injury, or the animal suffering pain. If the bladder is full, it may require catheterization to empty it, although in some instances *gentle* pressure through the abdominal wall will trigger urination. Catheterization is a relatively simple technique, but requires some degree of expertise, and it will usually be preferable to consult a veterinary surgeon or experienced animal technician. If catheterization is not possible, it may prove necessary to drain the bladder by direct puncture through the body wall. This procedure should only be attempted by individuals who have undergone training in the technique. Catheterization of the bladder of most laboratory species requires induction of a brief period of general anaesthesia, or heavy sedation.

Problems during the recovery period

The immediate recovery periods

The swallowing and cough reflexes are usually suppressed during anaesthesia, and these gradually return as the animal recovers consciousness. As mentioned earlier, if an endotracheal tube has been placed, it should be removed when the animal begins to swallow spontaneously or attempts to cough. Care must be taken that the tube is not pulled out too soon, for example, when the animal is repositioned as surgical drapes are removed.

In this immediate recovery period, use of a pulse oximeter to assess respiratory function is extremely useful, particularly in larger species (see Chapter 3). Changes in oxygen saturation after disconnection from the breathing system should be assessed. An observation period of approximately 2 min is usually sufficient to assess the fall in oxygen saturation that occurs when changing to breathing room air rather than the higher oxygen concentration in anaesthetic gases. If saturation falls below 85%, then oxygen should be administered, and ventilation supported or stimulated. If an endotracheal tube is in use, if it is a cuffed tube, deflate the cuff and gently remove the tube as the protective pharyngeal and laryngeal reflexes return. After removal of the endotracheal tube (if one has been used), maintain the animal on a face mask and administer oxygen. If respiratory movements and oxygen saturations are judged to be adequate, remove the mask, and continue to monitor the animal. Removal of the endotracheal tube often causes a fall in oxygen saturation, as the airway is not as well-maintained. Before removal of the tube, or if one is not used, before recovery of swallowing and cough reflexes, the mouth should be inspected, and any secretions removed using suction. A soft tipped catheter (e.g. a feeding tube) connected to a large syringe allows this to be carried out in small rodents. Monitoring of adequacy of ventilation can also be assessed using a capnograph, and this is particularly useful following prolonged periods of anaesthesia, especially if the animal's lungs have been mechanically ventilated.

During this initial recovery period, drapes and surgical equipment should be removed, together with any nonessential monitoring devices. This will allow the animal to be moved rapidly to a more comfortable environment if it regains consciousness more rapidly than expected.

The respiratory depression produced by most anaesthetic agents often persists into the postoperative period. The degree of depression may also increase postoperatively, and this may go unnoticed until severe hypercapnia and hypoxia have developed. For this reason, it may be advisable to continue monitoring the respiratory system, and the use of a pulse oximeter is ideal for this purpose, particularly in larger species (see Chapter 3). If not already in use, the probe can be attached to the animal in the operating theatre and a battery-operated instrument used to monitor the animal during movement to the recovery area. The probe can be left taped in place on the tail or on a digit until the animal has regained its righting reflex.

If a pulse oximeter is not available, then other forms of respiratory monitor can be used, for example, by positioning a sensor close to the animal's nose. At the very least, regular clinical observation of the animal should be made, and the respiratory rate recorded. If respiratory depression is noted, it should be treated using a respiratory stimulant such as doxapram and by the administration of oxygen. Since doxapram has a relatively short duration of action (10–15 min), it may be necessary to administer repeated doses or to establish a continuous infusion of the drug.

Many animals appear to benefit if oxygen administration is continued into the immediate postoperative period. This is relatively easy to achieve in small animals by piping the gas into an incubator, but in large animals, it is often more practicable to tape a small, soft-ended catheter at the external nares and use this to administer the gas (Fig. 5.10). Note that the catheter and oxygen supply

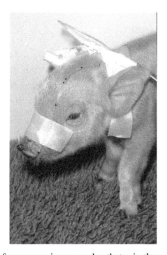

FIG. 5.10   Administration of oxygen using a nasal catheter in the postoperative period.

tubing should be connected to the anaesthetic machine without the use of a reservoir bag and pop-off valve, as the high resistance to flow of the nasal catheter will result in all the gas being diverted through the pressure relief valve.

Nonruminant species should be placed on their sides, with head and neck extended, to try to minimize the risk of airway obstruction. If the animal is recumbent for more than 4 h, then it should be repositioned to lie on its other side, to prevent passive congestion of the lungs and the development of hypostatic pneumonia. In large animals such as dogs and farm animals, it may be necessary to massage areas such as the elbow and hock, to prevent pressure sores developing. If prolonged recumbency is anticipated, it may be advisable to protect these areas with padded bandages.

If the animal begins to vomit, it should be positioned so that its head is below the level of the thorax and abdomen, to try to prevent aspiration of the vomit. If practicable, the mouth and pharynx should be cleared using a vacuum suction, or a piece of suitably sized tubing attached to a 50-mL syringe. Oxygen should be administered, and if inhalation of vomit could have occurred, corticosteroids should be administered (30 mg/kg iv of methyl prednisone), together with a broad-spectrum antibiotic.

Ruminants (sheep, goats, and cattle) can present problems during recovery from anaesthesia. They should be propped up on their sternums to minimize the risk of over-distension of the rumen with gas (rumenal tympany) and to reduce the risk of inhalation of regurgitated rumen contents. If rumenal tympany develops, it should be relieved immediately either by passing a stomach tube or by puncturing the rumen through the left abdominal wall with a large bore trochar. If a trochar is not available, the largest possible needle (preferably 12 SWG or larger) should be used. If the member of staff involved is not familiar with nor trained in this technique, veterinary advice should be sought immediately.

Food intake and bowel function

If the animal fails to pass faeces, this may be due simply to an absence of faecal material because of preoperative fasting. It may also be caused by a loss of normal peristalsis (ileus, see below), or the animal may be constipated and require administration of an enema (e.g. Microlax, SmithKline Beecham). Defaecation may be suppressed if the animal is in pain, particularly following a laparotomy.

Ileus (gut stasis) can be a serious postoperative complication and can be life-threatening in rabbits and Guinea pigs. Ileus is particularly common after laparotomy but can occur after any surgical procedure. Minimizing handling of the bowel can reduce the incidence of ileus following abdominal surgery. When displacing and handling the viscera is unavoidable, ensure they are kept moist and handled gently. Pigs seem particularly sensitive to handling of the intestines, and we have found 'bowel bags' designed for use in humans to protect the intestines during surgery to be of great value in preventing problems.

Management of ileus remains difficult in all species, including man (Buscail and Deraison, 2022). Pain must be controlled since this can increase the severity of ileus. The surgical notes should be reviewed to check that a swab was not inadvertently left in the abdomen. Motility stimulants (metoclopramide and cisapride) can be administered to stimulate gut function, but the dose rates and efficacy of these and other agents are often not well established in the target species. In rabbits, ranitidine (2–5 mg/kg by mouth, daily) has been used for managing postoperative inappetence and gut stasis as it promotes gut motility (Kounensis et al., 1992). Cisapride is widely used in rabbits in veterinary clinical practice, but one study showed no beneficial effects in this species (Feldman et al., 2021).

In some species (e.g. rabbits and Guinea pigs), inappetance due to other causes can lead to the development of ileus, since normal gut function appears to depend to some extent on regular intake of fibre. Supplemental feeding, using nasogastric tubes, if necessary, may be beneficial. A range of specialist dietary preparations is now available for veterinary use in 'exotic' companion species, and these can be of considerable benefit in laboratory animals.

It is important that food and water intake and the other observations described above are recorded carefully. It is helpful to provide a standardized paper or electronic record for each animal, which will encourage nursing staff to complete the required observations. It will also allow easy and rapid reference by staff who may be called in to deal with any problems that might arise. It is always preferable to obtain measures of preoperative body weight and, if possible, of food and water consumption, so that the progress of an animal can be assessed accurately in the postoperative period. Obtaining daily weights for 3–4 days preoperatively both familiarizes the animal with handling and provides a base-line growth curve to allow interpretation of postoperative changes.

Prevention of wound infection

Provided careful aseptic surgical techniques have been employed, it may be considered unnecessary to administer antibiotics routinely to animals in the postoperative period. In addition, some species appear to show a remarkable resistance to the development of wound sepsis and appear to tolerate standards of cleanliness that would be totally unacceptable in human medical practice. This apparent resistance to infection must not be used as an excuse for poor surgical standards, and every effort should be made to adopt aseptic techniques for all animal surgical procedures (www.procedureswithcare.org.uk). It has been demonstrated, for example, that rats are not only susceptible to infection but also show behavioural changes following the establishment of wound infections (Bradfield et al., 1992). It is therefore important that all animal species should be monitored carefully for any signs of infection (Morris, 1995).

Since animals will almost inevitably soil their wounds with faeces and urine, administration of prophylactic antibiotics may be useful in minimizing the risk of infection. One problem of providing perioperative treatment with antibacterials is the risk of inducing enterotoxaemia in some species, particularly the Guinea pig, hamster, and rabbit. The use of antibacterial agents in rodents and rabbits has been reviewed by (Morris, 1995) and provided care is taken in the choice of agent such problems can be avoided. Suggested dose rates of antibiotics for each species are given in Tables 5.2 and 5.3.

Unexpected side-effects of anaesthetics

Anaesthetic agents can sometimes cause unexpected adverse effects in the postoperative period. Older agents such as chloral hydrate can cause gut stasis in rats. Tribromoethanol (Avertin) can cause peritonitis in mice (see Chapter 2).

A relatively common side-effect of anaesthetic mixtures containing medetomidine or xylazine is the development of opacity in the eye, resembling cataract (Calderone et al., 1986). This is most often seen in mice but also occurs occasionally in rats. This change in appearance reverses within a few hours and appears to have no long-lasting consequences (Fig. 5.11). It is not related to a lack of protection of the eyes with eye ointment during anaesthesia. In both rats and mice, permanent corneal injury has been reported (Turner and Albassam, 2005; Koehn et al., 2015).

Management of postoperative pain

Pain in laboratory animals is a major animal welfare problem that must be addressed if we are to apply Russell and Burch's principle of refinement (Russell and Burch, 1959)—'to reduce to an absolute minimum the pain and distress experienced by those animals that are used' (in research procedures). To provide effective analgesia, it is essential that we have a good knowledge and understanding of animal pain. We need to know when pain might occur and how long it might last and assess how well it responds to therapy. We also need to consider the advantages and the disadvantages of the various methods of managing pain, and how we can best apply these in different situations. If we are to manage pain relief optimally, and monitor the effects of our therapy, then we will need to recognize the presence of pain and assess its severity. When developing our understanding of this area, we will also need some information about the basic mechanisms involved in pain perception. More fundamentally, we must accept that pain occurs in animals—that it can result in suffering, in a similar way to pain in humans—and so become convinced that its avoidance and alleviation need to be given a high priority.

Despite the emphasis given to humane treatment of laboratory animals in the national legislation of many countries, analgesics may still not be administered routinely in the postoperative period. This omission is particularly common

TABLE 5.2 Antibiotic and antibacterial drug doses for laboratory animals (small mammals).

	Mouse	Rat	Hamster	Gerbil	Guinea pig	Rabbit
Cephalexin	15 mg/kg im b.i.d.	15 mg/kg sc b.i.d.	–	25 mg/kg sc u.i.d.	15 mg/kg sc b.i.d.	15 mg/kg sc b.i.d.
Chloramphenicol	50 mg/kg sc b.i.d.	10 mg/kg im b.i.d.	30 mg/kg sc b.i.d.	30 mg/kg sc b.i.d.	20 mg/kg im b.i.d.	15 mg/kg im b.i.d.
Enrofloxacin	10 mg/kg sc b.i.d.	10 mg/kg sc b.i.d.	10 mg/kg sc b.i.d.	10 mg/kg sc b.i.d.	5–10 mg/kg sc b.i.d.	5–10 mg/kg sc b.i.d.
Neomycin	2 mg/mL in drinking water	2 mg/mL in drinking water	250 mg/kg per os in divided doses	100 mg/kg per os in divided doses	5 mg/kg per os b.i.d.	0.2–0.8 mg/mL in drinking water
Co-trimazine 40/200	30–50 mg/kg sc b.i.d.	30–50 mg/kg sc b.i.d.	30 mg/kg sc b.i.d.	30 mg/kg sc b.i.d.	30–50 mg/kg sc b.i.d.	30–50 mg/kg sc b.i.d.
Tylosin	–	10 mg/kg sc u.i.d.	10 mg/kg sc u.i.d.	10 mg/kg sc u.i.d.	–	–

Note that the majority of these doses are based solely on clinical experience, since only limited pharmacokinetic data are available for these species (with the exception of enrofloxacin). Before administering any of these compounds, research workers are strongly advised to consult their laboratory animal veterinarian for advice on drug selection and the duration of treatment. For a comprehensive review of the effects of antibiotics in laboratory species, see Morris (1995).

TABLE 5.3 Antibiotic and antibacterial drug doses for laboratory animals (larger animals).

	Ferret	Cat	Dog	Pig	Sheep	Primate
Amoxycillin	7 mg/kg sc u.i.d.	7 mg/kg sc u.i.d.	7 mg/kg sc u.i.d.	7 mg/kg im u.i.d.	7 mg/kg im u.i.d.	7 mg/kg sc u.i.d.
Cephalexin	10 mg/kg sc u.i.d.	10 mg/kg sc u.i.d.	10 mg/kg sc u.i.d.	10 mg/kg im u.i.d.	10 mg/kg im u.i.d.	10 mg/kg im b.i.d.
Chloramphenicol	25 mg/kg sc u.i.d.	25 mg/kg sc u.i.d.	50 mg/kg sc u.i.d.	11 mg/kg im u.i.d.	–	20 mg/kg im b.i.d.
Enrofloxacin	5–10 mg/kg sc b.i.d.	5 mg/kg sc u.i.d.	5 mg/kg sc u.i.d.	2.5 mg/kg sc u.i.d.	–	5 mg/kg sc b.i.d.
Neomycin	10 mg/kg per os u.i.d. in divided doses	10 mg/ml per os u.i.d. in divided doses	10 mg/kg per os u.i.d. in divided doses	11 mg/kg per os b.i.d.	11 mg/kg per os b.i.d.	10 mg/kg per os b.i.d.
Trimethoprim/sulphonamide	15–30 mg/kg sc b.i.d.	30 mg/kg sc u.i.d.	30 mg/kg sc u.i.d.	15–24 mg/kg im u.i.d.	15–24 mg/kg im u.i.d.	30 mg/kg sc u.i.d.

Note although some of these doses are based on manufacturer's recommendations, others are based solely on clinical experience, since pharmacokinetic data are not available for all agents in all species. Before administering any of these compounds, research workers are strongly advised to consult their laboratory animal veterinarian for advice on drug selection and the duration of treatment. For a comprehensive review of the effects of antibiotics in laboratory species, see Morris (1995).

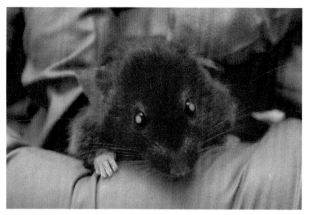

FIG. 5.11   Opacity of the eyes following use of medetomidine. This opacity reverses within 1–2 h following recovery from anaesthesia.

when the animals concerned are small rodents (Richardson and Flecknell, 2005; Coulter et al., 2009), but also has been noted with larger species (Bradbury et al., 2016). It is also difficult to assess current practice because of poor reporting of data in peer-reviewed publications (Carbone and Austin, 2016). Even when analgesics are given, the assessment of their efficacy in alleviating pain is often based on highly subjective criteria. In many instances, research workers simply assume that administering an analgesic at a recommended dose rate will provide effective pain relief and do not even attempt to assess the degree of pain relief provided. This approach in people was recognized as being one of the major factors in provision of poor postsurgical pain management, with over 50% of patients reporting inadequate analgesia (Smith, 1991; Gan et al., 2014), and is still a major barrier to effective pain control (Schug et al., 2020).

A lack of easy to use, reliable and objective method of assessing animal pain leads to use of subjective, often anthropomorphic approaches. Although starting from the assumption that pain in animals is similar to pain in people is appropriate, assuming that animals in pain will therefore behave like people in pain is rarely correct. Different species will behave in different ways when in pain, and this behaviour can be strongly influenced by the presence of a human observer (see 'Pain assessment'). But in order to manage pain effectively, we need to be able to assess it; otherwise, we cannot know if our analgesics have proved effective.

Pain in humans is defined as 'An unpleasant sensory and emotional experience associated with, or resembling that associated with, actual or potential tissue damage' (IASP, Raja et al., 2020).

So, pain in humans is a sensory and psychological experience with several components:

- Sensory discriminative—where the pain is, how intense it is, what type it is, and when it occurs.

- Affective and emotional—the 'feeling' of pain, which is unpleasant and distressing.
- Cognitive—people can think about what their pain means to them and what it could indicate ('Am I having a heart attack?' 'Do I have cancer?'), and this can change the intensity of pain (Jackson et al., 2014) and their need for analgesics.

All of these aspects of pain can cause behavioural responses.

The experience of pain is largely subjective, so different people will respond to similar causes of pain differently, have differing experiences and require different treatments. It seems likely that the subjective experience of pain in animals will differ from that in humans, and that different species of animals will experience pain in different ways. In order to accept that animals can experience pain, we have to accept that animals have a conscious awareness of their emotional states—in other words, that they have 'feelings' (Duncan, 1996).

This remains a controversial topic. We can demonstrate relatively easily that animals can experience the sensory components of pain—they have very similar mechanisms for detecting damaging or potentially damaging stimuli (with nociceptors), and this information is transmitted to spinal and higher brain centres in similar ways in animals and humans (Viñuela-Fernández et al., 2007). However, the demonstration of equivalent anatomical structures and physiological processes does not provide conclusive evidence that both the sensory and emotional components of the experience of pain are similar in animals and humans. It is possible that the relative significance, magnitude and duration of pain in response to particular types of injury may all vary in animals (Sneddon et al., 2014). Whether animals possess the same, or a similar capacity as humans, to experience emotions such as pain has been extensively debated for centuries. The main reason for the continued debate is that it is impossible to investigate such emotional states directly—we can only draw inferences from other, indirect measures, such as investigation of behavioural responses (Mason and Lavery, 2022). Some philosophers and scientists have firmly asserted that animals cannot experience pain but only respond to noxious stimuli, without being consciously aware (see Rollin, 2011). Others argue in support of the presence of emotional states such as pain (see for example (Duncan, 1996; Weary et al., 2006; Fraser, 2009; Panksepp, 2011). This uncertainty regarding animal pain is similar to that relating to pain in human neonates, a debate that still generates controversy especially in relation to preterm infants (Bowsher, 2006; Bartocci et al., 2006). The inferences drawn from neuroanatomy, neurophysiology, and behaviour that have been used to argue for the capacity of neonatal humans to experience pain (Simons and Tibboel, 2006) have clear parallels in the debate relating to animal pain.

Since pain is a subjective experience, it is doubtful that we will ever be able to demonstrate its presence in animals conclusively, but the growing body of evidence supporting conscious emotional states suggests we should assume a capacity for pain in animals. Certainly, most members of the public have no hesitation in stating that animals experience pain. On reflection, many would agree that the experience might not be exactly the same as the pain they might experience themselves, but nevertheless would have no doubt that it was 'pain'. This view is reflected in the legislation that controls our treatment of animals. Most recently, a comprehensive evaluation of the evidence for 'sentience' (the capacity to experience emotional states) has been produced as background to new UK legislation (Animal Welfare (Sentience) Act, 2022) (Birch et al., 2020). It is also clear that the affective, or emotional component of pain and other states can be demonstrated in animals (e.g. Corder et al., 2019; Jirkof et al., 2019).

Irrespective of whether animals experience pain or simply respond to activation of sensory nerve (nociceptor) pathways, this process results in major physiological and pathophysiological changes. Consequently, pain or nociception will represent a source of uncontrolled variation in research and may introduce specific confounding factors in some studies. We can therefore advocate the control or elimination of both pain and nociception on both scientific and welfare grounds (Gebhart et al., 2009). Although we would wish to alleviate pain either because of concerns for animal welfare or to reduce a potential confounding factor in a research project, several counterarguments have been advanced to justify withholding analgesics.

- 'Alleviation of postoperative pain will result in the animal injuring itself'

  Pain has a protective function and is of value in warning of tissue damage in an individual. Pain arising from injured tissues often results in the animal or human immobilizing the affected area since this will help to prevent further injury. However, this response is also harmful since the immobility and muscle spasm it produces can cause muscle wasting and weakness. Thoracic and abdominal pain may reduce ventilation and cause hypoxia and hypercapnia. Pain may also cause a marked reduction in food and water consumption (Liles and Flecknell, 1993). Pain in humans has been shown to prolong the metabolic response to surgery (Kehlet and Dahl, 2003), to increase the requirement for hospital care following operative procedures and to have a range of other detrimental effects (Breivik, 1994).

  Provided that surgery has been carried out competently, administration of analgesics to encourage resumption of normal activity by controlling pain rarely results in problems associated with the removal of pain's protective function. Claims that analgesic administration results in skin suture removal are unsubstantiated, and contrary to findings in our laboratory. In certain circumstances, for example, after major orthopaedic surgery, additional measures to protect and support the operative site may be required, but this is preferable to allowing an animal to experience unrelieved pain. All that is required in these circumstances is to temporarily reduce the animal's cage or pen size or to provide additional external fixation or support for the wound.

It must be emphasized that these measures are very rarely necessary, and in our institute, administration of analgesics to laboratory animals after a wide variety of surgical procedures has not resulted in any adverse clinical effects.

- 'Analgesic drugs have undesirable side-effects such as respiratory depression'

  In medical clinical practice, analgesic drugs were frequently withheld because of fears of their undesirable side-effects such as respiratory depression and addiction (Cousins et al., 2000). This attitude has changed significantly (Bonnet and Marret, 2007). It is also important to note that the side-effects of opioids, such as respiratory depression, are generally less marked in animals than in people and should rarely be a significant consideration when planning a postoperative care regimen. It is, however, important to consider the potential interactions between analgesic therapy and research protocols, and this is discussed in more detail below.

- 'We do not know the appropriate dose rates and dosage regimens'

  Another factor that may limit the use of analgesic drugs is a lack of knowledge of appropriate dose rates and dosage regimens. This is primarily a problem of poor dissemination of existing information. Virtually every available analgesic drug has undergone extensive testing in animals, both for safety, and for efficacy in a range of nociceptive tests (e.g. hot-plate and tail flick tests, see below). Safe dose rates are therefore available for a range of drugs in several common laboratory species (Flecknell, 1984; Liles and Flecknell, 1992). The main problem that we currently face is extrapolating available dose rates from one species to another and translating dose rates that are effective in nociceptive tests into those that are appropriate for clinical use. Nevertheless, in many instances, a reasonable guide as to a suitable, and safe, dose rate can be obtained. It is important to appreciate that many of the dose rates recommended in review articles and textbooks (including this one) provide only a guide to a likely effective dose. The appropriate dose is the dose rate that controls pain in that particular animal. This can only be established by applying effective means of pain assessment.

- 'Pain-relieving drugs might adversely affect the results of an experiment'

  Some research scientists are reluctant to administer pain-relieving drugs because their use might adversely affect the results of an experiment. Although there will be occasions when the use of one or other type of analgesic is contra-indicated, it is extremely unlikely that there will be no suitable analgesic that could be administered. More usually, the reluctance to administer analgesics is based upon the misconceived idea that the use of any additional medication in an experimental animal is undesirable. The influence of analgesic administration in a research protocol should be considered in the context of the overall response of the animal to anaesthesia and surgery. As discussed in Chapter 2, the responses to surgical stress may overshadow any possible adverse interactions associated with analgesic administration. In many instances the intraoperative support provided to animals fails to control variables such as body temperature, respiratory function, and blood pressure. It seems illogical to assume that these changes are unimportant, but that administration of an analgesic will be of overriding significance. It is an ethical and legal responsibility of a research worker to provide a reasoned, scientific justification if analgesic drugs are to be withheld (Carbone, 2019). It is also important to realize that the presence of pain can produce a range of undesirable physiological changes, which may radically alter the rate of recovery from surgical procedures, (Jirkof, 2017; Peterson et al., 2017; Baral et al., 2019). In animals, postsurgical pain can reduce food and water consumption, interfere with normal respiration (for example, after thoracotomy) and reduce a whole range of 'self-maintenance' behaviours. The immobility caused by pain can lead to muscle spasm, can cause atrophy of areas, and can slow healing. Prolonged immobility can also cause pressure sores, urine scalding, and faeces soiling and can greatly complicate animal care routines. Immobility in mice also results in a fall in body temperature (Refinetti and Menaker, 1992; Weinert and Waterhouse, 2007), and this can have significant and wide-ranging metabolic effects. Pain can also increase aggression between cage-mates (Khosravi et al., 2021). Positive effects of analgesics have also been reported, for example administration of NSAIDs improved outcomes from embryo transfer in mice (Schlapp et al., 2015).

A second major consideration is the magnitude of influence analgesics exert on a research variable of interest, in relation to the effect size that it is hoped will be detected as part of the study design. In many instances, effects that could confound research data occur only when high-dose rates of analgesic agents are administered for relatively prolonged periods (e.g. for more than the 1–3 days normally required for effective pain control following surgery). A series of review articles on specific research areas are available that address these issues, (Carpenter et al., 2019; DeMarco and Nunamaker, 2019; Huss et al., 2019; Larson et al., 2019; Taylor, 2019) as are several working party reports (Lidster et al., 2016; Percie du Sert et al., 2017) that also consider the broader issues of refinement of specific areas of research.

- Legal constraints

In many countries, the use of most opioids is controlled by legislation (e.g. the Misuse of Drugs Act in the UK). Complying with this legislation often requires careful record keeping of the purchase, storage, and dispensing of opioids and may restrict the persons who are able to dispense and administer these substances. In some countries, the degree of record keeping required can act as a strong disincentive to the use of these analgesics in animals. Legislative control, together with genuine safety concerns, may also limit the dispensing of this class of analgesics for use by investigators or technicians. These issues can be addressed by using nonopioid analgesics when these would be appropriate, and by evolving systems of prescribing and supply that make it easier to meet legislative requirements.

Pain assessment

The approach to animal pain based on comparative biology, outlined at the start of this chapter, leads naturally to the assumption that conditions which would cause pain in people would also cause pain in animals. When examining animals, we interpret certain clinical signs as suggesting the presence of pain. Following a surgical procedure, a dog might howl or whimper, perhaps guarding the surgical wound, and show signs of avoidance or aggression when the area is handled. These types of behaviour are easy to equate with the behaviour of humans in pain, so we readily diagnose animals showing these clinical signs as being in pain and may then give analgesics. Unfortunately, this anthropomorphic view of pain is flawed. Many animals do not respond to conditions and procedures that would cause pain in humans in a way that is immediately apparent as pain-related behaviour. For example, to an untrained observer, rats do not appear to show obvious signs of pain following routine laparotomy. This is an apparent contradiction of assumptions based on comparative biology—people do experience significant pain after abdominal surgery, most complain about their pain and most require opioids or other forms of analgesia. This discrepancy between the apparent behaviour of animals and the behaviour that would be predicted from human experience gives rise to the view that, although pain may occur in animals, it is less severe than that in people. It also leads to the assumption that the more resilient nature of animals results in more rapid recovery with less experience of pain. The natural consequence of this is to assume that animals do not require analgesics as frequently as people, and perhaps may not even require them at all. The key to introducing effective pain control is therefore to improve our methods of pain recognition and assessment. For example, in the laparotomy example mentioned earlier, if the animal is observed closely and its behaviour analysed carefully, then more subtle changes become apparent (Roughan and Flecknell, 2001). These changes may be normalized by administration of an analgesic, and this supports the view that they are related to the presence of postoperative pain.

Pain assessment is important not simply because it would encourage greater use of analgesics, but because it would also encourage more appropriate use of these drugs. In many animal research units, national legislation requires that pain is assessed based on the assumption that procedures that are painful in people will be equally painful in animals. But the choice of analgesic should be determined in some part by the degree of pain that is present, since inappropriate use of potent analgesics may lead to the undesirable side-effects of these agents outweighing any benefits arising from alleviation of pain (Blaha and Leon, 2008). Similarly, the use of low-potency agents in circumstances in which severe pain is present will result in insufficient pain relief. Simply assuming that after identical surgical procedures, the degree of pain present in all animal species and in people will be identical is highly unlikely to be correct. Even if this broad comparison were possible, it would also be necessary to assume that the duration of pain, and hence requirement for pain relief, was identical in all animal species and

humans in equivalent circumstances. It also fails to account for individual variation in response to analgesics. Following identical surgical procedures, different
human patients can have markedly different analgesic requirements (Yoshida
et al., 2015). This has become clearly apparent with the introduction of patient-
controlled analgesia, which removed some of the obstacles to analgesic administration (Skues et al., 1993). Although equivalent data in laboratory animals are
limited, data from nociceptive tests in research animals show similar variation
among individuals (Cowan et al., 1977a; Cowan et al., 1977b), and both age
and sex have been shown to influence the responses to analgesics (Frommel and
Joye, 1964; Kest et al., 2000). Major variations in the behavioural and endocrine
responses to surgery have been reported in mice (Wright-Williams et al., 2007),
and similar changes in nociceptive thresholds occur (Mogil et al., 1999; Mogil
et al., 2006). Different strains of rats and mice also differ in their responses to
different analgesics (Elmer et al., 1998; Morgan et al., 1999). Selection of an
arbitrary dose of analgesic will therefore almost certainly lead to overdosing of
some animals, and provision of inadequate analgesia for others. Development
of reliable methods of pain assessment would enable analgesic treatment to be
tailored to suit the needs of each individual animal.

This problem, of varying analgesic responses in different individuals is
encompassed in medical practice in the concept of 'number needed to treat'
(NNT) (McQuay et al., 2012). In the context of analgesic use, this is defined
as the number of patients that need to receive a particular analgesic in order
for one patient to experience a 50% reduction in pain. NNT is therefore a measure of the effectiveness of a particular analgesic. Rankings of analgesics based
on systematic reviews of controlled trials assigns NNTs ranging from 1.5 for
eterocoxib (an NSAID) to 17 for codeine. Morphine has an NNT of 2.9. NNT
is rarely reported in animal studies but applying the concept would help better
explain the variability seen in responses of individuals to pain procedures and
the effects of analgesics. This in turn would give a more realistic expectation of
outcomes, and most importantly it would reinforce the need for careful assessment of the efficacy of analgesic therapy. An animal that does not respond to
treatment requires either additional doses of the analgesic or administration of
a different analgesic.

Methods of assessing animal pain

Assessment of acute pain responses—nociceptive tests

During drug development programs, an acute noxious stimulus is often used to
determine the efficacy of different analgesics. The majority of these investigations have been carried out in rodents, and use mechanical, thermal, or electrical
stimuli to produce brief painful stimuli (reviewed by Le Bars et al., 2001). Most
studies are designed in such a way that the animal can terminate the stimulus.
These assessment methods enable determination of the analgesic potency of
different drugs, but the neurological mechanisms involved do not fully reflect

those involved in clinical pain. In addition, the dose rates required vary depending upon the test and the analgesic used (Sadler et al., 2022). Outcomes of nociceptive testing are also influenced by the species used, the genotype, and the environmental conditions in which the test is conducted. When inappropriate nociceptive tests are used to compare different classes of analgesics, misleading conclusions can be drawn as to the likely clinical efficacy of the analgesics. For example, NSAIDs are primarily antihyperalgesic agents and are relatively ineffective in tests using thermal and electrical stimuli, whereas most opioids are effective in both types of test. It is also difficult to relate the dose rates that are effective in these acute test systems with those that are needed to control clinical pain (Roughan and Flecknell, 2002). Results from these tests do indicate the likely broad range of effective doses in different strains and species of animal, and data from studies of adverse effects indicate the likely dose ranges that could cause significant clinical problems. Taken together, these results can be of some value in the initial evaluation of the likely efficacy of analgesics for control of postprocedural pain.

As outlined earlier, pain in humans is recognized to be a complex, multidimensional sensory and emotional experience. Although the nature of pain in animals almost certainly varies between species (Sneddon et al., 2014), methods of assessment should enable both the sensory and emotional components of pain to be identified. Newer techniques that attempt to assess the emotional component of pain in animals have been used in developing novel compounds intended for pain management in people, for example use of operant models, conditioned place preference and place avoidance and grimace scales (see Tappe-Theodor et al., 2019; Sadler et al., 2022 for reviews). Some of these measures are of practical value in assessing postsurgical pain in a range of species (see below) and for the establishment of appropriate analgesic dose rates for the control of pain resulting from research procedures.

Behaviour-based pain scoring systems
Abnormal behaviours after abdominal surgery

Behaviour-based schemes for assessing pain have been developed in a range of laboratory species, including rat (Roughan and Flecknell, 2001), mouse (Wright-Williams et al., 2007), rabbits (Leach et al., 2009), and Guinea pigs (Ellen et al., 2016) (see below).

Pain faces

The assessment of pain by evaluating facial expressions has been widely used in infants and children (Craig et al., 1993; Grunau et al., 1998). More recently, a means of analysing pain faces in mice, using a Mouse Grimace Scale, was described (Langford et al., 2010) and the method applied successfully to assess postsurgical pain (Matsumiya et al., 2012; Faller et al., 2015). Grimace scales have been described for the rat, rabbit, ferrets, cats, sheep, piglets, cattle, and horses (reviewed by McLennan et al., 2019; Mogil et al., 2020). In most species, a series of specific action units have been identified, and each of these is scored separately and then combined to produce an overall grimace score.

It is important to appreciate that use of this approach is still at a relatively early stage of development. It is not yet certain what factors other than pain can influence facial expression in many species, and sedation persisting after anaesthesia appears to have significant effects in increasing grimace scores (Miller et al., 2015, 2016). The validity and reliability of the scales varies in different species, with the rat and mouse grimace scales being the best validated and most widely used (Evangelista et al., 2022). When applying these scales in mice, it has been shown that different strains of mice have varying grimace scores when pain-free and varying degrees of response following surgery and handling (Miller et al., 2015; Miller and Leach, 2016).

Despite these reservations, grimace scoring can be used successfully to detect pain following a range of different procedures. It is currently the most effective method available, but it is important that it is applied with care, and that preprocedure measurements are made in the particular groups of animals that are being used. Whenever possible, use of grimace scoring should be combined with other methods of evaluating animals after surgery (Miller et al., 2022). Most studies using the technique have obtained high resolution images, and then scored them retrospectively, but initial work in several establishments has indicated that 'cage-side' assessment is possible. It has, for example, been used as a rapid means of determining the need for analgesic intervention (Oliver et al., 2014). It also has the advantage of being relatively unaffected in normal animals by opioid analgesics, that have been shown to markedly influence normal behaviour.

A very significant development in the use of grimace scores to assess pain has been the development of automated image analysis techniques (Tuttle et al., 2018). These approaches are being applied to several different species and may lead to pain scoring tools that can be used routinely to improve pain management in research facilities.

Other behavioural assessments

Unalleviated postoperative pain is likely to inhibit performance of a range of normal behaviours, and some highly motivated behaviours may be sensitive measures of the efficacy of analgesic use. Use of these measures is also at an early stage, but studies suggest that nest-building in mice (Arras et al., 2007), or the time to commence nest building (Jirkof et al., 2013; Rock et al., 2014), may be useful assessments. Similarly, burrowing behaviour has been shown to be both a measure of general welfare in rats and mice (Deacon, 2006; Deacon, 2009) and also, in rats, to be reduced in frequency by pain, with this effect reversed by analgesics (Andrews et al., 2012; Whittaker et al., 2014). Burrowing may also be a useful measure of postoperative pain in mice (Jirkof et al., 2010) and of pain associated with other procedures (Zhang et al., 2022). Wheel-running may also be reduced by pain (Häger et al., 2018). Although easy to assess using an exercise wheel placed in the animals' cage, extensive base-line data may be needed to interpret changes following procedures (Kandasamy and Morgan, 2021).

As with the other measures described above, a number of factors other than pain may influence both nest-building, burrowing, and wheel-running, and in mice considerable strain variation occurs (Deacon et al., 2007).

A problem with applying behaviour-based systems is that it relies on animals recovering relatively rapidly from anaesthesia. When recovery is delayed or is associated with prolonged sedation, then animals may fail to express pain behaviour. At present, it is not certain whether this is because the animals are not experiencing pain, or whether the heavy sedation prevents them showing signs of pain. The scoring system may also be influenced by other factors, such as fear and apprehension, and unexpected variations in behaviour between different strains of the animal may be encountered. Using any of the behaviour-based scoring systems as cage-side assessments will also be subject to observer bias. However, use of video recordings can help overcome this. Overall, validated behaviour-based scoring of pain represents a significant advance in pain management in laboratory animals. However, detailed, well-controlled studies are not available for all species, and where validated scoring systems are not available, use must be made of less reliable assessments.

Alterations in physiological variables

Pain generally causes changes in the respiration pattern and rate. This can be dramatic following thoracic surgery when the reduction in the depth of respiration can cause considerable concern. In other instances, the change may be less obvious and masked by the normal tendency of animals such as rodents or rabbits to respond to restraint or close observation with an increase in their respiratory rate. Pain may also affect the cardiovascular system. Frequently, the heart rate is increased, but the natural responses to handling may mask these changes. The other factors influencing these cardiorespiratory variables may render them of little use for routine assessment of postoperative pain (Conzemius et al., 1997; Ledowski et al., 2012). However severe pain may cause the development of circulatory failure (shock), with blanching and chilling of the extremities and a decrease in the strength of the peripheral pulse. As a research tool, measures of heart rate variability can be useful for monitoring pain and other stressors (Byrd et al., 2019) and be more effective than simple measures of heart rate.

Assessment of postoperative pain

Several different approaches to pain assessment in animals have been suggested and these are summarized for each of the most widely used laboratory species.

This is followed by general guidance based on clinical opinion that can assist in the assessment of species in which no validated pain assessment scheme has been developed.

Mouse

Following abdominal surgery, mice show a number of specific abnormal behaviours (Wright-Williams et al., 2007) (Table 5.4) and these can be used for cage-side assessment of pain. The mouse grimace scale (MGS, Langford et al., 2010)

TABLE 5.4 Behavioural signs associated with abdominal pain in rodents.

Species	Behaviours
Mouse[a]	• Writhing—contraction of abdominal muscles. • Belly-press—pressing of abdomen to cage floor, often associated with hindlimb extension. • Hind-limb lift—momentary lifting of rear paw, often associated with writhe or press. • Twitching—brief and rapid movement of the skin overlying the back. • Flinching—as in twitching, but also involving other areas of the body.
Rat[a]	• Back arching—vertical stretch from crouched position—similar to the stretch made by cats when waking. • Belly-press—muscular contraction where the ventral abdomen is pressed downwards onto the cage—occurs immediately prior to or during walking. • Fall or stagger—stagger or fall during walking or a rapid transition to crouch from high or low rear. More often a partial loss of balance during grooming, resulting in lateral lying position from which recovery to balanced crouched posture occurs almost immediately. • Writhing—contraction of flank abdominal muscles, usually when crouching but also during transient break in walking or grooming—often noticeable as a 'hollowing' of the abdomen. • Twitch—brief and rapid movement of the skin overlying the back
Guinea pig[b]	• Change in posture from standing to recumbency, often with one hind limb extended. • Hind leg lift • Writhing—slow contraction of flank abdominal muscles • Flinch—a whole body muscle movement

For further details, see Roughan and Flecknell (2003, 2004), Wright-Williams et al. (2007) and Ellen et al., 2016.
[a] *These observations should be combined with the use of the mouse and rat grimace scales.*
[b] *If any of these abnormal, pain related behaviours are seen, unalleviated pain may be present, but the behaviours occur very infrequently, so prolonged (20–30 min) observation periods may be needed in Guinea pigs. In rats and mice, a 5–10 min observation period is sufficient for an assessment.*

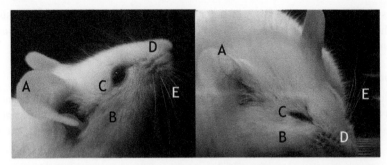

FIG. 5.12   Changes in facial expression associated with pain in mice. (A) In pain-free mice, the ears are held perpendicular to the head and directed forward. The ears themselves are rounded and gently concave. When in pain, the ears rotate outwards and/or back, away from the face. The space between the ears increases as they are pulled back, and they may lay flat against the head. (B) Mice normally have cheeks that form a smooth gently rounded profile. When mice are in pain, the underlying muscles contract, producing a more obviously rounded area. This extends over the area from the whiskers to just anterior to the ear. (C) Mice normally have slightly bulging eyes, that are wide open. When in pain, they develop a narrowing of the area around the eye, a tightly closed eyelid, or an eye squeeze. A wrinkle may be visible around the eye. (D) Mice normally have a smooth profile to their nose, with no obvious wrinkle between the whisker area and the cheek. When in pain, the muscles around the nose contract, producing a bulge on the bridge of the nose. Vertical wrinkles down the side of the nose from the bridge may also be seen. (E) The whiskers are normally held evenly spaced and swept slightly backwards from the nose. When in pain, the whiskers are either pulled back to lay flat against the cheek or pulled forward, so they appear to be 'standing on end'. They can also clump together.

has been used successfully to assess pain after a range of different procedures and should be used as a routine. The changes in facial expression that can be seen are illustrated in Fig. 5.12 and the full Mouse Grimace Scale in Fig. 5.13. Posters illustrating the mouse, rat, and rabbit grimace scales can be downloaded from www.nc3rs.org.uk.

Mice in pain reduce burrowing and nest-building, and when possible these behaviours should be assessed by including nesting material and burrowing opportunities within their cages (Deacon, 2012). For burrowing, a water bottle filled with food pellets provides an easy means of assessment in mice. Although more sophisticated means of using these assessments are likely to be developed, at present they can form a useful overall assessment of animals following surgery. For example, if a mouse was forming a good quality nest preoperatively (Fig. 5.14) and is failing to do so postsurgery, this should trigger careful evaluation. Similarly, a reduction in burrowing activity should give cause for concern.

Mice continue to express pain-related behaviours in the presence of an observer, so direct observations for cage-side scoring of pain is possible.

Rat

Measurements of body weight and food and water intake can be used as potential indicators of postoperative pain and the efficacy of analgesic therapy

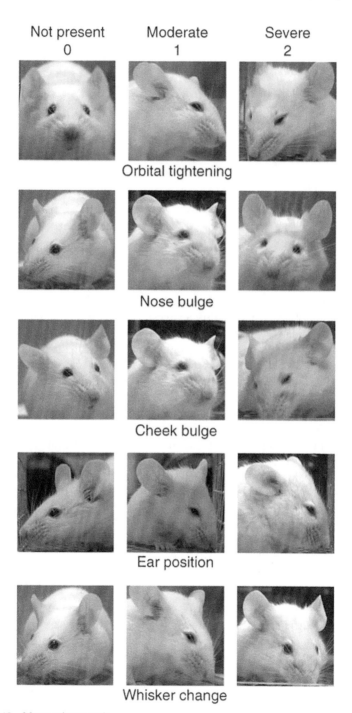

FIG. 5.13 Mouse grimace scale.

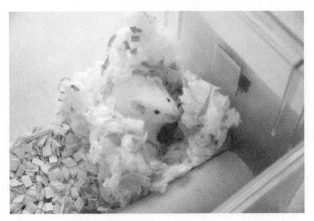

FIG. 5.14 Mouse with a well-formed nest.

(Liles and Flecknell, 1993) (Jacobsen et al., 2012). These measures are simple, objective, and easy to implement, but they are retrospective measures and so could not be used to modify analgesic therapy for a particular animal. They are also relatively nonspecific measures that can be influenced by numerous factors in addition to postoperative pain. They can, however, be used as a simple measure of postoperative recovery, and as a means of adjusting future analgesic and postoperative care regimens for similar animals undergoing similar surgical procedures.

When rats have undergone abdominal surgery, specific abnormal, pain-related behaviours can be observed (Roughan and Flecknell, 2001) (Table 5.4). Following all surgical procedures, use should be made of the rat grimace scale (RGS, Sotocinal et al., 2011). The type of changes in expression that can be associated with pain in rats are shown in Fig. 5.15 and the full Rat Grimace Scale in Fig. 5.16. When uncertain about the degree of pain or its duration, it can be helpful to include assessment of digging behaviour. Although this is not usually practicable as a routine, it provides another cage-side method of assessing pain (Andrews et al., 2012; Whittaker et al., 2014).

Rats, like mice, still express pain-related behaviours in the presence of an observer, so direct observations for cage-side scoring are possible.

Guinea pig

Although specific abnormal behaviours can be used to assess pain following abdominal surgery (Table 5.4), assessment takes 20–30 min as the behaviours occur relatively infrequently (Ellen et al., 2016). In addition, the response of Guinea pigs to any disturbance is to freeze, masking the abnormal behaviours (Oliver et al., 2017). Since there is no grimace score for Guinea pigs, pain assessment must rely on the general changes in behaviour described below.

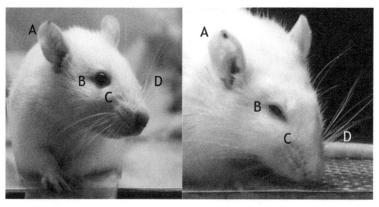

FIG. 5.15   Changes in facial expression associated with pain in rats. (A) In a pain-free rat, the ears are held perpendicular to the head, face forward and are angled slightly backward. The ears themselves are rounded and gently concave. When in pain, the ears tend to fold, curl inwards and angle forwards, resulting in a 'pointed' shape. The space between the ears appears wider than in pain-free animals. (B) In a pain-free rat, the eye is open and slightly protruding. When in pain, rats develop a narrowing of the area around the eye, a tightly closed eyelid, or an eye squeeze. (C) Rats normally have a slight bulge at the bridge of the nose and a clear demarcation of the whisker pads and the cheek. When in pain, the bridge of the nose flattens and elongates and the whisker pads flatten. As a result of this, the crease between the whisker pads and the cheek disappears. (D) In pain-free rats, the whiskers are relaxed and droop slightly downwards. When in pain, the whiskers angle back along the head. Contraction of the whisker pads causes the whiskers to bunch together.

Other small rodents

There is little published data related to pain assessment in gerbils, hamsters, and other small rodents used in research. An attempt to develop a modified grimace scale and other behavioural indicators of pain for Syrian hamsters was unsuccessful (Edmunson et al., 2021). This lack of objective assessments means that pain assessment must rely on general changes in behaviour.

Rabbits

Rabbits show abnormal behaviours following abdominal surgery (Leach et al., 2009) (Table 5.5), and a rabbit grimace scale has been developed (Keating et al., 2012). The Rabbit grimace scale consists of five action units: Orbital tightening, Cheek flattening, Pointed nose, Whisker change and Ear position and these are illustrated and described in Figs. 5.17A–5.17E. Both the behavioural changes and the grimace scale have been used to assess postoperative pain (Miller et al., 2022; Pinho et al., 2022). The latter publication includes video sequences illustrating all of the behaviours used in the study (Pinho et al., 2022). A more extensive pain assessment scheme has been developed combining the grimace scale with clinical observations (Banchi et al., 2020, 2022) and another behaviour-based scheme based on expert opinion (Benato et al., 2021).

Rabbits mask some pain-related behaviours in the presence of an observer (Leach et al., 2009; Pinho et al., 2022) so remote observation or video-monitoring

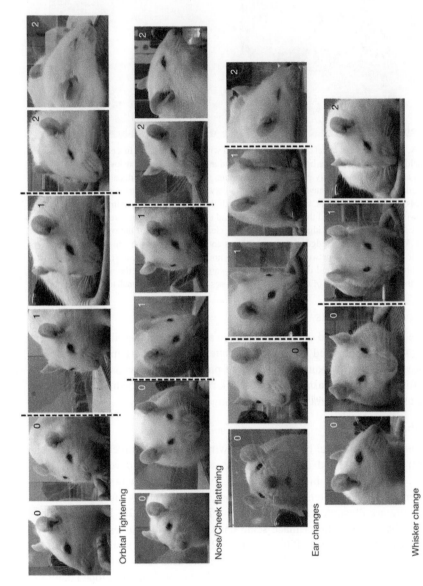

Orbital Tightening

Nose/Cheek flattening

Ear changes

Whisker change

FIG. 5.16 Rat grimace scale.

TABLE 5.5 Behavioural signs associated with abdominal pain in rabbits.

Behaviour

- Writhing—slow contraction of abdominal muscles, often noted as a 'hollowing' of the flanks
- Press—pressing of abdomen to cage floor.
- Arching—arching of the back upwards
- Hind-limb lift—momentary lifting of rear paw, often associated with writhe or press.
- Twitching—brief and rapid movement of the skin overlying the back.
- Flinching—body jerks upwards for no apparent reason
- Wince—rapid movement backwards with eye closing & swallowing
- Stagger—partial loss of balance
- Shuffle—walking at a slow pace, without stepping normally

These observations should be combined with the use of the rabbit grimace scale.
See Leach et al., 2009 and Pinho et al., 2022 for further details. The latter study includes video sequences illustrating some of these behaviours.

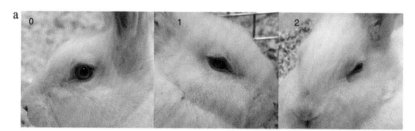

FIG. 5.17A   Rabbit grimace scale (all images provided by Dr Matt Leach, Newcastle University)—Orbital tightening: The eyelid is partially or completely closed. The eyes themselves may also be drawn in toward the head so that they protrude less. If the eye closure reduces the visibility of the eye by more than half, it would be scored as 2.

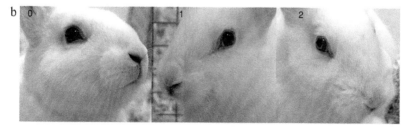

FIG. 5.17B   Rabbit grimace scale (all images provided by Dr Matt Leach, Newcastle University)—Cheek flattening: Contraction around the muzzle so that the whisker pads are pressed against the side of the face. The side contour of the face and nose is angular and the rounded appearance of the cheeks to either side of the nose is lost.

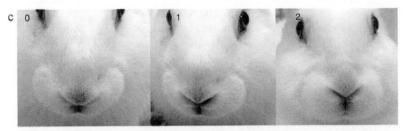

FIG. 5.17C Rabbit grimace scale (all images provided by Dr Matt Leach, Newcastle University)—pointed nose: The upper edges of the nostrils are drawn vertically creating a more pointed nose that resembles a 'V' more than the normal 'U' shape. The lower edge of nostrils loses its curved profile and increasingly becomes straighter and drawn vertically.

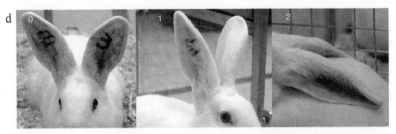

FIG. 5.17D Rabbit grimace scale (all images provided by Dr Matt Leach, Newcastle University)—Ear position: Normally the ears are held roughly perpendicular to the head, facing forward or to the side, in an upright position away from the back and sides of the body and with a more open and loosely curled shape. When a rabbit is in pain the ears rotate to face towards the hindquarters, tend to move backward and be held closer to the back or sides of the body. They also develop a more tightly folded or curled shape (i.e. more like a tube).

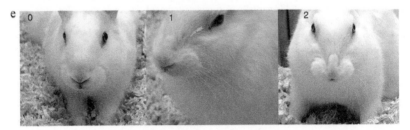

FIG. 5.17E Rabbit grimace scale (all images provided by Dr Matt Leach, Newcastle University)—Whisker position and shape: Normally the whiskers have a gentle downward curve. In rabbits in pain, the whiskers are straightened and become extended horizontally or are pulled back toward the cheeks.

is likely to provide more reliable and more rapid assessments of pain. The varying pain assessment schemes that have been published all have elements that can be readily adapted for assessing pain in particular circumstances. Incorporating grimace scoring with other behavioural measures is likely to provide the most effective scoring schemes (Banchi et al., 2020).

Pig

Although pigs are used relatively frequently for studies involving major surgical procedures, methods of pain assessment have not yet been fully validated for major surgical procedures (Steagall et al., 2021). Grimace scales for piglets have been developed and used successfully to evaluate piglets following painful procedures such as tail docking and castration (Viscardi and Turner, 2018) and combined with other behavioural measures to produce a multidimensional scale for use in piglets (Baysinger et al., 2021). A grimace scale for adult swine has been described but not evaluated following surgical procedures (Navarro et al., 2020). Suggestions for signs of pain from experienced clinicians include changes in temperament, loss of appetite, and changes in posture, activity, and demeanour (see Ison et al., 2016 for a comprehensive review). In the absence of more objective measures, these assessments can be used to evaluate pain (Royal et al., 2013; Goutchtat et al., 2021) and more structured assessments made using the approach described by Morton and Griffiths (1985, see below) (Harvey-Clark et al., 2000).

Sheep

Behavioural scoring of pain in sheep have not been fully validated for major surgical procedures, but pain scoring following laparotomy has been described (Silva et al., 2020), and grimace scale has been developed (McLennan et al., 2016; Häger et al., 2017). However, there are very few reports of the use of the grimace scale in adult sheep, or of the use of other behaviour-based scales, since most studies have focussed on pain related with agricultural practices. General changes in behaviour have been used to assess pain and guide analgesic use following thoracotomy in sheep (Izer et al., 2018) and a combination of measures following lapaparotomy (Viscardi et al., 2021). Behaviours that are thought to be associated with pain in sheep include reduced feed intake and reduced rumination, reluctance to move, altered posture, and altered social interactions. It is likely that behaviour-based scores, combined with use of the sheep grimace scale, can be developed and applied to most studies involving surgical procedures in sheep.

Cattle

A behaviour-based pain scoring scheme, including development of a grimace scale for cattle, has been developed (Gleerup et al., 2015) and used to assess pain associated with lameness and other production disease in dairy cattle. Pain following orchidectomy has used to develop and validate a behaviour-based scoring system (Oliver et al., 2014), and a series of studies have assessed behavioural changes following other husbandry procedures such as disbudding (dehorning), castration (Molony et al., 1995), branding (Müller et al., 2019), and spaying (Yu et al., 2020). Some of the behavioural and other methods used to assess pain following husbandry procedures (reviewed by Tschoner, 2021) may be applicable to assessing pain following experimental procedures. As with other species, use of grimace scales may be the most widely applicable approach.

Nonhuman primates

Attempts to evaluate behavioural signs of pain in primates, and use of facial expression to assess pain, have been largely unsuccessful (Descovich et al., 2019). This is surprising, given that a Facial Action Coding system (MaqFACS) was developed and applied successfully to assess other emotional states in macaques (Parr et al., 2010; Morozov et al., 2021). The lack of success in validating pain assessment schemes may be due to study limitations, for example lack of negative controls (i.e. animals receiving no analgesics after a surgical procedure) because of ethical concerns. Although this means reliance must be placed on general behavioural assessments, when primates are used on long-term studies their individual behaviour and temperament are often very familiar to animal care staff. This enables relatively subtle behavioural cues and indicators of pain or poor welfare to be used in these species, provided sufficient time is allocated for these interactions. A survey of veterinarians working with primates indicated that guarding of the surgical site, abnormal posture, reluctance to move, and decreased appetite were considered the most important signs of pain, but a wide range of other behavioural changes were also used (Miyabe-Nishiwaki et al., 2021).

Cats and dogs

Numerous publications are available describing pain assessment and pain management in dogs and cats and validated pain scales are readily available for use following a range of potentially painful procedures (see Hernandez-Avalos et al., 2019; Reid et al., 2018).

Birds

Most information relating to pain assessment in birds has been obtained in domestic poultry in an agricultural setting (e.g. Tahamtani et al., 2021). Although these studies have focussed on pain associated with lameness, other production diseases and husbandry procedures such as debeaking, the information obtained on analgesic dose rates and efficacy may be applicable to postoperative pain control (Malik and Valentine, 2018). General signs of poor health and welfare are usually relied upon to indicate potential postprocedure pain—for example abnormal posture and activity, and ruffled feathers (Hawkins et al., 2016).

Fish, reptiles, amphibia, and cephalopods

Pain assessment in these groups of animals is particularly challenging. Some information related to signs of pain in fish is available, although these behaviours are mainly related to experimental studies using defined noxious stimuli

(Sneddon, 2020). Laboratory-based studies of nociceptive responses have been undertaken in reptiles and amphibia (Coble et al., 2011; Stevens, 2011; Vachon, 2014) and cephalopods (Crook et al., 2013, reviewed by Walters, 2018) and more complex behavioural responses measured in octopus (Crook, 2021). However, assessment of postprocedure pain remains highly subjective (Fiorito et al., 2015; Lambert et al., 2019; Whittaker et al., 2021; Williams et al., 2019).

A practical approach to pain assessment

If a validated pain scoring system is available for the species and the type of procedure, it should be implemented. This requires time both for implementation of the scoring system, but also to train staff in its use (Roughan and Flecknell, 2006). The results of specific pain assessments should be integrated into an overall postprocedure scoring system that assesses the impact of the procedure on the animals' health and welfare. Using a nonspecific scoring scheme is even more important if species-specific, validated scoring methods are not available.

The general approach to scoring animal health and welfare is usually based a modification of the scoring scheme developed by Morton and Griffiths (1985). When applied carefully, the Morton and Griffiths scheme provides a structured method for assessing animals and can be a useful aid in monitoring animals following both surgical and nonsurgical procedures. The scheme assesses a range of clinical signs and rather than simply noting whether they are normal or abnormal, a score is assigned from 0 (completely normal) or 3 (the most abnormal you could anticipate). A range of clinical signs could be scored, but only those that show changes during the duration of the procedure should be included in a scoresheet. The most useful signs are those that identify when the adverse effects of a particular procedure are becoming worse. These can then be used to trigger interventions such as additional fluids or analgesics or could trigger a decision to humanely kill the animal.

Some general assessments of behaviour can be made in most species and included in a scoring system. It is important to note that these are not reliable indicators of pain but are helpful in assessing general health and well-being. When assessed following surgery, some will be helpful indicators of analgesic efficacy.

Activity

As mentioned above, the overall level of activity of an animal suffering pain is often reduced, and most laboratory species will tend to remain motionless in a corner of their cage. Occasionally, an animal may show unusual restlessness and may seem unable to relax. When the animal moves, its posture or gait may be altered. This is most obviously seen when limb pain is present, but is often noted following laparotomy, when the back may be arched to reduce tension on the abdominal muscles. This altered posture, coupled with a tendency to shorten the length of each stride, can be seen both in rodents and rabbits, and in dogs, cats, and farm animals. Pain from an abdominal incision may also affect the frequency of urination and defaecation in species in which this process requires marked abdominal muscle contraction. Behaviours such as climbing, rearing up onto the hindlimbs, stretching, and scratching may also be affected, but careful observation by an experienced assessor may be necessary before such changes are noticed. A further complication in assessing behaviour is that the animal may change its responses in the presence of an unfamiliar observer. In addition, some species are nocturnal, and observation of normal behaviour will require attendance during the dark phase of its photoperiod. Both problems can be solved to some extent by using video cameras to monitor the animal's behaviour.

Appearance

Even when at rest, the animal's overall appearance may be altered. The animal may adopt a hunched-up posture and position itself in a corner of its cage or pen. Pain may result in a reduction in grooming activity, which leads to the development of an unkempt appearance of the coat and soiling of the anus. Lack of grooming may also lead to the build-up of an encrusted discharge around the eyes, nose, and mouth. Rats may develop dark encrustations around the eyes or nose. This material is porphyrin excreted from the Harderian glands, and if wiped with moist cotton wool, it has a red colour. The presence of porphyrin staining is a nonspecific stress response but should alert the observer to the possibility that the stress involved may be pain (Fig. 5.18).

Temperament

Changes in temperament may occur in animals experiencing pain. Previously tractable animals may become uncharacteristically aggressive and may bite or scratch. Alternatively, a previously active animal that showed obvious interest

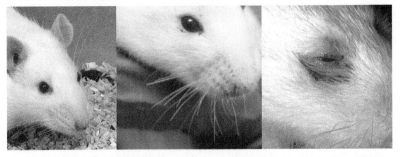

FIG. 5.18 Rat with porphyrin staining around the eyes and nose (right), with very slight accumulation around the eye (the blackish material, centre) and a normal rat (left). Porphyrin staining or accumulation is a non-specific stress response, but can be associated with the presence of pain.

in its handler may appear completely apathetic. The animal may cower away from the handler and attempt to avoid being restrained. The interpretation of any of these types of behaviour will require not only a knowledge of the normal predicted behaviour of an animal of that age, sex, and species, but also prior knowledge of the normal behaviour of that individual. Clearly, close liaison with animal care staff is essential in attempting to assess the behaviour of an animal in the postoperative period.

Vocalizations

Acute pain can make an animal cry out and handling an animal that is in pain may provoke such a response. The pitch of the cry may be abnormal and may be accompanied by attempts to bite the handler or to escape. Animals in pain rarely cry continuously, although on occasions dogs may howl or whimper for long periods and sheep and cattle may also make prolonged vocalization. When assessing pain in rodents, it is important to appreciate that many of their cries are at high sound frequencies that are inaudible to humans.

Feeding behaviour

Food and water intake are often markedly reduced if an animal is in pain. Severe pain is often associated with a complete cessation of eating and drinking. These changes in feeding may go unnoticed if the animal is fed ad libitum from a hopper or if other animals that are feeding normally are present in the cage or pen. A reduction in body weight because of this inappetence can usually be readily detected, but normal day-to-day variations in body weight must also be appreciated. To improve the detection of changes in food and water intake, weighed quantities of food and water should be dispensed and daily intake measured. Weighing the food hopper and the water bottle provides a satisfactory means of monitoring intake in larger rodents. Care must be taken that spillage of food by the animal does not result in intake being erroneously assessed as normal. In addition to recording food consumption, the animal should be weighed each day to determine any changes in body weight.

A reduction in food and water intake will also be reflected in a reduction in faecal and urine output, but the latter may be difficult to detect. The onset of dehydration will be reflected in the clinical appearance of the animal. Loss of skin tone will cause it to tent and tend to remain elevated when a fold is twisted between the fingers.

Developing scoresheets

Each of the measures that we think might be of value can be included in a score sheet, with each measure scored, and the total score used to monitor the progress of the animal. This could use the 0–3 scale originally proposed by Morton and Griffiths or could score signs as simply being present or absent (0/1 or +/−). Alternatively, extended grading could be used, for example with scales of 0–5 or 0–10.

A range of different metrics can be used, for example:

- External appearance, which could be further broken down to include the appearance of the eyes, ears, nose, coat etc.
- Posture, movement and spontaneous behaviour (see above).
- Response to handling.
- Food and water consumption.
- Bodyweight.

When possible, pain scoring, e.g. the results of grimace scoring can be added to the scoresheet.

There are many approaches, the key issue is to be sure the score sheet is suitable for the procedure, and that it assists in monitoring the welfare of the animals on the study. The actions to be taken can also be specified in advance, and these may be triggered either by a change in the total score or can be related to specific signs. For example, an increase in grimace score could result in administration of additional analgesia, a change in skin tone with 'tenting' of the skin could be the result of dehydration and require administration of fluids.

Many of the changes that will be observed are primarily indicators of 'abnormality' and are not necessarily indicative of pain—they could be caused by the general response to surgery or anaesthesia or could be the result of dehydration, hypothermia or other factors. However, noting a positive response to analgesic therapy helps indicate which measures can be useful, but remember that some analgesics (e.g. opioids) can alter behaviour.

Developing and using scoring systems requires a team effort, to make use of the range of expertise of different staff members in an animal facility. It is important to involve all of those who may carry out the assessments, so that a standardized approach can be developed. If several staff assess the same animal together, then grading of the degree of abnormality will become more consistent. This approach is particularly valuable when different staff are involved in assessments on different occasions. It is also important that the terminology used is understood by all of those who will be using the score sheets. Further detailed guidance on developing and using scoresheets is provided by Bugnon et al. (2016).

Applying a scoring scheme, once it has been developed, also takes time, and the staffing resources needed should be included in the general infrastructure of the facility or the specific budget for each research project.

Scoresheets should be widely used following all types of experimental procedures. The key points to note are:

- The type of scoring will depend on the species, the strain and the procedure being carried out.
- The different measures included may need to be weighted (i.e. a high score in one specific sign would carry more weight than a high score in another sign)—but it is usually best not to rely on one single measure to determine a humane endpoint or other intervention.

- Ease of use is an important factor—score sheets with too many measures will be both too time consuming to use, and likely to contain irrelevant measures.
- Score sheets should also include signs of positive welfare.
- Scoring systems need to be reviewed regularly.
- Clinical signs that are noted infrequently can be removed unless they are important for indicating that a humane endpoint has been reached.
- At the end of a procedure, assessing the correlation with clinical outcomes (e.g. death, the onset of severe signs) and pathological findings can be used to validate and improve scoring schemes.
- All score sheets should include a section where other observations can be recorded. This enables any new signs that are noted frequently to be incorporated into a revised score sheet.
- Automated technologies are becoming more widely available and can be used to speed the on-going assessment of animals.

Implementing effective pain assessment and use of score sheets is particularly challenging in small rodents, since often relatively large numbers of animals undergo surgery in a single day. Although we might be able to include an initial assessment of the animals immediately postsurgery, we need to continue to monitor them. If we do not do this, then we will not detect when additional doses of analgesic might be needed, and we will not know when treatment can be stopped.

Pain assessment and use of score sheets will be facilitated by:

- A good knowledge of the species-specific behaviours of the animal being assessed.
- A knowledge and comparison of the individual animal's behaviour and appearance before and after the onset of pain (e.g. pre- and postoperatively).
- The use of palpation or manipulation of the affected area and assessment of the responses obtained.
- Examination of the level of function of the affected area, for example, leg use following injury or limb surgery, together with a knowledge of any mechanical interference with function.
- The use of analgesic regimens or dose rates that have been shown to be effective in controlled clinical studies, and evaluation of the changes in behaviour this brings about.
- A knowledge of the nonspecific effects of any analgesic, anaesthetic, or other drugs that have been administered.

Further practical recommendations are summarized in Table 5.6.

Pain scoring systems are almost certainly still under-used in most facilities (Herrmann and Flecknell, 2019, additional data collected by author, 2018–22). We know that analgesic agents are not always effective, that the dose required will vary depending upon the age, strain, and sex of the animal and will be influenced by numerous other factors.

TABLE 5.6 Key points for implementing pain assessment methods and pain management in laboratory animals.

1. Be familiar with the normal appearance and behaviour of the species you are working with and with that of the specific group of animals involved in your project.

2. Be sure that all of those who may be needed to assist with your project are aware of the scheduling of key events such as surgery and the proposed protocol for pain assessment and pain management. Avoid scheduling studies such that additional support could be needed at weekends or outside normal working hours unless this can be specifically arranged.

3. Wherever possible, we should use multiple measures to assess pain, as they all have potential limitations, and one method can often compensate for the limitation in another.

4. Perform baseline assessments of your animals using the assessment methods you plan to use. Carry out at least one assessment 30–60 min after recovery from anaesthesia. This will enable adjustments to the analgesic regimen if necessary.

5. Agree in advance whether only individuals assessed as needing additional analgesia are treated, or whether treatments need to be standardized across all animals in the study.

6. Repeat pain assessments before administering additional analgesics, or when deciding to end analgesic treatment.

7. Agree in advance a 'plan b'—an alternate or additional analgesic regimen that can be adopted if the initial protocol is not sufficiently effective. Check that any protocol approvals, e.g. by an ethical review body or regulator, include the option to modify the analgesic regimen in this way.

8. At the conclusion of each study, review the effectiveness of the protocol of pain management and pain assessment, and make refinements for future studies.

9. Be sure to incorporate pain assessment and pain management into an overall scheme for monitoring the animals (for example, using a scoresheet) and refinement of the procedure.

Assessing pain accurately and frequently is therefore fundamental to the selection of an appropriate analgesic regimen and evaluating and then modifying that regimen according to the response of the animals being treated.

Pain relief

Leaving aside the problems of pain assessment, empirical treatment of presumed painful conditions will continue, and it is not unreasonable to assume that analgesic therapies shown to be effective in people are also likely to be effective in animals. A growing body of data from well-controlled trials of analgesic efficacy in most laboratory species is now also becoming available, but even when these have not been completed, results of nociceptive tests can be used to guide dosing regimens. Analgesics can be broadly divided into two main groups, the opioids or narcotic analgesics and the NSAIDs such as aspirin. Local anaesthetics can also make an important contribution to the management of postoperative pain relief by blocking all sensation from the affected area. Details of individual agents are given in Chapter 2. Suggested dose rates of analgesics are provided in Tables 5.7–5.10. A practical approach to formulating analgesic protocols is provided at the end of this chapter.

Pain relief—Practical difficulties of providing continued analgesic treatment

Several practical issues need to be considered when analgesics are administered to control postoperative pain. An important consideration is the short duration of action of most of the opioid (narcotic) analgesics in many species. Maintenance of effective analgesia with, for example, pethidine (meperidine) may require administration every 1–3 h, depending upon the species. Continuation of such a regimen overnight can cause practical difficulties. One method of avoiding this difficulty is to use buprenorphine as the analgesic, since there is good evidence in humans, rodents, rabbits, and pigs that it has a duration of action of 4–8 h, depending upon the dose administered (Cowan et al., 1977a; Dum and Herz, 1981; Hermansen et al., 1986 Flecknell and Liles, 1990; Sramek et al., 2015; Andrews et al., 2020; Fabian et al., 2021). Its duration of action in the sheep appears to be considerably less, although of longer duration than pethidine and morphine (Nolan et al., 1987). Considerably longer analgesia can be provided by using slow-release formulations of buprenorphine (see Chapter 2) or other opioids. Several slow-release preparations of analgesics have been marketed for use in humans (e.g. morphine, oxycodone, hydromorphone). These may be useful in larger species but should be used with caution pending establishment of the pharmacokinetics of these agents in the particular species. In smaller animals, the tablets and the capsules would need to be divided into smaller doses, and in most instances, this results in a loss of the slow-release properties of the formulation. An exception appears to be an oral morphine preparation ('Oramorph SR', Boehringer Ingelheim) which has been shown to produce prolonged antinociception in rats (Leach et al., 2010a).

Several slow-release preparations have been developed specifically for use in laboratory animals. Slow-release formulations of buprenorphine are now available (see Chapter 2), and these can provide effective plasma concentrations of analgesics for up to 3 days (Chum et al., 2014). These formulations may be particularly valuable when prolonged moderate to severe pain is anticipated. Although less potent than opioids, NSAIDs may be sufficient to control pain effectively after some surgical procedures, especially when combined with use of local anaesthetics. Several NSAIDs have a prolonged

TABLE 5.7 Suggested dose rates for nonsteroidal antiinflammatory drugs in laboratory animals (smaller species).

Drug	Mouse	Rat	Guinea pig	Rabbit	Ferret
Aspirin	120 mg/kg per os	100 mg/kg per os	87 mg/kg per os	100 mg/kg per os	200 mg/kg per os
Carprofen	5 mg/kg sc	5 mg/kg sc	4 mg/kg sc? once daily	1.5 mg/kg per os u.i.d., 4 mg/kg sc u.i.d.	4 mg/kg sc u.i.d.
Diclofenac	8 mg/kg per os	10 mg/kg per os	2.1 mg/kg per os	–	–
Flunixin	2.5 mg/kg sc or im? 12 hourly	2.5 mg/kg sc or im? 12 hourly	2.5 mg/kg sc or im? 12 hourly	1–2 mg/kg sc im? 12 hourly	0.5–2 mg/kg sc 12–24 hourly
Ibuprofen	30 mg/kg per os	15 mg/kg per os	10 mg/kg im?4 hourly	10 mg/kg iv? 4 hourly	–
Indomethacin	1 mg/kg per os	2 mg/kg per os	8 mg/kg per os	12.5 mg/kg per os	–
Ketoprofen	5 mg/kg sc	5 mg/kg sc	–	3 mg/kg im	3 mg/kg im
Meloxicam	5 mg/kg sc or per os	1 mg/kg sc or per os	0.1–0.3 mg/kg sc or per os every 24 h	0.6–1 mg/kg sc or per os	0.1–0.2 mg/kg sc or per os
Paracetamol (acetominophen)	200 mg/kg per os, 30–100 mg/kg ip	200 mg/kg per os	–	–	–

Note that considerable individual and strain variation in response may be encountered and that it is therefore essential to assess the analgesic effect in each individual animal.

TABLE 5.8 Suggested dose rates for nonsteroidal antiinflammatory drugs in laboratory animals (larger species).

Drug	Pig	Sheep	Primate	Dog	Cat
Aspirin	10–20 mg/kg per os, 4–6 hourly	50–100 mg/kg per os, 6–12 hourly	20 mg/kg per os, 6–8 hourly	10–25 mg/kg per os, 8 hourly	10–25 mg/kg per os, every 48 h
Carprofen	2–4 mg/kg iv or sc, once daily	2–4 mg/kg sc or iv, once daily (? 2–3 days)	3–4 mg/kg sc u.i.d.	4 mg/kg iv or sc, once daily 1–2 mg/kg b.i.d. per os, for 7 days	4 mg/kg sc or iv
Flunixin	1–2 mg/kg iv or sc, once daily	2 mg/kg iv or sc, once daily	0.5–2 mg/kg sc or iv daily	1 mg/kg iv or im, 12 hourly 1 mg/kg per os, daily for up to 3 days	1 mg/kg sc, daily for up to 5 days
Ibuprofen	–	–	7 mg/kg per os	10 mg/kg per os, 24 hourly	–
Ketoprofen	1–3 mg/kg iv, im, sc, per os, 12 hourly	–	2 mg/kg sc daily	2 mg/kg sc, im or iv, once daily for up to 3 days 1 mg/kg per os, daily for 5 days	1 mg/kg sc, once daily for up to 3 days 1 mg/kg per os, once daily for up to 5 days
Meloxicam	0.4 mg/kg sc, once daily	0.5 mg/kg iv, sc up to b.i.d. for 1 day, then 0.5 mg/kg per os u.i.d. for 5 days	0.1–0.2 mg/kg u.i.d. sc or per os	0.2 mg/kg u.i.d. sc or per os, then 0.1 mg/kg sc or per os	0.2 mg/kg u.i.d. sc or 0.3 mg/kg per os, then 0.1 mg/kg sc or per os
Tolfenamic acid	–	–	–	4 mg/kg sc daily for 2 days	4 mg/kg sc daily for 2 days
Paracetamol (acetominophen)	–	–	–	15 mg/kg per os, 6–8 hourly	Contra-indicated

Note that considerable individual and strain variation in response may be encountered, and that it is therefore essential to assess the analgesic effect in each individual animal.

TABLE 5.9 Suggested dose rates for opioid analgesics in laboratory animals (smaller species).

Drug	Mouse	Rat	Guinea pig	Rabbit	Ferret
Buprenorphine	0.05–0.1 mg/kg sc 12 hourly	0.01–0.05 mg/kg sc or iv, 8–12 hourly 0.1–0.25 mg/kg per os, 8–12 hourly	0.05 mg/kg sc, 8–12 hourly	0.01–0.05 mg/kg sc or iv, 8–12 hourly	0.01–0.03 mg/kg iv, im or sc, 8–12 hourly
Buprenorphine extended-release[a]	2.5 mL/kg (3.35 mg/kg) can be repeated after 3 days	0.5 mL/kg (0.65 mg/kg) can be repeated after 3 days	–	–	–
Butorphanol	1–2 mg/kg sc, 1–2 hourly	1–2 mg/kg sc, 1–2 hourly	1–2 mg/kg sc, 1–2 hourly	0.1 – 0.5 mg/kg iv, 1–2 hourly	0.4 mg/kg im, 2–3 hourly
Hydromorphone	–	–	–	0.1–0.2 mg/kg ? 6–8 hourly	0.1–0.2 mg/kg? 6–8 hourly
Morphine	2.5 mg/kg sc, 2–4 hourly	2.5 mg/kg sc, 2–4 hourly	2–5 mg/kg sc or im, 4 hourly	2–5 mg/kg sc or im, 2–4 hourly	0.5–2 mg/kg im or sc, 6 hourly
Nalbuphine	2–4 mg/kg im? 4 hourly	1–2 mg/kg im, 3 hourly	1–2 mg/kg iv, ip or im	1–2 mg/kg iv, 4–5 hourly	–
Oxymorphone	0.2–0.5 mg/kg sc? 4 hourly	0.2–0.5 mg/kg sc? 4 hourly	0.2–0.5 mg/kg sc ? 4 hourly	0.05–0.2 mg/kg sc? 6–8 hourly	0.05–0.2 mg/kg sc? 6–8 hourly
Pentazocine	5–10 mg/kg sc 3–4 hourly	5–10 mg/kg sc, 3–4 hourly	–	5–10 mg/kg sc, im or iv, 4 hourly	–
Pethidine (Meperidine)	10–20/kg sc or im, 2–3 hourly	10–20 mg/kg sc or im, 2–3 hourly	10–20 mg/kg sc or im, 2–3 hourly	5–10 mg/kg sc or im, 2–3 hourly	5–10 mg/kg im or sc, 2–4 hourly
Tramadol	5 mg/kg sc, ip?	5 mg/kg sc, ip?	–	–	–

Note that considerable individual and strain variation in response may be encountered, and that it is therefore essential to assess the analgesic effect in each animal.? 5 duration of action uncertain.

[a] Manufacturer recommended dose for 'Ethiqa XR' see text for recommendations for other species.

TABLE 5.10 Suggested dose rates for opioid analgesics in laboratory animals (larger species).

Drug	Pig	Sheep	Primate	Dog	Cat
Buprenorphine[a]	0.01–0.05 mg/kg im or iv, 6–12 hourly	0.005–0.01 mg/kg im or iv, 4 hourly	0.005–0.01 mg/kg im or iv, 6–12 hourly	0.005–0.02 mg/kg im, sc or iv, 6–12 hourly	0.005–0.01 mg/kg sc or iv, 8–12 hourly
Butorphanol	0.1–0.3 mg/kg im or iv, 1–2 hourly	0.5 mg/kg im or iv, 1–2 hourly	0.01 mg/kg iv,? 2–3 hourly	0.2–0.4 mg/kg sc or im, 1–2 hourly	0.4 mg/kg sc, 1–2 hourly
Hydromorphone	–	–	–	0.05–0.2 mg/kg im, sc 2–4 hourly	0.1 mg/kg im, sc 0.2 2–4 hourly
Morphine	0.2–1 mg/kg im,? 4 hourly	0.2–0.5 mg/kg im,? 4 hourly	1–2 mg/kg sc or im, 4 hourly	0.5–5 mg/kg sc or im, 4 hourly	0.3 mg/kg sc, 4 hourly
Nalbuphine	–	–	–	0.5–2.0 mg/kg sc or im, 3–4 hourly	1.5–3.0 mg/kg iv, 3 hourly
Oxymorphone	0.15 mg/kg im 4 hourly	–	0.15 mg/kg im 4–6 hourly	0.05–0.22 mg/kg, sc or iv, 2–4 hourly	0.2 mg/kg sc or iv
Pentazocine	2 mg/kg im or iv, 4 hourly	–	2–5 mg/kg im or iv, 4 hourly	2 mg/kg im or iv, 4 hourly	–
Pethidine (meperidine)	2 mg/kg im or iv, 2–4 hourly	2 mg/kg im or iv, 2–4 hourly	2–4 mg/kg im or iv, 2–4 hourly	10 mg/kg im, 2–3 hourly	2–10 mg/kg sc or im, 2–3 hourly
Tramadol	–	–	? 1–2 mg/kg sc or iv, 2 mg/kg orally? b.i.d.	2–5 mg/kg iv or sc, 2–5 mg/kg orally t.i.d.	2–4 mg/kg sc

Note that considerable individual and strain variation in response may be encountered, and that it is therefore essential to assess the analgesic effect in each animal.? 5 duration of action uncertain.

[a] See text for suggested dose rates for extended release buprenorphine.

duration of action (8–24 h) which facilitates maintenance of effective analgesia (see Chapter 2).

An alternative approach is to adopt the well-established clinical technique used in people, of administering analgesics as a continuous infusion. Infusions of analgesics have the advantage of maintaining effective plasma levels of the analgesic, and so providing continuous pain relief. This contrasts with intermittent injections, where pain may return before the next dose of analgesic is administered. This technique obviously poses some methodological difficulties in animals, but if an indwelling catheter and harness and swivel apparatus are available, then this can be arranged quite simply. In larger species (>3–4 kg body weight), a light-weight infusion pump (Smiths Medical, Appendix 4) can be bandaged directly to the animal and continuous infusion made simply by means of a butterfly-type needle anchored subcutaneously or intramuscularly. When analgesics are to be administered by continuous infusion, the infusion rate can be calculated from knowledge of the pharmacokinetics of the analgesic to be used (Chapter 4). If these data are not readily available, an approximation that appears successful in clinical use is as follows: calculate the total dose required over the period of infusion, reduce this by half and set the pump infusion rate; accordingly, administer a single, normal dose of the drug as an initial loading dose and start the infusion. The rate can then be adjusted depending upon the animal's responses.

Prolonged analgesia can also be provided using slow-release patches that are placed on the animal's skin. Both fentanyl and buprenorphine patches are available, and they have been used with some success in a range of species (Harvey-Clark et al., 2000; Shafford et al., 2004; Malavasi et al., 2006; Egger et al., 2007; Thiede et al., 2014). The patches are manufactured for use in humans, so the rate of drug release varies in different animal species (Riviere and Papich, 2001; Mills and Cross, 2006; Heikkinen et al., 2015). Measurement of plasma concentrations of drugs has shown that considerable individual variation occurs (Davidson et al., 2004). For this reason, it is best to consider these patches as providing basal analgesia, and to assess the animal regularly to ensure sufficient analgesia is being provided. Patches need to be placed on the skin for approximately 24 h before adequate plasma concentrations of analgesic are attained. Lidocaine patches have also been used in dog, cat, and horse, with the patch placed close to the site of the surgical wound. Relatively little efficacy data are available, and the use of this approach is likely to be restricted to larger species (Ko et al., 2007; Ko et al., 2008; Andreoni and Giorgi, 2009).

Administration in food and water

The need for repeated injections of analgesics is time consuming and may be distressing to the animal, particularly smaller species that require firm physical restraint to enable an injection to be given safely and effectively. In addition, the need for repeated injections requires veterinary or other staff to attend the animal overnight. To circumvent this problem, analgesics may be incorporated

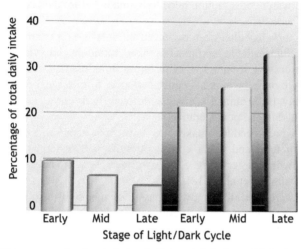

FIG. 5.19   Water consumption in rats during the light and dark phase of their photoperiod. *Data redrawn from Burwell, R.D., et al., 1992. Effects of aging on the diurnal pattern of water intake in rats. Behav. Neural Biol. 58 (3), 196–203.*

into the food or water on the assumption that animals will self-administer the agent. This approach is often used in laboratory rodents, but several practical problems can make it relatively ineffective:

- Some animals eat and drink relatively infrequently or may only do so in the dark phase of their photoperiod (Fig. 5.19). This may result in no analgesic being ingested in the light phase of the photoperiod, and inadequate pain relief being provided.
- Food and water intake varies markedly between different strains of rodents (Bachmanov et al., 2002; Tordoff et al., 2007, 2008) (Fig. 5.20) and are influenced by husbandry conditions (such as type of cage) so measurements of

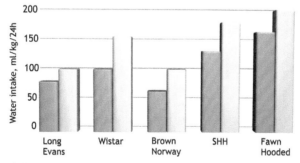

FIG. 5.20   Variation in water consumption in different strains of rat, male, *dark blue* and female, *light blue*. Data redrawn from Tordoff et al. 2008.

food and water consumption need to be made before the procedure in each group of animals.

- Other factors may alter postoperative fluid intake—for example some components of anaesthetic mixtures (e.g. medetomidine and xylazine) cause diuresis (excessive urination). The resulting fluid loss may result in increased fluid intake once the animal begins to recover from surgery and anaesthesia. Conversely, if the animal is given additional fluids during surgery, this may reduce fluid intake postoperatively.
- Although preprocedure intake may have been measured to calculate intake, both food and water consumption are often depressed for several days following surgery (Fig. 5.21), so effective dosing may not be achieved (Evangelista-Vaz et al., 2018).
- If opioids are used, the high first-pass liver metabolism following oral administration requires that high-dose rates are given, and this can represent a significant cost if all the animals' drinking water or food is medicated.
- There may be problems of palatability (Speth et al., 2001; Bauer et al., 2003) and the stability of the analgesic in food or water needs to be established (Ingrao et al., 2013).
- Since animals will consume small quantities of analgesic at each bout of eating or drinking, it will take a considerable time to achieve effective plasma concentrations of the drug.

Despite these problems, encouraging results have been obtained with paracetamol (acetominophen) in rats (Mickley et al., 2006), and with buprenorphine (Kalliokoski et al., 2011) and the approach deserves further evaluation in a range of different circumstances. It is also important to provide effective analgesia by other means in the period before the animal commences eating or drinking (Christy et al., 2014).

Finally, it is important to note that the bioavailability of drugs, particularly those that undergo high first pass metabolism, may vary greatly between ani-

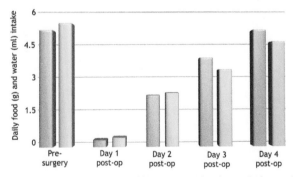

FIG. 5.21 Food (*yellow/brown*) and water (*blue*) consumption in rats before and after surgery. *Data redrawn from Hayes, K.E., et al., 2000. An evaluation of analgesic regimens for abdominal surgery in mice. Contemp. Topics Lab. Anim. Sci./Am. Assoc. Lab. Anim. Sci. 39 (6), 18–23.*

mals. For example, the oral dose of buprenorphine required to produce analgesia equivalent to the recommended subcutaneous dose is too high to be clinically useful (Martin et al., 2001; Thompson et al., 2004). In contrast, other studies have indicated oral administration is effective (Flecknell et al., 1999b; Roughan and Flecknell, 2004; Godlkuhl et al., 2010). It is clear that in some animals, this route of administration is likely to be ineffective, so it should only be used if a reliable pain assessment system is in place (Leach et al., 2010a).

If analgesics are to be given in the food or water:

- Check the analgesic is stable in solution, or in the food. Using a commercial formulation of palatable gel helps ensure this.
- Check the animals eat or drink sufficiently to obtain an effective dose.
- Provide additional analgesia immediately postoperatively, to ensure effective pain relief until 'lights out'.
- Assess postoperative pain to check the analgesic regimen is proving to be effective.

An alternative approach is to administer of small quantities of medicated food at regular intervals. This does not avoid the need for repeated attendance overnight but does remove the need for repeated subcutaneous or intramuscular injections in small rodents. With all medicated foodstuffs, rats are initially cautious of the novel formulation, but once some has been consumed, subsequent palatable 'treats' are eaten as soon as they are offered. It is therefore advisable to commence administering the foodstuff, which does not contain analgesic, 2–3 days before surgery. After surgery, analgesic-containing foodstuff can be given. If using jelly ('jello'), the flavoured gelatin used is domestic fruit-flavoured jelly, reconstituted at double the recommended strength. Other highly palatable foodstuffs, e.g. Nutella (Abelson et al., 2012) or standard pelleted diet (Molina-Cimadevila et al., 2014) have also been shown to be suitable vehicles for oral analgesic administration.

Techniques for administration of food pellets at intervals to experimental animals are well established, and it would be a relatively simple procedure to introduce an automated means of delivering pellets at appropriate time intervals. The technique could also be used with larger species, and need not be restricted to opioids, or indeed analgesics. Provided that the animal is eating or drinking, small quantities of highly palatable material could be provided at appropriate intervals. Simple timer devices to achieve this are already marketed for delayed feeding of pet dogs and cats.

Epidural and intrathecal opioids: Epidural and intrathecal opioids have been shown to have a prolonged effect in humans and to provide effective analgesia (Glynn, 1987). In animals, both clinical and experimental studies have indicated that the technique can be used in a number of species (Duke, 2000; Pablo, 1993; Pascoe and Dyson, 1993; Popilskis et al., 1993). The necessary techniques of epidural or intrathecal injection have been described in rabbits (Kero et al., 1981; Hughes et al., 1993), Guinea pigs (Thomasson et al., 1974), and small rodents (Mestre et al., 1994), (Fairbanks, 2003). In larger species such as the cat, dog, sheep, and pig, descriptions of the injection technique can be found in most veterinary anaesthesia texts and a number of other publications (e.g. Grimm et al., 2015). Intrathecal morphine has been shown to be effective in rats following orthopaedic surgery (Thomas et al., 2016) and has been used extensively in studies of experimental pain. It has the advantage of requiring lower total doses of opioid, which may be of benefit in reducing the potential interactions with research protocols.

Additional considerations in pain relief: Although the use of analgesic drugs remains the most important technique for reducing postoperative pain, the use of these drugs must be integrated into a total scheme for perioperative care (Carli and Asenjo, 2003; Kohn et al., 2007). As discussed in Chapter 2, pain relief in the immediate recovery period can be provided by including an analgesic drug in any preanaesthetic medication. Alternatively, if a neuroleptanalgesic combination has been used to produce anaesthesia, it can be reversed using buprenorphine, nalbuphine, or butorphanol, rather than naloxone. These agents have been shown not only to reverse the respiratory depressant effects of opioids such as fentanyl but, in contrast to naloxone, to provide effective prolonged analgesia (Flecknell et al., 1989b).

The expertise of the surgeon can also greatly influence the degree of postoperative pain. A good surgical technique that minimizes tissue trauma and the prevention of tension on suture lines can considerably reduce postoperative pain. The use of bandages to pad and protect traumatized tissue must not be overlooked and forms an essential adjunct to the use of analgesic drugs.

Pain and affective state

Aside from measures directed towards alleviating or preventing pain, it is important to consider the overall care of the animal and the prevention of distress. Distress is used in this context to describe conditions which are not in themselves painful, but which are unpleasant and which the animal would normally choose to avoid. For example, recovering from anaesthesia on wet, uncomfortable bedding in a cold, unfamiliar environment would be likely to cause distress to many animals. These factors, and others, that may reduce stress or distress can have a direct effect on pain perception. In people, numerous studies have shown that fear and anxiety increase pain and increase the requirement for analgesics (Schug et al., 2020). In animals, stress has been shown to modify nociceptive thresholds (Imbe et al., 2006). It therefore seems reasonable to make every effort to reduce the stress associated with experimental procedures that could cause pain. We should also consider going further and attempt to induce a positive affective state in animals, since positive emotional states are associated with reduced pain perception in people (Bushnell et al., 2013). This can be done in several ways, for example by use of environmental enrichment (Brydges et al., 2011; Nguyen et al., 2020), and in some species by positive interactions with a handler (LaFollette et al., 2018). Induction of a positive emotional state can reduce the impact of aversive procedures (Hinchcliffe et al., 2022), including acute and chronic pain (Kimura et al., 2022).

Recommendations

Which analgesic to use, when to give it, and when to repeat treatments, needs to be based on an assessment of the likely intensity of the pain and the effectiveness of the analgesic regimen. Since the efficacy of specific analgesics will vary between individuals, fixed dose analgesic protocols are only a starting point for effective pain management. The following general guidance is provided as a starting point for developing analgesic protocols:

- Implement measures to reduce stress and anxiety and aim to induce a positive affective state in animals before undertaking surgery or other procedures that could cause pain.
- Administer analgesics preemptively or preventatively (see Chapter 2) when possible. If there are concerns related to interactions with anaesthetic and surgical protocols, administer analgesics so that they are effective before the animal recovers consciousness.
- Use multimodal analgesic regimens since this will provide more effective pain relief (see Chapter 2).
- Use a method of pain assessment whenever possible, carry out assessments preprocedure, and use the results of your assessment to modify analgesic protocols.
- Always have a 'Plan B'—an analgesic regimen agreed with all involved in the care of the animals, that can be implemented in the event of problems arising in relation to pain control or adverse drug reactions.

Surgery involving significant tissue trauma, for example orthopaedic procedures, laparotomy or thoracotomy, is likely to require inclusion of opioids in the analgesic protocol. If the procedure is conducted skilfully, then in some circumstances an NSAID and local anaesthesia may be sufficient, but this can be confirmed by use of pain assessment. If validated assessment methods are not available, then it is preferable to include at least one dose of opioid.

If the procedure is relatively minor, for example, jugular or carotid cannulation, then only a single dose of analgesic may be required. In some circumstances, a potent NSAID, such as meloxicam or carprofen, may be used as an alternative to buprenorphine. Whenever possible, local anaesthetics administered by local infiltration or as a 'splash block' should also be used.

The duration of treatment should be based on the duration of pain. Following more invasive surgical procedures, such as laparotomy, orthopaedic surgery or craniotomy, opioid administration should be continued for 8–48 h, depending upon the species and the expertise of the surgeon (since this has a major influence on the degree of tissue trauma). When undertaking major surgery, particularly in larger species when the degree of tissue trauma tends to be greater, analgesic administration may continue for 72 h. In addition, local anaesthetics

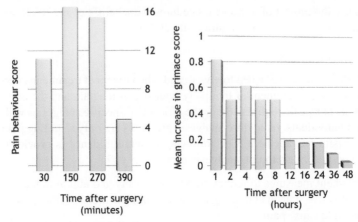

FIG. 5.22 Pain intensity after abdominal surgery in rats (left) and mice (right) assessed using behavioural scoring (rats) and grimace scores (mouse). *Data redrawn from Roughan, J.V., Flecknell, P.A., 2004. Behaviour-based assessment of the duration of laparotomy-induced abdominal pain and the analgesic effects of carprofen and buprenorphine in rats. Behav. Pharmacol. 15 (7), 461 (rats) and Matsumiya, L.C., et al., 2012. Using the mouse grimace scale to reevaluate the efficacy of postoperative analgesics in laboratory mice. J. Am. Assoc. Lab. Anim. Sci. 51 (1), 42–49 (mice).*

(e.g. bupivacaine combined with lidocaine) may be infiltrated into the wound margins or used to provide a localized nerve block of the area.

The intensity of pain gradually reduces, for example in rodents, pain following laparotomy reduced rapidly within 6–48 h, depending upon the assessment method used (Fig. 5.22). Analgesic protocols can be tailored to match the likely pain intensity. For example, an opioid (e.g. buprenorphine) can be administered in combination with an NSAID for 8–24 h, followed by an NSAID alone for a further 24–72 h (see Tables 5.7–5.10 for suggested dose rates). Alternatively, a slow-release formulation of analgesic (e.g. buprenorphine) could be given if opioid treatment for a prolonged period is required. The duration of treatment, and the decision as to whether to continue with opioid administration should be based on pain assessments.

This approach reduces the likelihood both of undesirable effects of analgesics and potential interactions with research protocols.

Conclusions

Attention to the suggestions made in this chapter concerning postoperative care can have a dramatic effect on the speed with which animals return to normality following surgical procedures. It has been repeatedly demonstrated in humans that the provision of effective analgesia reduces the time taken for postoperative recovery (Joshi and Ogunnaike, 2005; Schug et al., 2020). The provision of good postoperative care should therefore be considered essential not only because of a concern for the animal's welfare but also because it is good scientific practice.

Chapter 6

Anaesthesia of common laboratory species: Special considerations

Laboratory animals are anaesthetized either to provide humane restraint while relatively atraumatic procedures are carried out or to eliminate the perception of pain during surgical operations. Several factors influence the selection of a method of anaesthesia—concern for the welfare of the animal, the constraints imposed by specific types of research and the expertise of the anaesthetist. An anaesthetic technique should therefore:

- cause a minimum of distress,
- provide an appropriate degree of analgesia, and
- result in an uneventful recovery, free from unpleasant side-effects.

Ideally, the technique should also be easy to implement, should have a high success rate and use anaesthetic agents that have a minimum influence on the experimental work that is being undertaken. These factors have been considered carefully when selecting the methods recommended for each species in this chapter. The primary consideration has been the well-being of the animal, coupled with ease of use and safety of the drug or drug combination. For a more extensive discussion of selecting an anaesthetic agent, see Chapter 2.

Alternative anaesthetic regimens are included since some research protocols will preclude the use of the drugs recommended and in addition some anaesthetic agents may not be readily available in certain laboratories. A comprehensive listing of anaesthetic drug dose rates for each species is also provided.

It is particularly important to read the general sections on intraoperative care in conjunction with the notes below on anaesthetic techniques for different species. The dose rates recommended in this chapter are those that have been found effective in the majority of individuals of the species concerned. The response to an anaesthetic drug can vary considerably and may be influenced by the strain of animal, sex, age, and environmental conditions in which the animal is housed (Lovell, 1986a, b) Strain variations may also become apparent only during recovery from anaesthesia; for example, different inbred strains of mice have shown varying degree of respiratory depression immediately after isoflurane

Laboratory Animal Anaesthesia and Analgesia. https://doi.org/10.1016/B978-0-12-818268-0.00010-3

anaesthesia (Groeben, 2003). When using a drug or drug combination for the first time, or when anaesthetizing a different strain of animal, it is advisable to proceed cautiously. For example, assess the safety and efficacy of the regimen on only one or two animals, before proceeding to anaesthetize larger numbers. As experience is gained, a dose rate appropriate to the particular strain, sex, age, and weight of animal can be established.

In order to provide some guidance as to the predicted effects of the different anaesthetics and their duration of action, the dose rate tables for each species includes an estimate of the likely depth of anaesthesia, its duration, and the anticipated duration of loss of the animal's righting reflex. It is important to note that considerable variation in response is to be expected. With many agents, a range of dose rates is given with a corresponding range of anticipated effects (e.g. light–deep anaesthesia). The terminology used is as follows:

- *Sedation (light, medium, or heavy):* the animal will have reduced activity and may become completely immobile but is easily aroused, particularly by painful stimuli.
- *Analgesia:* some pain-alleviating effect is present.
- *Immobilization:* the animal is immobilized but still responds to painful stimuli.
- *Light anaesthesia:* the animal is immobile and unconscious, but still responsive to even minor surgical procedures.
- *Medium anaesthesia:* most surgical procedures (e.g. laparotomy) may be carried out without causing any response, but the animal may still respond to major surgical stimuli (e.g. orthopaedic surgery).
- *Deep anaesthesia:* the animal is unresponsive to all surgical stimuli.

These terms are used to provide a general guide, but in all instances the depth of anaesthesia produced in a particular animal should be assessed before commencing surgery (see Chapter 3).

Small rodents

The problems arise when anaesthetizing rodents are related primarily to their small body size. Their high surface area to body weight ratio makes them particularly susceptible to the development of hypothermia; intravenous drug administration is limited by the size of the superficial veins, and the small and relatively inaccessible larynx makes endotracheal intubation difficult. A further consequence of the small size of these species is that the volumes of anaesthetic required may be very small. This can make accurate dosing of individual animals difficult. In addition, although the volumes are small, they are often still large relative to the muscle mass of the animal. For example, administering ketamine at 100 mg/kg to a mouse requires a volume of 0.03 mL (30 μL) of anaesthetic. This seems a small volume, but is equivalent to 70 mL administered to an adult person. As described in in 'Routes of administration', Chapter 1, injection of relatively high volumes of agents by the intramuscular route can result in muscle damage, pain on injection, and the material. The route is therefore best avoided and the intraperitoneal route used—even though this is associated with a relatively high partial failure rate (Das and North, 2007). Information is becoming available regarding use of the subcutaneous route of administration of anaesthetics and analgesics in small rodents, and this may prove a more reliable technique. Because of the small volume of undiluted drug needed, it is often convenient to mix together the required compounds and dilute them with saline or sterile water for injection. Preparing these diluted mixtures also facilitates accurate dosing of individual animals. Suggested dilutions are given in Appendix 3.

Given these practical constraints, it is often simplest to select an inhalational anaesthetic agent, as induction can be achieved smoothly and rapidly in an anaesthetic chamber, and anaesthesia maintained using a suitable breathing system.

The incidence of spontaneous disease in colonies of laboratory animals has greatly reduced, but some still have endemic respiratory infections. The disease may not cause obvious clinical signs, but may cause respiratory failure during the period of anaesthesia or result in the development of severe clinical respiratory disease in the postoperative period.

It is unnecessary to withhold food and water before induction of anaesthesia since vomiting on induction or recovery does not occur in any of the small rodents (see 'preanaesthetic fasting', Chapter 1). As mentioned earlier (Chapter 1), problems may be seen with some guinea pigs that retain food in their pharynx after being anaesthetized. If this occurs then a short period of preanaesthetic fasting (3–4 h) may be introduced.

Rats

Preanaesthetic medication

Most rats can easily be restrained humanely to enable the subcutaneous, intraperitoneal, or intramuscular injection anaesthetic agents, provided they have become accustomed to being handled. One simple way to achieve this is to weigh the animal daily during its acclimatization period (see Chapter 1). This also provides useful information on its normal growth pattern and ensures that it has recovered from the stress associated with transportation. In general, intraperitoneal and subcutaneous injections are tolerated better than intramuscular injections as they cause less pain to the animal. Preanaesthetic medication to sedate the animal is not usually required as many protocols only require a single injection of a mixture of two or more agents. If an intravenous induction agent is to be used, initial sedation with a tranquillizer or sedative/analgesic is recommended, unless positive reinforcement training has been used to accustom the animal to restraint for the procedure.

The following drugs can be used to produce sedation and are listed in order of preference (see Table 6.1):

1. Hypnorm (fentanyl/fluanisone; Janssen) (0.3–0.6 mL/kg ip). At the lower dose rate, sedation and some analgesia is produced. The higher dose rate produces sufficient analgesia to enable procedures such as skin biopsy or cardiac puncture to be carried out (Green, 1975). Occasionally, marked respiratory depression is seen when the drug is administered at the higher dose rate. If this produces severe cyanosis, it can be reversed with nalbuphine, butorphanol, or naloxone.

2. Medetomidine (30–100 μg/kg sc) and Dexmedetomidine (15–50 μg/kg) produces light to heavy sedation, and at the higher dose rate, many animals will lose their righting reflex. Some strains require significantly higher dose rates (Medetomidine 300 μg/kg, Dexmedetomidine 150 μg/kg) before becoming sedated and losing their righting reflex. The degree of analgesia produced is insufficient for anything other than very minor procedures, but is suitable for nonpainful manipulations such as

TABLE 6.1 Sedatives, tranquillizers and other preanaesthetic medication for use in the rat.

Drug	Dose rate	Comments
Acepromazine	2.5 mg/kg im, ip	Light sedation
Atropine	0.05 mg/kg ip, sc	Anticholinergic
Dexmedetomidine	15–50 μg/kg sc, ip	Light to heavy sedation, mild to moderate analgesia
Diazepam	2.5–5.0 mg/kg ip, im	Light sedation
Fentanyl/dropiderol (Innovar-Vet)	0.3–0.5 mL/kg im	Immobilization/analgesia
Fentanyl/fluanisone (Hypnorm)	0.2–0.5 mL/kg im 0.3–0.6 mL/kg ip	Light/moderate sedation, moderate analgesia
Glycopyrrolate	0.5 mg/kg im	Anticholinergic
Ketamine	50–100 mg/kg im, ip	Deep sedation, immobilization, mild to moderate analgesia
Medetomidine	30–100 μg/kg sc, ip	Light to heavy sedation, mild to moderate analgesia
Midazolam	5 mg/kg ip	Light sedation
Xylazine	1–3 mg/kg im, ip	Light to heavy sedation, mild to moderate analgesia

Considerable variation in effect occurs between different strains.

radiography (Virtanen, 1988). Medetomidine and Dexmedetomidine markedly potentiate the effects of other anaesthetic agents. For example, the concentration of volatile agent needed to produce surgical anaesthesia may be reduced by more than 60%. The degree of sedation can be increased by combining Medetomidine with butorphanol and midazolam (Bellini et al., 2014).

3. Xylazine (1–3 mg/kg ip) produces mild to moderate sedation. Although the drug provides little analgesia when used alone, it markedly potentiates the effects of other anaesthetic agents.
4. Ketamine (50–100 mg/kg ip) produces deep sedation. The degree of muscle relaxation is poor, and the level of analgesia is insufficient for even superficial surgery (Green et al., 1981a).
5. Acepromazine (2.5/kg ip) produces moderate sedation, but has no analgesic action. Administration will potentiate the effects of other anaesthetic agents.
6. Diazepam or midazolam (2.5–5 mg/kg ip) produces light sedation, but neither drug has any analgesic action. Administration will potentiate the effects of other anaesthetic agents.

Atropine (0.05 mg/kg ip or sc) or glycopyrrolate (0.5 mg/kg im) (Olson et al., 1994) can be administered to reduce salivary and bronchial secretions and protect the heart from vagal inhibition.

Appropriate preanaesthetic medication will reduce the stress caused by induction of anaesthesia and also ease handling and restraint. In addition, it will reduce the amount of other anaesthetic agents required to produce general anaesthesia. The dose rates of anaesthetic drugs quoted in Table 6.2 apply to rats that have received no preanaesthetic medication unless otherwise stated. Generally, these dosages can be reduced by at least 30%–50% if one of the drugs listed above has been administered.

General anaesthesia

Injectable agents

The small body size of the rat makes intravenous injection difficult; hence, drugs are usually administered by the intraperitoneal, subcutaneous, or intramuscular routes. If these routes are used, it is not possible to administer the drug gradually to effect and the anaesthetic must be given as a single, calculated dose. Because of the wide variation in drug response between different strains of rat, between male and female animals and between individuals, it is best to use a drug or drug combination that provides a wide margin of safety. Intraperitoneal administration is also associated with a relatively high (5%–10%) partial failure rate (Das and North, 2007, see Chapter 1). Anaesthetic dose rates are summarized in Table 6.2.

Neuroleptanalgesic combinations Fentanyl/fluanisone (Hypnorm, Janssen) together with diazepam or midazolam (0.6 mL/kg ip 'Hypnorm', and diazepam 2.5 mg/kg ip) provides safe and effective anaesthesia in rats. When using

TABLE 6.2 Anaesthetic dose rates in the rat.

Drug	Dose rate	Effect	Duration of anaesthesia (min)	Sleep time (min)
Alphaxalone	2–5 mg/kg iv	Surgical anaesthesia	5	10
Alphaxalone/dexmedetomidine	30 mg/kg + 0.05 mg/kg ip	Surgical anaesthesia	45–60	50–70
Chloral hydrate	400 mg/kg ip	Light/surgical anaesthesia	60–120	120–180
Alpha-chloralose	55–65 mg/kg ip	Light anaesthesia	480–600	Nonrecovery only
Etorphine/methotrimeprazine (Immobilon) + midazolam	0.5 ml/kg sc[a]	Surgical anaesthesia	60–70	120–240
Fentanyl/fluanisone + diazepam	0.6 ml/kg ip + 2.5 mg/kg ip	Surgical anaesthesia	20–40	120–240
Fentanyl/fluanisone/midazolam	2.7 ml/kg ip[b]	Surgical anaesthesia	30–40	120–240
Fentanyl + medetomidine	300 μg/kg + 300 μg/kg ip	Surgical anaesthesia	60–70	240–360
Inactin (thiobutobarbital)	80 mg/kg ip	Surgical anaesthesia	60–240	120–300
Ketamine + acepromazine	75 mg/kg + 2.5 mg/kg ip	Light anaesthesia	20–30	120
Ketamine + dexmedetomidine	75 mg/kg + 0.25 mg/kg ip	Surgical anaesthesia	20–30	120–240
Ketamine + diazepam	75 mg/kg + 5 mg/kg ip	Light anaesthesia	20–30	120
Ketamine + medetomidine	75 mg/kg + 0.5 mg/kg ip	Surgical anaesthesia	20–30	120–240
Ketamine + midazolam	75 mg/kg + 5 mg/kg ip	Light anaesthesia	20–30	120

Ketamine + xylazine	75–100 mg/kg + 10 mg/kg ip	Surgical anaesthesia	20–30	120–240
Ketamine + xylazine + acepromazine	40–50 mg/kg + 2.5 mg/kg + 0.75 mg/kg im	Surgical anaesthesia	60–70 min	120–160
Medetomidine + midazolam + butorphanol	0.15 mg/kg + 2.0 mg/kg + 2.5 mg/kg sc	Surgical anaesthesia	40–60	50–70[a]
Medetomidine + Midazolam + Fentanyl	0.15 mg/kg + 2 mg/kg + 5 µg/kg sc	Surgical anaesthesia	25–30	10–15[a]
Pentobarbital	40–50 mg/kg ip	Light anaesthesia	15–60	120–240
Propofol	10 mg/kg iv	Surgical anaesthesia	5	10
Propofol/medetomidine/fentanyl	100 mg/kg + 0.1 mg/kg + 100 µg/kg	Surgical anaesthesia	30	30[a]
Thiopental	30 mg/kg iv	Surgical anaesthesia	10	15
Tiletamine/zolezepam	40 mg/kg ip	Light anaesthesia	15–25	60–120
Urethane	1000 mg/kg ip	Surgical anaesthesia	360–480	Nonrecovery only

Duration of anaesthesia and sleep time (loss of righting reflex) are provided only as a general guide, since considerable between-animal variation occurs. For recommended techniques, see text.

Dose in millilitres per kilogram of a mixture of one part 'Immobilon', one part midazolam (5 mg/mL initial concentration) and two parts water for injection.

Doses of combinations using medetomidine or dexmedetomidine are provided using the agent used in the relevant publication (see text).

[a] After reversal, see text.

[b] Dose in millilitres per kilogram of a mixture of one part 'Hypnorm' plus two parts water for injection, and one part midazolam (5 mg/mL initial concentration).

midazolam the components are mixed together with water for injection (see Appendix 3). These combinations provide good surgical anaesthesia with excellent muscle relaxation lasting about 20–40 min (Flecknell and Mitchell, 1984). Longer periods of anaesthesia can be achieved by the administration of additional doses of Hypnorm (about 0.1 mL/kg im every 30–40 min). Following the completion of surgery, the anaesthesia can be reversed using nalbuphine (0.1 mg/kg iv, 1.0 mg/kg ip or sc) or butorphanol (0.1 mg/kg iv, 2 mg/kg ip or sc). Unfortunately, 'Hypnorm' has only been available intermittently as a commercial product, and it is not possible to obtain the components and produce a substitute combination.

Ketamine combinations A second effective alternative is to administer medetomidine (0.5 mg/kg ip), dexmedetomidine (0.25 mg/kg), or xylazine (10 mg/kg ip) in combination with ketamine (75 mg/kg ip). The two compounds can be mixed in the same syringe and administered to provide good surgical anaesthesia, although the depth of anaesthesia may be insufficient for major surgery in some animals (Van Pelt, 1977; Green et al., 1981a; Hsu et al., 1986; Wixson et al., 1987; Nevalainen et al., 1988; Jang et al., 2009; Wellington et al., 2013; Callahan et al., 2014). These combinations provide about 30 min of surgical anaesthesia. The combinations can all be partially reversed using atipamezole (1 mg/kg sc or ip), but early reversal (10–20 min after induction) may be associated with undesirable behavioural disturbances due to the effects of ketamine (Morris, personal communication). Ketamine/xylazine has been reported to cause an increased incidence of postanaesthetic corneal ulceration, although the incidence can be reduced by reversal of xylazine (Turner and Albassam, 2005). Ketamine and xylazine can also be administered in combination with acepromazine, enabling the use of lower doses of the individual components (Welberg et al., 2006). Some rats may develop a reversible ocular opacity, but the incidence is much lower than in mice (see below). Ketamine administration by the intramuscular route can cause muscle damage in rats (see Chapter 1) so the combinations are best administered intraperitoneally. Even when administered by this route, there is clear evidence of local irritation, with ketamine/xylazine resulting in more irritation than ketamine/dexmedetomidine (Wellington et al., 2013). Mixtures of ketamine with acepromazine, midazolam, or diazepam can produce surgical anaesthesia in some strains of rats, but they are generally less effective than the combinations with the alpha-2 agonists (Green et al., 1981a; Molina et al., 2015).

Opioids and medetomidine Several mixtures of opioids and medetomidine can be used to produce effective surgical anaesthesia in rats. Fentanyl (300 µg/kg ip) and medetomidine (300 µg/kg ip) can be mixed and administered as a single injection to provide about 60 min of surgical anaesthesia (Hu et al., 1992). Sufentanil (40 µg/kg) and medetomidine (150 µg/kg), mixed and administered subcutaneously as a single injection, may also be used (Hedenqvist et al., 2000). Both combinations produce respiratory depression and this can be severe, so administration of oxygen is strongly recommended. However, recovery is very rapid provided anaesthesia is reversed by administration of atipamezole (1 mg/kg sc or ip) (to reverse medetomidine) and either nalbuphine (0.1 mg/kg iv, 1.0 mg/kg ip or sc), butorphanol (0.1 mg/kg iv, 2 mg/kg ip or sc), or another mixed agonist/antagonist opioid analgesic (see Tables 6.5–6.8 and Table 6.3). Experience has shown that the quality of induction and recovery with this method of anaesthesia is greatly improved by allowing the rats to acclimatize for 1–2 h after movement into the room in which the procedure is undertaken (Drage, personal communication).

TABLE 6.3 Antagonists to anaesthetic regimens for use in rodents and rabbits.

Compound	Anaesthetic regimen	Dose rate	Comments
Atipamezole	Any regimen using xylazine, medetomidine, or dexmedetomidine	0.1–1 mg/kg im, ip, sc, or iv	Highly specific alpha2 adrenoreceptor antagonist; dose required varies depending on dose of xylazine, medetomidine, or dexmedetomidine administered
Buprenorphine	Any regimen using u opioids (e.g. fentanyl)	See Table 14c	Slower onset than butorphanol and nalbuphine, but longer-acting analgesia
Doxapram	All anaesthetics	5–10 mg/kg im, iv, or ip	General respiratory stimulant
Flumazenil	Benzodiazepine (e.g. midazolam)	0.1–10 mg/kg	Dose varies depending upon dose of benzodiazepine; resedation may occur
Butorphanol	Any regimen using u opioids (e.g. fentanyl)	See Table 14c	Almost as rapid-acting as naloxone, maintains postoperative analgesia
Naloxone	Any regimen using u opioids (e.g. fentanyl)	0.01–0.1 mg/kg iv, im, or ip	Reverses analgesia as well as respiratory depression
Yohimbine	Any regimen using xylazine, medetomidine, or dexmedetomidine	0.2 mg/kg iv 0.5 mg/kg im	Relatively nonspecific antagonist; not recommended

Dexmedetomidine can be substituted for medetomidine at 50% of these dose rates. The dose of fentanyl required can be greatly reduced by adding midazolam (medetomidine, 0.15 mg/kg, midazolam, 2.0 mg/kg, and fentanyl 5 μg/kg) and this combination also provides an effective and reversible anaesthetic regimen for rats (Albrecht et al., 2014), with reversal provided by atipamezole (0.75 mg/kg), flumazenil (0.2 mg/kg), and butorphanol (2.5 mg/kg). Medetomidine (0.15 mg/kg), midazolam (2 mg/kg) and butorphanol (2.5 mg/kg), mixed and administered sc, have also been reported as providing effective anaesthesia in rats. This combination can also be reversed by administration of atipamezole (0.75 mg/kg) (Shibuta et al., 2019).

Propofol and alphaxalone If intravenous administration of drugs is feasible, then propofol (10 mg/kg iv) (Glen, 1980; Brammer et al., 1993; Cockshott et al., 1992) or alphaxalone (2–5 mg/kg iv) (Lau et al., 2013; Goodchild et al., 2015) produce surgical anaesthesia, and both compounds are especially useful for administering by continuous infusion to provide stable, long-lasting anaesthesia. Prolonged anaesthesia with alphaxalone can be produced using continuous infusions at $1.67 \text{ mg/kg min}^{-1}$ for 2.5 min, followed by $0.75 \text{ mg/kg min}^{-1}$ (White et al., 2017). The maintenance dose of propofol (0.5–1.0 mg/kg, see Table 4.3) can be markedly reduced if buprenorphine is administered as preanaesthetic medication (Penderis and Franklin, 2005). When administered by the intraperitoneal route the effects are less predictable and these drugs can only be relied upon to produce light anaesthesia (Arenillas and Gomez de Segura, 2018) but combining alphaxalone (30 mg/kg) with dexmedetomidine (0.05 mg/kg) can produce a surgical plane of anaesthesia (West et al., 2020). These studies showed a marked difference in response between male and female rats, confirmed by detailed pharmacokinetic studies (White et al., 2022). Similarly, combining propofol with fentanyl and medetomidine, all administered intraperitoneally produced surgical anaesthesia (Alves et al., 2010).

Other agents Tiletamine/zolazepam generally only produces light anaesthesia, but surgical planes of anaesthesia can be produced in some strains of rat. In these animals, the degree of cardiovascular system depression seemed less than with other anaesthetic agents (Saha et al., 2007).

Pentobarbital should be diluted to provide a 30 mg/mL solution and up to 40–50 mg/kg administered intraperitoneally. Severe respiratory depression invariably accompanies the onset of surgical anaesthesia and this agent has a narrow safety margin. Until an appropriate dose rate is established, both inadequate and excessively deep anaesthesia may result, so this drug is best avoided in rats. Intraperitoneal administration of pentobarbital may cause pain, as a result of the high pH of the solution (Svendsen et al., 2007). Formulations of pentobarbital for anaesthesia are no longer available in many geographical regions, and it is not advisable to attempt to dilute preparations intended as euthanasia solutions since these often contain other constituents, and may not be prepared in a sterile manner.

Inhalational agents

The most convenient method of inducing anaesthesia in the rat is to use an anaesthetic chamber. This should be constructed from clear materials (e.g. Perspex), so that the animal can be observed during induction. Anaesthetic vapour should be supplied from an anaesthetic machine, and the chamber should be designed so that excess anaesthetic gas can be ducted to a gas-scavenging device or removed from the room via the ventilation system. Following induction of anaesthesia, the rat should be removed from the chamber and anaesthesia maintained using a small face mask connected to the anaesthetic machine (see Chapter 1). Extensive data on potency and effects of inhalational agents in rats is readily available (e.g. Orliaguet et al., 2001; Hofstetter et al., 2007; Stratmann et al., 2009; Callaway et al., 2012; Shih et al., 2012).

Endotracheal intubation

The major disadvantage of using a standard face mask for connection of the animal to the anaesthetic gas supply is that it is difficult to assist ventilation should this prove necessary. However, since rats are obligate nose-breathers, ventilation can be assisted effectively using a purpose-designed mask (see Chapter 4, 'mechanical ventilation'). Endotracheal intubation, together with use of an appropriate anaesthetic breathing system allows easy control of ventilation. Intubation is not a difficult procedure to master, especially if specialized apparatus is purchased. Further details of the technique are given in Chapter 1.

Mechanical ventilation

Several different ventilators are available for use in rats, with a variety of mechanisms of action. All aim to achieve controlled ventilation of the lungs by means of the application of intermittent positive pressure to the patient's airway. Several manufacturers produce both volume-cycled and pressure-cycled ventilators for rodents (see Chapter 4). Few of these ventilators have facilities for humidification of anaesthetic gases, but this can be achieved quite readily by bubbling the gases through a water bottle. An economic approach is to purchase a human infant feed bottle warmer, fill it with water and pipe anaesthetic gases through a glass aerator placed in the unit.

Anaesthetic management is particularly important to prevent the development of hypothermia in rats. Ideally, the rat should be placed on a thermostatically controlled heating blanket or alternatively, heating lamps can be used. Both measures can be combined with the use of insulating material such as cotton wool, aluminium foil, or bubble packing (Chapter 3). These measures must be continued in the postoperative recovery period.

Mice

Preanaesthetic medication

Mice are easily restrained humanely and it will rarely be necessary to produce sedation before induction of anaesthesia. If sedation is required, the following drugs can be used (Table 6.4):

1. Hypnorm (Janssen; 0.1–0.3 mL/kg ip) provides sedation and sufficient analgesia for superficial procedures such as ear punching (Green, 1975). The drug is most conveniently administered as a 1:10 dilution of the commercial preparation. The effects of this mixture can be partially reversed using nalbuphine (4 mg/kg sc or ip) or butorphanol (2 mg/kg ip or sc).
2. Medetomidine (30–100 μg/kg ip) and dexmedetomidine (15–50 μg/kg ip) produce light to deep sedation. As with the rat, considerable strain variation may occur. Sedation can be completely reversed using atipamezole (1 mg/kg ip).
3. Xylazine (5–10 mg/kg ip) produces sedation but appears to have little analgesic action when used alone in mice.
4. Acepromazine (2–5 mg/kg ip) produces sedation but has no analgesic action (Chu et al., 2014).
5. Diazepam (5 mg/kg ip) or midazolam (5 mg/kg ip) produces sedation but no analgesia.

TABLE 6.4 Sedatives, tranquillizers, and other preanaesthetic medication for use in the mouse.

Drug	Dose rate	Comments
Acepromazine	2–5 mg/kg ip, sc	Light sedation
Atropine	0.04 mg/kg sc	Anticholinergic
Dexmedetomidine	15–50 μg/kg sc	Light to deep sedation, mild to moderate
Diazepam	5 mg/kg im, ip	Light sedation
Fentanyl/dropiderol (Innovar-Vet)	0.5 mL/kg im	Immobilization, analgesia
Fentanyl/fluanisone (Hypnorm)	0.1–0.3 mL/kg ip	Light sedation, moderate analgesia
Ketamine	100–200 mg/kg im	Deep sedation, mild to moderate analgesia
Medetomidine	30–100 μg/kg sc	Light to deep sedation, mild to moderate
Midazolam	5 mg/kg im, ip	Light to moderate sedation
Xylazine	5–10 mg/kg ip	Light sedation, mild to moderate analgesia

Considerable variation in effects occurs between different strains.

Atropine (0.04 mg/kg sc or ip) can be administered to reduce salivary gland bronchial secretions. Dose rates for general anaesthetics given below should be reduced by 30%–50% if one of the sedative drugs listed above has been administered.

General anaesthesia

Injectable agents

As with rats, drugs are most conveniently administered by the intraperitoneal route, but it is likely that a similarly high partial failure rate will be encountered (see Chapter 1). A number of agents such as ketamine/dexmedetomidine and ketamine/xylazine can be given subcutaneously, and the onset of action is equally rapid as the ip route (Burnside et al., 2013; Levin-Arama et al., 2016). Dose rates of anaesthetic agents are summarized in Table 6.5.

Neuroleptanalgesic combinations Fentanyl/fluanisone (Hypnorm, Janssen) together with midazolam or diazepam (0.4 mL/kg ip 'Hypnorm' and diazepam 5 mg/kg ip) produces stable and effective surgical planes of anaesthesia in most strains of mice. When using midazolam the components are mixed together with water for injection (see Appendix 3). These combinations provide surgical anaesthesia lasting about 20–40 min (Flecknell and Mitchell, 1984). Anaesthesia can be prolonged by the administration of additional doses of Hypnorm (0.5 mL/kg every 30–40 min). Following the completion of surgery, anaesthesia can be partially reversed by the administration of nalbuphine (4 mg/kg ip or sc) or butorphanol (2.0 mg/kg sc or ip).

Ketamine combinations A combination of ketamine (75 mg/kg ip or sc) and medetomidine (1.0 mg/kg ip or sc) or dexmedetomidine (0.5 mg/kg) produces moderate surgical anaesthesia in most strains of mice. In some strains, however, the degree of analgesia is insufficient for major surgery (e.g. laparotomy) (Voipio et al., 1990; Cruz et al., 1998). In some strains, this dose of medetomidine caused increased mortality and better results were obtained with a dose of 0.25 mg/kg medetomidine and 100 mg/kg ketamine (Kilic and Henke, 2004). This illustrates the importance of assessing the effects of injectable anaesthetics in the particular strain, age, and sex of mouse that is to be used.

An alternative combination is that of ketamine (80–100 mg/kg ip) and xylazine (10 mg/kg ip). It provides 20–30 min of anaesthesia, but the depth of anaesthesia may be insufficient to enable major surgery to be carried out humanely (Mulder and Mulder, 1979; Green et al., 1981a; Erhardt et al., 1984). The depth and duration of anaesthesia can be increased by the addition of acepromazine (ketamine 100 mg/kg, xylazine 10 mg/kg, acepromazine 3 mg/kg, all administered ip) (Arras et al., 2001; Buitrago et al., 2008), or additional analgesia at the surgical site provided using local anaesthetics. The addition of lidocaine administered

TABLE 6.5 Anaesthetic dose rates in the mouse.

Drug	Dose rate	Effect	Duration of anaesthesia (min)	Sleep time (min)
Alphachoralose	100–120 mg/kg ip	Light anaesthesia	300–420	Nonrecovery only
Alphaxalone	10 mg/kg iv	Surgical anaesthesia	5	10
Alphaxalone + Dexmedetomidine	30 mg/kg + 0.3 mg/kg ip	Surgical anaesthesia	30	40[a]
Chloral hydrate	400 mg/kg ip	Light anaesthesia	30	60–90
Fentanyl/fluanisone (Hypnorm) + diazepam	0.4 mL/kg ip + 5 mg/kg ip	Surgical anaesthesia	30–40	120–240
Fentanyl/fluanisone (Hypnorm)/midazolam	10.0 mL/kg ip[a]	Surgical anaesthesia	30–40	120–240
Ketamine + acepromazine	100 mg/kg + 5 mg/kg ip	Immobilization/anaesthesia	20–30	40–120
Ketamine + dexmedetomidine	75 mg/kg + 1.0 mg/kg ip	Surgical anaesthesia	20–30	60–120
Ketamine + diazepam	100 mg/kg + 5 mg/kg ip	Immobilization/anaesthesia	20–30	60–120
Ketamine + medetomidine	75 mg/kg + 1.0 mg/kg ip	Surgical anaesthesia	20–30	60–120
Ketamine + midazolam	100 mg/kg + 5 mg/kg ip	Immobilization/anaesthesia	20–30	60–120
Ketamine + xylazine	80–100 mg/kg + 10 mg/kg ip	Surgical anaesthesia	20–30	60–120
Ketamine + xylazine + acepromazine	80–100 mg/kg + 10 mg/kg ip + 3 mg/kg ip	Surgical anaesthesia	30–40	60–120

Medetomidine + midazolam + butorphanol	0.2 mg/kg + 6.0 mg/kg + 10 mg/kg	Surgical anaesthesia	40	50–60[a]
Medetomidine + midazolam + fentanyl	0.5 mg/kg + 5 mg/kg + 50 µg/kg sc	Surgical anaesthesia	25–30	30–35[a]
Pentobarbital	40–50 mg/kg ip	Immobilization/anaesthesia	20–40	120–180
Propofol	26 mg/kg iv	Surgical anaesthesia	5–10	10–15
Propofol + medetomidine + fentanyl	75 mg/kg + 1 mg/kg + 0.2 mg/kg	Surgical anaesthesia	15	30[a]
Thiopental	30–40 mg/kg iv	Surgical anaesthesia	5–10	10–15
Tiletamine/zolezepam	80 mg/kg ip	Immobilization	5–10	60–120
Tribromoethanol	240 mg/kg ip	Surgical anaesthesia	15–45	60–120

Duration of anaesthesia and sleep time (loss of righting reflex) are provided only as a general guide, since considerable between-animal variation occurs. For recommended techniques, see text.

Dose in millilitres per kilogram of a mixture of one part 'Hypnorm' plus two parts water for injection, and one part midazolam (5 mg/mL initial concentration).

Doses of combinations using medetomidine or dexmedetomidine are provided using the agent used in the relevant publication (see text).

[a] After reversal, see text.

intraperitoneally, as part of the anaesthetic mixture (ketamine 95 mg/kg, xylazine 7 mg/kg, lidocaine, 16 mg/kg) produced more rapid induction and deeper anaesthesia in outbred mice (Dholakia et al., 2017) and might be a useful alternative in strains in which the depth of anaesthesia of ketamine/xylazine alone is insufficient.

The combinations of ketamine/medetomidine or dexmedetomidine and ketamine/xylazine can be premixed in the correct proportions and administered as a single intraperitoneal injection or subcutaneous injection ((Burnside et al., 2013, Levin-Arama et al., 2016). Anaesthesia can be partially reversed by administration of atipamezole (1 mg/kg sc). Urethral obstruction following use of medetomidine and dexmedetomidine has been reported, but not with xylazine (Wells et al., 2009). Although the risk of this side-effect is low (3%), it can reach levels of 66% in some strains of mice (Cagle et al., 2017).

Opioids and medetomidine The combination of fentanyl (50 µg/kg), midazolam (5 mg/kg), and medetomidine (0.5 mg/kg), mixed and given as a single injection ip produced a surgical plane of anaesthesia, which could be reversed using flumazenil (0.5 mg/kg), atipamezole (2.5 mg/kg), and naloxone (1.2 mg/kg) (Fleischmann et al., 2016). Since this approach leads to complete reversal of analgesia, it would be preferable to reverse the fentanyl with butorphanol (2.5 mg/kg).

Medetomidine (0.2 mg/kg), midazolam (6.0 mg/kg), and butorphanol (10 mg/kg) produces a surgical plane of anaesthesia in mice and can be partially reversed with atipamezole (1 mg/kg) (Tashiro and Tohei, 2022).

The combination of metomidate (60 mg/kg) and fentanyl (0.06 mg/kg) produces stable surgical anaesthesia in mice (Green et al., 1981b). The two drugs are combined and given as a single subcutaneous injection.

Propofol and alfaxalone If the technique of intravenous injection can be mastered, then either propofol (26 mg/kg iv) (Glen, 1980) or alphaxalone/ alphadolone (10–15 mg/kg iv) (Child et al., 1971; Green et al., 1978) can be used to provide short periods (5–10 min) of anaesthesia. An advantage of these compounds is that repeated administration to prolong anaesthesia is not associated with prolongation of the recovery period (see section 'long-term anaesthesia' in Chapter 4). It is likely that alphaxalone has properties similar to those of alphaxalone/alphadolone. Intraperitoneal administration of propofol, either alone or together with opioid analgesics, has unpredictable effects and is not recommended in this species (Alves et al., 2007), however the addition of medetomidine resulted in surgical anaesthesia (Alves et al., 2009). Similar results have been obtained with combinations of alphaxalone (30 mg/kg) and dexmedetomidine (0.3 mg/kg), mixed and given ip (Ferrini et al., 2020). A combination of alphaxalone and xylazine (10 mg/kg) produced less consistent results and required higher dose rates of alphaxalone (80-120 mg/kg), with males requiring higher doses than females (Erickson et al., 2019).

Other agents Tribromoethanol ('Avertin')—this agent has been widely used, particularly for embryo transfer, at dose rates of 250 mg/kg ip. Because of the risk of anaesthetic-related complications and mortality (see Chapter 2), it is better to use alternative techniques (Norton et al., 2016).

Pentobarbital—this agent has a very narrow margin of safety in mice, especially when attempting to produce a surgical plane of anaesthesia. The variation of effect in different strains of mice is very considerable, sleep times ranging from 10 to 300 min (Lovell, 1986b) with identical doses of anaesthetic (45 mg/kg), so that over- or underdosage with this drug frequently occurs. As mentioned earlier, formulations of pentobarbital for anaesthesia are no longer available in some countries. If pentobarbital is to be used, it should be diluted to provide a 6 mg/mL solution and administered at a dosage of 40–50 mg/kg ip.

Inhalational agents

Induction of anaesthesia using an anaesthetic chamber is simple and convenient. Maintenance using a face mask is straightforward, but requires a suitably sized mask to be constructed, see Chapter 1. Extensive data on potency and effects of inhalational agents in mice is readily available and all of the currently available agents can be used safely and effectively in mice (see Chapter 2). The rapid recovery following use of inhalational agents is particularly valuable in mice, because of the increased risk of hypothermia in this species. Using inhalational agents also overcomes much of the variability seen with injectable agents in different strains of mice (Sonner et al., 2000) and in males and females (Eger et al., 2003).

Endotracheal intubation

Endotracheal intubation is technically difficult to carry out in mice and requires the use of a purpose-built laryngoscope (Costa et al., 1986) or construction or purchase of specialist apparatus (see Chapter 1).

Mechanical ventilation

Mechanical ventilation can be carried out using one of a number of purpose-designed ventilators (Schwarte et al., 2000; Schwarte and Ince, 2003) (Chapter 4). Normal respiratory parameters of mice are available (Glaab et al., 2001, 2007).

Anaesthetic management

Mice are even more prone than rats to develop hypothermia, and it is essential to take measures to maintain body temperature (see Chapter 3). Following use of injectable anaesthetic combinations, even with reversal, thermal support may be required for several hours (Tashiro et al., 2020).

Hamsters

Preanaesthetic medication

Hamsters are easily restrained humanely and preanaesthetic sedation is rarely necessary. If restraint is a problem, an anaesthetic chamber should be used for induction of anaesthesia. If sedation is required, the following drugs can be used (see also Table 6.6):

1. Hypnorm (0.2–0.5 mL/kg ip) provides sufficient analgesia for superficial procedures.
2. Medetomidine (30–100 μg/kg sc) or Dexmedetomidine (15–50 μg/kg sc) produces moderate sedation in hamsters, but animals do not lose their righting reflex even at high dose rates.
3. Diazepam (5 mg/kg ip) or midazolam (5 mg/kg ip) produces sedation but no analgesia.

Atropine (0.04 mg/kg sc, im, or ip) can be administered to reduce salivary and bronchial secretions. Dose rates for general anaesthesia given below should

TABLE 6.6 Sedatives, tranquillizers, and other preanaesthetic medication for use in the hamster.

Drug	Dose rate	Comments
Acepromazine	2.5 mg/kg ip	Light sedation
Atropine	0.04 mg/kg sc	Anticholinergic
Dexmedetomidine	15–50 μg/kg sc, ip	Light to heavy sedation, mild to moderate analgesia
Diazepam	5 mg/kg im, ip	Light to moderate sedation
Fentanyl/dropiderol (Innovar-Vet)	0.9 mL/kg im	Analgesia; unpredictable degree of sedation
Fentanyl/fluanisone (Hypnorm)	0.2–0.5 mL/kg im 0.3–0.6 mL/kg ip	Light/moderate sedation, moderate analgesia
Glycopyrrolate	0.5 mg/kg im	Anticholinergic
Ketamine	50–100 mg/kg ip	Deep sedation, immobilization, mild to moderate analgesia
Medetomidine	30–100 μg/kg sc, ip	Light to heavy sedation, mild to moderate analgesia
Midazolam	5 mg/kg ip	Light sedation
Xylazine	1–5 mg/kg im, ip	Light to heavy sedation, mild to moderate analgesia

Considerable variation in effects occurs between different strains.

be reduced by 30%–50% if one of the sedative drugs listed above has been administered.

General anaesthesia

Injectable agents

Neuroleptanalgesic combinations As with other small rodents, drugs are most conveniently administered by intraperitoneal injection (see also Table 6.7). Most published information relates to anaesthesia of Syrian hamsters (*Mesocricetus auratus*). This species can be anaesthetized safely and effectively with fentanyl/fluanisone with midazolam or diazepam (1.0 mL/kg ip 'Hypnorm' and diazepam 5 mg/kg ip). When using midazolam the components are mixed together with water for injection (see Appendix 3). These combinations provide good surgical anaesthesia lasting about 20–40 min (Flecknell and Mitchell, 1984) and can be partially reversed with nalbuphine (2 mg/kg sc) or butorphanol (2.0 mg/kg sc).

Ketamine combinations An alternative, equally satisfactory combination in the Syrian hamster is ketamine (100–200 mg/kg ip) and xylazine (10 mg/kg ip), which in this species appears to reliably produce surgical anaesthesia (Curl and Peters, 1983). Ketamine (100 mg/kg) mixed with medetomidine (0.25 mg/kg) or dexmedetomidine (0.125 mg/kg) also appears to produce effective surgical anaesthesia (Erhardt et al., 2001; Kilic et al., 2004). Anaesthesia with all of these combinations can be partially reversed using atipamezole (1 mg/kg). As in other species, the combination can produce marked respiratory depression (Kilic et al., 2004).

Opioids and medetomidine A mixture of medetomidine (0.15 mg/kg), midazolam (2.0 mg/kg), and butorphanol (2.5 mg/kg) administered im provides a surgical plane of anaesthesia in hamsters (Nakamura et al., 2017). Administration of atipamezole (0.15 mg/kg) resulted in more rapid recovery from anaesthesia. Administration by the intraperitoneal route also appears to be effective (Sumikawa et al., 2017).

The use of pentobarbital (50–90 mg/kg ip) in hamsters is particularly hazardous and a high mortality often occurs. If pentobarbital is to be used in any small rodent, it is best to administer a dose sufficient to produce light anaesthesia (50 mg/kg ip) and then administer a volatile anaesthetic to produce full surgical anaesthesia.

Inhalational agents

Induction of anaesthesia using an anaesthetic chamber is simple and convenient, and halothane, isoflurane, and methoxyflurane provide effective and safe anaesthesia. A suitably sized mask may need to be constructed for anaesthetic maintenance, or a commercially available system purchased (e.g. IMS). Potency of inhalational anaesthetics are similar to other rodents (Vivien et al., 1999).

TABLE 6.7 Anaesthetic dose rates in the hamster.

Drug	Dose rate	Effect	Duration of anaesthesia (min)	Sleep time (min)
Alpha-chloralose	80–100 mg/kg ip	Immobilization	20–40	180–240
Fentanyl/fluanisone (Hypnorm) + diazepam	1 mL/kg im or ip + 5 mg/kg ip	Surgical anaesthesia	20–40	60–90
Fentanyl/fluanisone (Hypnorm)/midazolam	4.0 mL/kg ip[a]	Surgical anaesthesia	45–120	60–90
Ketamine/acepromazine	150 mg/kg + 5 mg/kg ip	Immobilization/anaesthesia	30–60	75–180
Ketamine/dexmedetomidine	100 mg/kg + 0.125 mg/kg ip	Surgical anaesthesia	30–45	60–120
Ketamine/diazepam	70 mg/kg + 2 mg/kg ip	Immobilization/anaesthesia	30–60	90–120
Ketamine/medetomidine	100 mg/kg + 0.25 mg/kg ip	Surgical anaesthesia	30–60	60–120
Ketamine/xylazine	200 mg/kg + 10 mg/kg ip	Surgical anaesthesia	75–120	90–150
Medetomidine + midazolam + butorphanol	0.15 mg/kg + 2.0 mg/kg + 2.5 mg/kg	Surgical anaesthesia	30–60	95–140[a]
Pentobarbital	50–90 mg/kg ip	Immobilization/anaesthesia	20–30	120–180
Tiletamine/zolezepam	50–80 mg/kg ip	Immobilization/anaesthesia	30	30–60
Tiletamine/zolezepam + xylazine	30 mg/kg + 10 mg/kg ip	Surgical anaesthesia	360–480	40–60
Urethane	1000–2000 mg/kg ip	Surgical anaesthesia		Nonrecovery only

Duration of anaesthesia and sleep time (loss of righting reflex) are provided only as a general guide, since considerable between-animal variation occurs. For recommended techniques, see text.
[a] Dose in millilitres per kilogram of a mixture of one part 'Hypnorm' plus two parts water for injection, and one part midazolam (5 mg/mL initial concentration).

Endotracheal intubation

Endotracheal intubation is difficult to carry out in hamsters and requires the use of a purpose-built laryngoscope (Costa et al., 1986) or specialist apparatus (see Chapter 1).

Mechanical ventilation

Mechanical ventilation can be carried out using a purpose-designed rodent ventilator (Chapter 4).

Anaesthetic management

As with other small rodents, prevention of hypothermia is of critical importance (see Chapter 3).

Gerbils

Preanaesthetic medication

Initial restraint of gerbils for intraperitoneal administration of anaesthetics is reasonably simple, but young or particularly active individuals may be better anaesthetized using an anaesthetic chamber.

Information on the effects of sedative agents is limited in gerbils, but the following agents appear reasonably effective in this species (see also Table 6.8).

1. Hypnorm (0.5–1.0 mL/kg ip) provides sufficient analgesia for superficial procedures. Partial reversal is possible using nalbuphine (4 mg/kg ip or sc) or butorphanol (2 mg/kg ip or sc).
2. Diazepam (5 mg/kg ip) or midazolam (5 mg/kg ip) produces sedation but no analgesia.

Atropine (0.04 mg/kg sc, im, or ip) can be administered to reduce salivary and bronchial secretions.

Dose rates for general anaesthesia given below should be reduced by 30%–50% if one of the sedative drugs listed above has been administered.

General anaesthesia

Injectable agents

Drugs are most conveniently administered by intraperitoneal injection in gerbils (see also Table 6.9), however injectable agents appear to have less predictable effects in gerbils (Flecknell et al., 1983) so balanced anaesthesia with lower dose injectable agents supplemented with inhalant agents may be particularly useful in these species.

Neuroleptanalgesic combinations Fentanyl/fluanisone with midazolam or diazepam (0.3 mL/kg ip 'Hypnorm' and diazepam 5 mg/kg ip) is less satisfactory

TABLE 6.8 Sedatives, tranquillizers, and other preanaesthetic medication for use in the gerbil.

Drug	Dose rate	Comments
Acepromazine	3 mg/kg im	Light sedation
Atropine	0.04 mg/kg sc	Anticholinergic
Dexmedetomidine	50–100 μg/kg ip	Light to heavy sedation, mild to moderate analgesia
Diazepam	5 mg/kg im, ip	Light sedation
Fentanyl/fluanisone (Hypnorm)	0.5–1.0 mL/kg im, ip	Moderate sedation, moderate analgesia
Ketamine	100–200 mg/kg im	Heavy sedation, mild to moderate analgesia
Medetomidine	100–200 μg/kg ip	Light to heavy sedation, mild to moderate analgesia
Midazolam	5 mg/kg im, ip	Light/moderate sedation
Xylazine	2 mg/kg im	Light sedation, mild to moderate analgesia

Considerable variation in effect occurs between different strains.

in gerbils than in other rodents, and only light anaesthesia may be produced. When using midazolam the components are mixed together with water for injection (see Appendix 3).

Ketamine combinations Ketamine (75 mg/kg) and medetomidine (0.5 mg/kg) (Perez-Garcia et al., 2003), or dexmedetomidine (0.25 mg/kg), mixed together and administered by intraperitoneal injection, produce medium planes of anaesthesia in gerbils. The medetomidine or dexmedetomidine may be reversed using atipamezole (1 mg/kg sc or ip).

Opioids and medetomidine The combination of fentanyl (0.05 mg/kg sc) and metomidate (50 mg/kg sc) appears most reliable in producing general anaesthesia in gerbils (Flecknell et al., 1983). Use of fentanyl (30 μg/kg), medetomidine (0.15 mg/kg), and midazolam (7.5 mg/kg) has been reported but it is unclear if this combination produced a surgical plane of anaesthesia (Kessler et al., 2018).

Other agents As in hamsters, the use of pentobarbital in gerbils is particularly hazardous and a high mortality often occurs if this drug is used to produce

TABLE 6.9 Anaesthetic dose rates in the gerbil.

Drug	Dose rate	Effect	Duration of anaesthesia (min)	Sleep time (min)
Alphaxalone/alphadolone	80–120 mg/kg ip	Immobilization	–	60–90
Fentanyl/fluanisone (Hypnorm) + diazepam	0.3 mL/kg im or ip + 5 mg/kg ip	Surgical anaesthesia	20	60–90
Fentanyl/fluanisone (Hypnorm)/midazolam	8.0 mL/kg ip[a]	Surgical anaesthesia	20	60–90
Ketamine/acepromazine	75 mg/kg + 3 mg/kg ip	Immobilization	–	60–90
Ketamine/dexmedetomidine	75 mg/kg + 0.25 mg/kg ip	Medium anaesthesia	20–30	90–120
Ketamine/diazepam	50 mg/kg + 5 mg/kg ip	Immobilization	–	30–60
Ketamine/medetomidine	75 mg/kg + 0.5 mg/kg ip	Medium anaesthesia	20–30	90–120
Ketamine/xylazine	50 mg/kg + 2 mg/kg ip	Immobilization	–	20–60
Pentobarbital	60–80 mg/kg ip	Immobilization/anaesthesia	20	60–90
Tribromoethanol	250–300 mg/kg ip	Surgical anaesthesia	15–30	30–90

Duration of anaesthesia and sleep time (loss of righting reflex) are provided only as a general guide, since considerable between-animal variation occurs. For recommended techniques, see text.

[a] Dose in millilitres per kilogram of a mixture of one part 'Hypnorm' plus two parts water for injection, and one part midazolam (5 mg/mL initial concentration).

surgical anaesthesia (80 mg/kg ip). Lower dose rates (60 mg/kg ip) produce light anaesthesia that can be deepened using low concentrations of volatile anaesthetics (e.g. 0.5% isoflurane).

Inhalational agents

Sevoflurane (Henke et al., 2004), halothane, isoflurane, and methoxyflurane can be used to provide effective and safe anaesthesia. Induction using an anaesthetic chamber is simple and convenient, followed by maintenance if required using a face mask, as with other small rodents. MAC determinations indicate that the potency of inhalational agents is slightly higher in gerbils in comparison to other rodents (de Segura et al., 2009).

Endotracheal intubation

Endotracheal intubation requires the use of a purpose-built laryngoscope (Costa et al., 1986) or specialist apparatus (see Chapter 1).

Mechanical ventilation

Mechanical ventilation can be carried out using a purpose-made ventilator (Chapter 4).

Anaesthetic management

Like other small rodents, gerbils are especially prone to develop hypothermia, and heating pads or lamps should be used to prevent this (see Chapter 3).

Guinea pigs

Guinea pigs are among the most difficult rodents to achieve safe and effective anaesthesia. Their response to many injectable anaesthetics is highly variable, and postanaesthetic complications such as respiratory infections, digestive disturbances, and generalized depression and inappetance are frequently seen. Many of these problems can be avoided by careful selection of anaesthetic agents and a high standard of intra- and postoperative nursing care. Use of balanced anaesthetic regimens as described in Chapter 2, is often safer and provides more stable planes of anaesthesia.

Preanaesthetic medication

Guinea pigs are nonaggressive animals that are generally easy to handle and restrain. When frightened they run around their cage at high speed, making safe handling difficult. It is important to approach guinea pigs quietly and handle them gently but firmly. They should be picked up around the shoulders and thorax and the hindquarters supported as they are lifted clear of their cage. Intramuscular or intraperitoneal injection of anaesthetic agents can then be carried out. Preanaesthetic medication is therefore not usually required but, if an anaesthetic is to be administered by intravenous injection into an ear vein, cephalic vein, or medial saphenous vein, initial sedation is advantageous.

The following drugs can be used to produce sedation and restraint (see also Table 6.10):

1. Fentanyl/fluanisone (Hypnorm, Janssen) (1.0 mL/kg im or ip) will produce restraint, sedation, and sufficient analgesia for minor procedures such as skin biopsy.
2. Alfaxalone (5–20 mg/kg sc) produces sedation and, at higher doses, immobility (Sixtus et al., 2021; Doerning et al., 2018).
3. Ketamine (100 mg/kg im) immobilizes guinea pigs but does not produce good analgesia.
4. Medetomidine, dexmedetomidine, and xylazine administered alone have very little sedative effect in guinea pigs, but do potentiate the effects of other anaesthetic agents (see below).
5. Diazepam (5 mg/kg ip) or midazolam (5 mg/kg ip or im) produces heavy sedation and immobility, but no analgesia. The animal is easily roused by painful stimuli or other disturbances such as noise. This agent can be useful in providing sufficient sedation to allow local anaesthetic techniques to be used humanely.

TABLE 6.10 Sedatives, tranquillizers, and other preanaesthetic medication for use in the guinea pig.

Drug	Dose rate	Comments
Acepromazine	0.5–1.0 mg/kg im	Light to moderate sedation
Alphaxalone/alphadolone	40 mg/kg im, ip	Heavy sedation, mild analgesia
Atropine	0.05 mg/kg sc	Anticholinergic
Dexmedetomidine	0.25 mg/kg sc	Sedation
Diazepam	2.5 mg/kg ip, im	Heavy sedation
Fentanyl/dropiderol (Innovar-Vet)	0.44–0.8 mL/kg im	Sedation, analgesia
Fentanyl/fluanisone (Hypnorm)	1.0 mL/kg im, ip	Moderate sedation, moderate analgesia
Ketamine	100 mg/kg im, ip	Heavy sedation, light analgesia
Medetomidine	0.5 mg/kg sc	Sedation
Midazolam	5 mg/kg im, ip	Heavy sedation

Considerable variation in effects occurs between different strains.

Atropine (0.05 mg/kg sc) should be administered to minimize the volume of bronchial and salivary secretions. It is particularly useful in guinea pigs because of their relatively narrow airways, which are prone to obstruction.

The dose rates of drugs listed below apply to guinea pigs that have received no preanaesthetic medication unless otherwise stated. The dosages of general anaesthetics should be reduced by 30%–50% if one of the drugs listed above has been administered.

General anaesthesia

Injectable agents

Intravenous administration of anaesthetics is difficult to achieve in guinea pigs, and drugs are usually administered by the intraperitoneal, subcutaneous, or intramuscular route. The animals should be carefully weighed and dose rates calculated accurately. Anaesthetic dose rates are summarized in Table 6.11.

Neuroleptanalgesic combinations Fentanyl/fluanisone (Hypnorm, Janssen) together with midazolam or diazepam (1.0 mL/kg ip 'Hypnorm', and diazepam 2.5 mg/kg ip) provides stable surgical anaesthesia lasting about 45 min (Flecknell and Mitchell, 1984). When using midazolam the components are mixed together with water for injection (see Appendix 3). If a longer period of anaesthesia is required, further doses of Hypnorm can be given (approximately 0.5 mL/kg im every 20–30 min). Following the completion of surgery the anaesthesia can be partially reversed using nalbuphine (1 mg/kg ip or sc), butorphanol (1 mg/kg ip or sc), or buprenorphine (0.01 mg/kg iv or 0.05 mg/kg ip).

Ketamine combinations An effective alternative is to administer ketamine (40 mg/kg im) and xylazine (5 mg/kg sc). This combination provides about 30 min of surgical anaesthesia, although the degree of analgesia may be insufficient to carry out major surgery in some animals (D'Alleinne and Mann, 1982; Hart et al., 1984; (Barzago et al., 1994). Recovery from anaesthesia, even after reversal of the xylazine with atipamezole, is prolonged (approx. 1 h) (Ketamine (40 mg/kg ip) and medetomidine (0.5 mg/kg ip) (Nevalainen et al., 1988) or dexmedetomidine (0.25 mg/kg ip) in combination produces light surgical anaesthesia. Anaesthesia can be partially reversed using atipamezole (1 mg/kg ip).

Opioids and medetomidine The mixture of medetomidine (0.2 mg/kg), midazolam (1.0 mg/kg), and fentanyl (0.025 mg/kg) administered im produced 40 min of surgical anaesthesia. As in other species, the effects of this combination could be reversed with atipamezole (1.0 mg/kg), flumazenil (0.1 mg/kg), and naloxone (0.03 mg/kg) (Schmitz et al., 2017). If postanaesthetic pain is likely, then naloxone should be avoided and butorphanol (2.0 mg/kg) used to reverse the effects of fentanyl.

TABLE 6.11 Injectable anaesthetic dose rates in the guinea pig.

Drug	Dose rate	Effect	Duration of anaesthesia (min)	Sleep time (min)
Alphaxalone/alphadolone	40 mg/kg ip	Immobilization	–	90–120
Alphachloralose	70 mg/kg ip	Light to medium anaesthesia	180–600	Nonrecovery only
Fentanyl/climazolam/xylazine	0.05 mg/kg + 2.0 mg/kg + 2.0 mg/kg im	Surgical anaesthesia		
Fentanyl/fluanisone (Hypnorm) + diazepam	1.0 mL/kg im or ip + 2.5 mg/kg ip	Surgical anaesthesia	45–60	120–180
Fentanyl/fluanisone (Hypnorm)/midazolam	8.0 mL kg ip[a]	Surgical anaesthesia	45–60	120–180
Ketamine/acepromazine	100 mg/kg + 5 mg/kg im	Immobilization/anaesthesia	45–120	90–180
Ketamine/dexmedetomidine	40 mg/kg + 0.25 mg/kg ip	Moderate anaesthesia	30–40	90–120
Ketamine/diazepam	100 mg/kg + 5 mg/kg im	Immobilization/anaesthesia	30–45	90–120
Ketamine/medetomidine	40 mg/kg + 0.5 mg/kg ip	Moderate anaesthesia	30–40	90–120
Ketamine/xylazine	40 mg/kg + 5 mg/kg ip	Surgical anaesthesia	30	90–120
Medetomidine + midazolam + butorphanol	0.2 mg/kg + 1.0 mg/kg + 2 mg/kg im	Surgical anaesthesia	40	50–60[a]
Medetomidine + midazolam + fentanyl	0.2 mg/kg + 1 mg/kg + 25 μg/kg sc	Surgical anaesthesia	40	45–50[a]
Pentobarbital	37 mg/kg ip	Surgical anaesthesia	60–90	240–300
Tiletamine/zolezepam	40–60 mg/kg im	Immobilization	–	70–160
Urethane	1500 mg/kg iv, ip	Surgical anaesthesia	300–480	Nonrecovery only

Duration of anaesthesia and sleep time (loss of righting reflex) are provided only as a general guide, since considerable between-animal variation occurs. For recommended techniques, see text.
[a] Dose in millilitres per kilogram of a mixture of one part 'Hypnorm' plus two parts water for injection, and one part midazolam (5 mg/mL initial concentration).

Medetomidine (0.2 mg/kg), midazolam (1.0 mg/kg), and butorphanol (2.0 mg/kg) (all im) produced sufficient anaesthesia for surgery (Nogawa et al., 2022).

Propofol and alphaxalone Alphaxalone produces only light surgical anaesthesia even when administered by the intravenous route. If additional anaesthetic is administered, severe respiratory depression frequently ensues. Alfaxalone (20 mg/kg), in combination with dexmedetomidine (0.25 mg/kg) and buprenorphine (0.05 mg/kg), administered as a single sc injection, immobilized guinea pigs but did not produce a plane of anaesthesia (Doerning et al., 2018).

Other agents If pentobarbital is to be used this is best administered at a dose of 25 mg/kg ip to sedate and immobilize the animal; anaesthesia should then be deepened using a volatile agent such as isoflurane. Use of higher dose rates of pentobarbital (37 mg/kg ip), which are needed to produce surgical anaesthesia, are frequently associated with an unacceptably high mortality.

Inhalational agents

Anaesthesia can be induced either by use of an anaesthetic chamber or by administration via a small face mask. Following induction, it is usually most convenient to maintain anaesthesia using a face mask, since endotracheal intubation is an extremely difficult technique to carry out in guinea pigs. If it is necessary to intubate the animal, use can be made of a purpose-made laryngoscope (Costa et al., 1986; Blouin and Cormier, 1987) or using specialist apparatus. Alternatively, the larynx can be visualized by transilluminating the neck and placing an otoscope speculum in the oral cavity (see Chapter 1). A soft-tipped wire introducer is then used to insert a catheter into the larynx.

Isoflurane and sevoflurane can also be used successfully, but hypotension may be produced. Both agents appear more irritant to guinea pigs than to other rodents; animals may rub their face and eyes, and lacrimate during induction of anaesthesia. It may therefore be preferable to administer a preanaesthetic agent to reduce any distress caused by the procedure.

Halothane can be used successfully and is nonirritant, but can produce profound hypotension even at normal maintenance concentrations. Prolonged halothane anaesthesia (4 h) has been reported to cause liver toxicity (Lunam et al., 1985).

Ether is unsuitable for use in guinea pigs since it is highly irritant to the respiratory tract, producing increased bronchial secretions that tend to occlude the narrow airways. In addition, bronchospasm may be produced during induction of anaesthesia with ether.

Local anaesthetics

Intrathecal (spinal) anaesthesia using local anaesthetics has been described in guinea pigs (Thomasson et al., 1974), and this technique coupled with the use of sedatives or low doses of other anaesthetic agents for restraint may be a useful technique in some circumstances. As in other species, infiltration of the surgical site with local anaesthetics can allow safer, balanced anaesthesia to be undertaken.

Anaesthetic management

Care must be taken to prevent the development of hypothermia, using the methods described in Chapter 3. It is advisable to suction the oropharynx after induction of anaesthesia as small quantities of food are often present. Preanaesthetic fasting is not recommended because of the greater risks of gastrointestinal disturbance in this species.

Mean arterial blood pressure has been reported as being lower in guinea pigs compared with other species (Brown et al., 1989; Kapoor and Matthews, 2005). Although high standards of postoperative care are required for all species, this is particularly important in guinea pigs.

Postoperative recovery is aided by administering 10–15 mL of warmed dextrose–saline (0.18% saline, 4% dextrose) subcutaneously to correct any fluid deficit. A warm (25–30°C) recovery area should be provided and the animal must be given additional subcutaneous fluid for the next few days if its appetite is depressed. It may also be advisable to administer metoclopramide (0.2–1.0 mg/kg po, sc, im, and iv q 6–12 h) and/or cisapride (0.5–1 mg/kg po q 8–24 h) to stimulate gut motility, particularly after abdominal surgery. Palatable foods should be provided to encourage an early return of appetite. For example, the animal can be provided with hay (autoclaved if needed for disease control reasons) that can provide both insulation and security, and a source of food.

Rabbits

Rabbits are easily stressed by inexpert preoperative handling and by induction of anaesthesia with volatile anaesthetics. The combined effects of stress and anaesthesia can result in cardiac and respiratory arrest. In addition, some laboratory colonies may have endemic infection with *Pasteurella multocida*, and the consequent subclinical respiratory disease may result in respiratory failure during the period of anaesthesia. Recovery from anaesthesia is often slow, particularly following the use of barbiturates, and the prolonged inappetance that is a frequent postoperative complication can result in gastrointestinal disturbances.

The incidence of these potentially serious problems can be minimized by obtaining rabbits only from sources that are free from infectious diseases, by carefully selecting the anaesthetic regimen, by avoiding stress both preoperatively and postoperatively and by maintaining high standards of intra- and postoperative care. It is unnecessary to withhold food and water prior to induction of anaesthesia since vomiting during induction or recovery does not occur in this species. The large caecum in this species and the occurrence of coprophagy also make preoperative fasting relatively ineffective in reducing the mass of abdominal viscera prior to abdominal surgery. Since normal gut motility is dependent on a continued supply of ingesta, fasting may exacerbate postsurgical ileus. Rabbits, like guinea pigs, are prone to develop enterotoxaemia following gut stasis (see below), so whenever possible, preoperative withholding of food should be avoided.

Preanaesthetic medication

As mentioned earlier, rabbits are easily stressed, so, whenever possible, a tranquillizer or sedative should be administered while the animal is still in its familiar surroundings. The rabbit can then be transported to the operating theatre when sedated, hence minimizing the stress caused by such manipulations. A wide variety of tranquillizers can be used successfully in rabbits, and these are listed in order of preference below (see also Table 6.12).

1. Hypnorm (fentanyl/fluanisone; Janssen) (0.2–0.5 mL/kg im). At the lower dose rate, sedation and some analgesia is produced (Green, 1975). The higher dose rate produces sufficient analgesia to enable procedures such as draining and cleaning of subcutaneous abscesses to be carried out. Occasionally marked respiratory depression is seen when the drug is administered at the higher dose rate. If this produces marked cyanosis, oxygen should be administered and the fentanyl component of the mixture reversed by the administration of nalbuphine (1 mg/kg sc or ip), butorphanol (1 mg/kg sc or ip), or buprenorphine (0.05 mg/kg sc or ip) (Flecknell et al., 1989b).

2. Medetomidine (0.25 mg/kg im) and Dexmedetomidine (0.125 mg/kg) also produce safe and effective sedation. At higher doses (0.5 mg/kg im, 0.25 mg/kg, respectively) animals lose their righting reflex. Only minimal analgesia is produced when medetomidine or dexmedetomidine are administered alone. Sedation is completely reversed by administration of atipamezole (0.2 mg/kg iv, 1.0 mg/kg im).

3. Xylazine (2–5 mg/kg im) produces light to heavy sedation but appears to have little analgesic action when used alone in rabbits. Sedation can be reversed using atipamezole (1.0 mg/kg im) (Lipman et al., 1987).

4. Acepromazine (1 mg/kg im) produces moderate sedation but has no analgesic action (Flecknell and Liles, 1996). Combining acepromazine (0.5 mg/kg) and butorphanol (0.5 mg/kg) produces good sedation combined with moderate analgesia.

5. Diazepam or midazolam (0.5–2 mg/kg iv, im, or ip) produces good sedation, but neither drug has any analgesic action. Sedation can be reversed using flumazenil (0.01–0.1 mg/kg iv), but the animal may become sedated again a few hours later.

6. Ketamine (25–50 mg/kg im) produces deep sedation. As with other species the degree of muscle relaxation is poor and the level of analgesia is insufficient for even superficial surgery.

7. Glycopyrrolate (0.01 mg/kg iv, 0.1 mg/kg sc or im) (Olson et al., 1994) may be administered to reduce salivary and bronchial secretions and protect the

TABLE 6.12 Sedatives, tranquillizers, and other preanaesthetic medication for use in the rabbit.

Drug	Dose rate	Comments
Acepromazine	1 mg/kg im	Moderate sedation
Acepromazine + butorphanol	0.5 mg/kg + 0.5 mg/kg im	Moderate to heavy sedation, moderate analgesia
Alphaxalone/alphadolone	9–12 mg/kg im	Moderate to heavy sedation, little analgesia
Atropine	0.05 mg/kg im	Very short acting in some rabbits
Dexmedetomidine	0.05–0.25 mg/kg im, sc	Light to heavy sedation, mild to moderate analgesia
Diazepam	0.5–2.0 mg/kg iv, im, ip	Light to moderate sedation
Fentanyl/dropiderol (Innovar-Vet)	0.22 mL/kg im	Immobilization, analgesia
Fentanyl/fluanisone (Hypnorm)	0.2–0.5 mL/kg im	Light to heavy sedation, light to deep analgesia
Glycopyrrolate	0.01 mg/kg iv, 0.1 mg/kg im sc	Anticholinergic
Ketamine	25–50 mg/kg im	Moderate to heavy sedation, mild to moderate analgesia
Medetomidine	0.1–0.5 mg/kg im, sc	Light to heavy sedation, mild to moderate analgesia
Midazolam	0.5–2 mg/kg iv, im, ip	Light to moderate sedation
Xylazine	2–5 mg/kg im	Light to moderate sedation, mild to moderate analgesia

Considerable variation in effects occurs between different strains.

heart from vagal inhibition. Atropine is relatively ineffective in many strains of rabbits because of high levels of atropinase in the liver, and repeated doses are usually required if this drug is used.

In addition to reducing the stress caused by induction of anaesthesia and easing handling and restraint, the use of appropriate preanaesthetic medication reduces the amount of other anaesthetic agents required to produce general anaesthesia. The dose rates quoted in Tables 6.12 and 6.13 apply to rabbits that have received no preanaesthetic medication unless otherwise stated. The dose rates for intravenous induction agents can be reduced by 30%–50% if one of the drugs listed above has been administered.

General anaesthesia

Injectable agents

Intravenous injection can be carried out relatively easily using the marginal ear vein, but use can also be made of the cephalic, saphenous, or mammary vessels. In small rabbits, the jugular vein may be more accessible. Injection is made even easier if the ear is treated with EMLA cream to produce local anaesthesia 45 min prior to injection (see Chapter 1). Anaesthetic dose rates are summarized in Table 6.13.

A number of anaesthetic options can be recommended for routine use in rabbits. Fentanyl/fluanisone (Hypnorm) (0.3 mL/kg im) and midazolam or diazepam (2 mg/kg im, iv, or ip) (Flecknell et al., 1983; Flecknell and Mitchell, 1984) provides good surgical anaesthesia with excellent muscle relaxation for about 20–40 min. It is recommended that fentanyl/fluanisone be administered first and 10–15 min allowed so that the animal becomes sedated. The rabbit can then be transferred to the operating theatre or procedure room without causing any distress. Since marked analgesia is produced, the animal will be unresponsive to the pain of intravenous injection, and the vasodilatation caused by 'Hypnorm' also aids placement of an intravenous needle or over-the-needle catheter. Midazolam or diazepam can then be administered to effect to produce loss of consciousness and relaxation. This usually requires a lower dose of the benzodiazepine (typically 0.5 mg/kg) and so recovery tends to be more rapid.

Longer periods of anaesthesia can be achieved by the administration of additional doses of Hypnorm (approximately 0.1 mL/kg im every 30–40 min). This is best achieved by diluting the commercial preparation 1:10 with water for injection. Use of saline results in precipitation of one of the components of 'Hypnorm'. If anaesthesia of several hours duration is required, it is preferable to administer fentanyl (30–100 μg/kg/h) alone, to avoid undue accumulation of the fluanisone component of 'Hypnorm'.

Following the completion of surgery the anaesthesia can be reversed using nalbuphine (0.1 mg/kg iv) or buprenorphine (0.01 mg/kg iv).

TABLE 6.13 Anaesthetic dose rates in the rabbit.

Drug	Dose rate	Effect	Duration of anaesthesia (min)	Sleep time (min)
Alphaxalone	4 mg/kg iv	Light anaesthesia	5–10	10–20
Alpha-chloralose	80–100 mg/kg iv	Light to surgical anaesthesia	360–600	Nonrecovery only
Etorphine/methotrimeprazine (Immobilon SA)	0.025–0.05 mL/kg im	Immobilization, analgesia	60 (analgesia)	120–240
Etorphine/methotrimeprazine (Immobilon SA) + midazolam	0.05 mL/kg im + 1 mg/kg iv	Surgical anaesthesia (severe respiratory depression, see text)	50–100	180–240
Fentanyl/fluanisone (Hypnorm) + diazepam	0.3 mL/kg im + 1–2 mg/kg iv, im, or ip	Surgical anaesthesia	20–40	60–120
Fentanyl/fluanisone (Hypnorm) + midazolam	0.3 mL/kg im + 1–2 mg/kg iv or ip	Surgical anaesthesia	20–40	60–120
Fentanyl + medetomidine	8 µg/kg iv + 330 µg/kg iv	Surgical anaesthesia	30–40	60–120
Fentanyl + medetomidine + midazolam	20 µg/kg iv + 0.2 mg/kg + 1.0 mg/kg i/m	Surgical anaesthesia	30–40	60–120
Ketamine/acepromazine	50 mg/kg imft + 1 mg/kg im	Surgical anaesthesia	20–30	60–90
Ketamine/dexmedetomidine	15 mg/kg im + 0.125 mg/kg sc, im	Surgical anaesthesia	20–30	60–90
Ketamine/diazepam	25 mg/kg im + 5 mg/kg im	Surgical anaesthesia	20–30	60–90
Ketamine/medetomidine	15 mg/kgsc + 0.25 mg/kg sc	Surgical anaesthesia	20–30	60–90
Ketamine/xylazine	35 mg/kg im + 5 mg/kg im	Surgical anaesthesia	25–40	60–120
	10 mg/kg iv + 3 mg/kg iv	Surgical anaesthesia	20–30	60–90

Continued

TABLE 6.13 Anaesthetic dose rates in the rabbit—cont'd

Drug	Dose rate	Effect	Duration of anaesthesia (min)	Sleep time (min)
Ketamine/xylazine/acepromazine	35 mg/kg im + 5 mg/kg im + 1.0 mg/kg im, sc	Surgical anaesthesia	45–75	100–150
Ketamine/xylazine/butorphanol	35 mg/kg im + 5 mg/kg im + 0.1 mg/kg im	Surgical anaesthesia	60–90	120–180
Pentobarbital	30–45 mg/kg iv	Light to medium anaesthesia	20–30	60–120
Propofol	10 mg/kg iv	Light anaesthesia	5–10	10–15
Thiopental	30 mg/kg iv	Surgical anaesthesia	5–10	10–15
Urethane	1000–2000 mg/kg iv	Surgical anaesthesia	360–480	Nonrecovery only

Duration of anaesthesia and sleep time (loss of righting reflex) are provided only as a general guide, since considerable between-animal variation occurs. For recommended techniques, see text.

A useful alternative is to administer ketamine (15 mg/kg sc) and medetomidine (0.5 mg/kg sc) or dexmedetomidine (0.25 mg/kg) (Orr et al., 2005), or ketamine (35 mg/kg im) and xylazine 5 mg/kg im) which all provide about 30 min of surgical anaesthesia (White and Holmes, 1976; Lipman et al., 1990; Difilippo et al., 2004). Stress can be reduced by initial administration of medetomidine (0.15–0.25 mg/kg sc) or dexmedetomidine (0.075–0.125 mg/kg) to sedate the animal. Five minutes later, oxygen can be given by mask to the animal, followed by ketamine (10–15 mg/kg sc or im). Alternatively, the two drugs can be mixed and administered as a single injection. Subcutaneous administration is better tolerated than the intramuscular injection of a relatively high volume of drug (0.4 mL/kg at the upper dose rate). Rabbits lose consciousness within 5–10 min of receiving both drugs after subcutaneous administration and 2–5 min after intramuscular administration (Orr et al., 2005). The upper dose rates can be used safely in healthy animals and will produce a sufficient depth of anaesthesia for surgical procedures such as laparotomy. The lower dose rates should be used for rabbits that are considered at higher risk. These lower dose rates are usually sufficient to allow endotracheal intubation, as laryngeal relaxation is good, but the degree of analgesia may be insufficient for major surgery. Adding a low concentration of a volatile anaesthetic, for example, 0.5%–1% isoflurane, enables the depth of anaesthesia to be deepened if this proves necessary.

Administration of medetomidine (or dexmedetomidine or xylazine) produces moderate peripheral vasoconstriction, so placement of an over-the-needle catheter is more difficult than when other regimens are used. The peripheral vasoconstriction also produces a pale and bluish colouration of the mucous membranes, even when oxygen is being administered. If oxygen is not provided, severe hypoxia will contribute to the rabbit's appearance (Hedenqvist et al., 2001). Only moderate hypercapnia develops after anaesthesia with this technique and this is easily corrected by intubation and assisted ventilation if anaesthesia is to be prolonged.

In most animals, surgical anaesthesia is produced for 30–60 min. The duration of anaesthesia can be prolonged by the addition of butorphanol (0.1 mg/kg) or buprenorphine (0.03 mg/kg) to the ketamine/medetomidine regimen, resulting in approximately 80 min of surgical anaesthesia (Hedenqvist et al., 2002; Murphy et al., 2010). If insufficient analgesia is produced, or an animal becomes too lightly anaesthetized during a prolonged procedure, it is possible to deepen anaesthesia by administration of additional ketamine and medetomidine, at approximately one-third of the original dose. However, this is not advisable. It is preferable to provide additional analgesia either by using 0.5%–1% of sevoflurane or isoflurane or by infiltrating the surgical site with local anaesthetic. If additional ketamine and medetomidine is to be used to prolong anaesthesia, then administer approximately one-tenth of the original dose, diluted 1:10 with water for injection, by slow intravenous injection until the desired effect is achieved. Dexmedetomidine at 50% of these dose rates can be used as an alternative to medetomidine.

This regimen has the particular advantage of being partially reversed when atipamezole is administered (0.5–1.0 mg/kg sc). Ketamine, at the dose rates used, produces immobility and a mild degree of analgesia, and has a marked effect for only approximately 45 min, so recovery is rapid, especially if reversal occurs after 30 or 40 min. It is this feature that makes the combination so attractive, but since severe hypoxia is almost always produced, oxygen should always be administered to prevent this. It is worth noting that the agent's effects are clearly dose dependent, so the mixture can be used to provide light anaesthesia for radiography (medetomidine 0.2 mg/kg, ketamine 10 mg/kg sc), or initial sedation and immobilization followed by use of low concentrations of inhalant agents to produce full surgical anaesthesia.

Ketamine (35 mg/kg im) combined with xylazine (5 mg/kg im) can be used in much the same way, but the degree of analgesia produced is slightly less than when medetomidine is administered (White and Holmes, 1976; Lipman et al., 1990). The duration of anaesthesia can be prolonged by the addition of butorphanol (0.1 mg) to the ketamine/xylazine regimen, resulting in approximately 80 min of surgical anaesthesia (Marini et al., 1992) As with medetomidine, anaesthesia can be partially reversed using atipamezole (1 mg/kg sc or iv).

Ketamine (25 mg/kg) can also be combined with midazolam (5 mg/kg) (Dupras et al., 2001) or acepromazine (Amarpal et al., 2010) to produce light to medium planes of anaesthesia. Lower dose rates (15 mg/kg/3 mg/kg im) can be sufficient to allow intubation (Grint and Murison, 2008). Anaesthesia can then be deepened if necessary using an inhalational agent.

Propofol (10 mg/kg iv) is less effective in the rabbit than in other species, and only light anaesthesia is produced at this dose rate. Higher doses (15–20 mg/kg) can cause respiratory arrest, however slow administration (over 30–90 s) allows anaesthesia to be induced with a sufficient level of relaxation to allow endotracheal intubation. Anaesthesia can then be maintained with a volatile agent. If sevoflurane is used, recovery is particularly smooth and rapid (Allweiler et al., 2010). Attempts to produce prolonged anaesthesia with propofol have been less successful in rabbits than in other species (Glen, 1980; Blake et al., 1988; Ko et al., 1992; Aeschbacher and Webb, 1993). However, adding an opioid, and supporting ventilation, does allow the agent to be used successfully (Baumgartner et al., 2011). Similar effects to propofol are seen with alphaxalone (4 mg/kg iv) which produces light general anaesthesia, but at the higher dose rates necessary to produce medium or deep surgical anaesthesia, it can cause sudden apnoea. Alphaxalone (2–3 mg/kg iv) administered after buprenorphine premedication (0.03 mg/kg) provides sufficient depth of anaesthesia to allow endotracheal intubation, and anaesthesia can then be prolonged using inhalational agents (Grint et al., 2008).

Fentanyl (8 µg/kg) and medetomidine (0.33 mg/kg) administered in combination by intravenous injection produces good surgical anaesthesia in rabbits, but some animals may make spontaneous movements in response to nonpainful stimuli, and in general this combination is less satisfactory than it is in rats. An advantage of the combination is that it can be completely reversed using atipamezole (1 mg/kg iv) and nalbuphine (1 mg/kg iv). It is important that the rabbit is placed in a suitable recovery cage immediately once anaesthesia is reversed, as full recovery may occur in less than 1 min. A similar, reversible, combination of fentanyl, medetomidine, and midazolam can also be used to provide surgical anaesthesia in rabbits (Henke et al., 2005). Sufentanil and midazolam as a continuous infusion, with assisted ventilation, can also be used to provide surgical anaesthesia (Hedenqvist et al., 2014).

Pentobarbital (30–45 mg/kg iv), if it must be used, should be diluted to provide a 30 mg/mL solution and administered slowly to effect. Considerable skill and extensive practical experience is required to use this drug effectively in the rabbit. Respiratory arrest frequently occurs before the onset of surgical anaesthesia, and because of the consequent high mortality, this drug is best avoided in this species (Peeters et al., 1988).

Intravenous administration of anaesthetics is best made after placing an over-the-needle catheter, which provides secure venous access. The marginal ear vein, cephalic vein, and recurrent tarsal vein are all suitable. Application of EMLA or similar topical local anaesthetic products reduces the risk of the rabbit moving in response to catheter placement (see Chapter 2).

Inhalational agents

It is possible to induce anaesthesia in rabbits using only inhalational agents, but this is usually stressful for both the patient and the anaesthetist. Induction is made more hazardous by a breath-holding response in the rabbit (Flecknell and Liles, 1996). Exposure to even low concentrations of halothane, isoflurane, or sevoflurane, delivered either by face mask or via an anaesthetic chamber, caused apnoea for periods of up to 2 min (Flecknell and Liles, 1996; Flecknell et al., 1999a). Administration of medetomidine, midazolam, or acepromazine does not block this response (Flecknell and Liles, 1996). It is therefore generally preferable to induce anaesthesia with an injectable agent and maintain the rabbit on an inhalational anaesthetic. If induction with an inhalational agent is required, a sedative (e.g. acepromazine, midazolam, fentanyl/fluanisone, or medetomidine) should be administered, and after 5–10 min, the animal should receive 100% oxygen for 2 min, followed by a gradually rising concentration of volatile anaesthetic. Use of the sedative allows induction to proceed with minimal physical restraint, so respiratory movements can be observed easily. Most rabbits will stop breathing during induction, and to avoid prolonged apnoea, the face mask should be removed temporarily. The rabbit will commence normal respiration, and the mask can then be replaced. This process may need to be repeated before the animal loses consciousness. The breath holding occurs in response to all of the commonly used volatile anaesthetics, but not to administration of oxygen. However, if the anaesthetic circuit has previously been used to deliver volatile anaesthetic, significant concentrations of anaesthetic, sufficient to trigger breath holding, can be released for some time (e.g. 30 min) even after the vaporizer has been turned off.

Because anaesthesia lightens rapidly when the face mask is removed, endotracheal intubation needs to be carried out very rapidly; it is better to gain experience of this technique when using an injectable anaesthetic combination. Recovery from anaesthesia is rapid, and anaesthetic depth can be altered easily.

Ether is an unsuitable agent for use in rabbits; its irritant nature can result in laryngospasm if used for induction, and it frequently exacerbates preexisting respiratory disease. Its irritant properties also result in profuse bronchial and salivary secretions. It is also explosive when mixed with oxygen or air, which makes it a serious safety hazard.

Endotracheal intubation

Endotracheal intubation can be carried out by a number of different techniques, using a 3–4mm endotracheal tube (see Chapter 1).

The most useful breathing systems for rabbits are the Ayre's T-piece and the Bain's coaxial system (Chapter 1).

Postoperative care

Providing continued monitoring and support in the postoperative period can be of critical importance in rabbits. A suitable recovery area should be established as part of the preoperative preparations, so that it can be stabilized at an appropriate temperature. Small rabbits will continue to be susceptible to hypothermia until they regain normal activity, so initially a temperature of approximately 35°C should be maintained. This can be lowered to 26–28°C as the animal recovers consciousness. Animals should be provided with warm, comfortable bedding. Once the animal has regained activity it can be transferred to a cage or pen containing good-quality hay or straw. This type of bedding allows the animal to surround itself with insulating material, which provides both warmth and a sense of security, and provides an immediate source of food.

Since many rabbits will have a reduced fluid intake postoperatively, even when good analgesia is provided, it is usually advisable to administer warmed (37°C) subcutaneous or intraperitoneal dextrose–saline at the end of surgery to provide some fluid supplementation in the immediate postoperative period.

Rabbits should be encouraged to eat as soon as possible after recovery from anaesthesia, as this reduces the incidence of digestive disturbances. Normal gastrointestinal function is more likely if effective postoperative analgesia is provided. Use of motility stimulants—metoclopramide (0.2–1.0mg/kg p/o, sc, im every 6–12h), cisapride (0.5–1mg/kg p/o every 12–24h), or ranitidine (2–5mg/kg p/o every 12h)—may be advisable.

Cats

Preanaesthetic medication

The majority of cats respond well to firm but gentle physical restraint, enabling intravenous administration of anaesthetics into the cephalic vein on the forelimb. Prior application of EMLA cream can prevent any struggling in response to intravenous injection (Flecknell et al., 1990b) (see Chapter 1). If an experienced assistant is not available, it may be more convenient to administer drugs by the subcutaneous or intramuscular route. Some preanaesthetic agents such as medetomidine can produce complete relaxation and loss of consciousness at higher doses (see also Table 6.14).

Cats should be fasted for 12 h prior to induction of anaesthesia to minimize the risk of vomiting during induction or the recovery period. In an emergency if fasting is possible, then medetomidine can be administered since this drug causes vomiting prior to sedation. The drugs listed below can all be used to produce sedation and will ease handling and restraint. Some of the agents can produce a sufficient depth of anaesthesia to enable minor procedures to be carried out. An extensive review of feline anaesthesia is given in Grimm et al. (2015).

1. Ketamine (5–30 mg/kg im) produces moderate analgesia and sedation, and the higher dose rate will immobilize a cat for about 30–45 min. Skeletal muscle tone is increased making minor manipulations difficult, but since pharyngeal and laryngeal reflexes are maintained, the drug is particularly useful if the animal has not been fasted.

   The palpebral and corneal blink reflexes are lost, and if prolonged anaesthesia is anticipated, the eyes should be filled with a bland ophthalmic ointment to prevent damage to the cornea through desiccation. Although the volume of injection is small, the low pH of the solution makes intramuscular injection painful.

2. Medetomidine (0.05–0.15 mg/kg im or sc) or dexmedetomidine (0.04 mg/kg sc) (Granholm et al., 2006) produces light to deep sedation, lasting 60–90 min. Sedation can be completely and rapidly reversed with atipamezole (100–600 μg/kg sc, im, or iv). Cats commonly vomit during the onset of sedation. The degree of analgesia is sufficient for minor procedures, such as percutaneous passage of a large-gauge over-the-needle catheter, but insufficient for surgical procedures.

3. Xylazine (1–2 mg/kg im or sc) produces good sedation lasting 30–40 min. Vomiting occurs commonly during the onset of sedation. The degree of sedation is sufficient to enable minor manipulation to be carried out, but the analgesic effects of the drug are variable. Reversal of sedation can be achieved by administration of atipamezole (100–600 μg/kg sc, im, or iv).

4. Acepromazine (0.05–0.2 mg/kg im) tranquillizes cats prior to induction of anaesthesia and eliminates the excitement associated with recovery from barbiturate anaesthesia.

5. Alphaxalone (5 mg/kg im) produces heavy sedation sufficient to carry out minor, nonpainful, manipulative procedures. Administering additional drug by the intravenous route can produce full surgical anaesthesia. Use of alphaxalone alone may require a high volume of drug to be injected, so it

TABLE 6.14 Sedatives, tranquillizers, and other preanaesthetic medication for the cat.

Drug	Dose rate	Comments
Acepromazine	0.05–0.2 mg/kg im	Light to moderate sedation
Acepromazine + buprenorphine	0.05 mg/kg im + 0.01 mg/kg im	Heavy sedation immobilization
Acepromazine + morphine	0.05 mg/kg im + 0.1 mg/kg im	Heavy sedation immobilization
Alphaxalone	5 mg/kg im	Moderate to heavy sedation
Atropine	0.05 mg/kg im, sc	Anticholinergic
Dexmedetomidine	40 µg/kg sc	Light to heavy sedation, mild to moderate analgesia
Glycopyrrolate	0.01 mg/kg iv, 0.05 mg/kg im	Anticholinergic
Ketamine	5–30 mg/kg im, 10–20 mg/kg per os	Light to heavy sedation, mild to moderate analgesia, immobilization at higher dose im
Medetomidine	10–150 µg/kg im or sc	Light to heavy sedation, mild to moderate analgesia
Pethidine	3–5 mg/kg im or sc	Light sedation, mild analgesia
Xylazine	1–2 mg/kg im or sc	Light to moderate sedation, mild to moderate analgesia

may be preferable to combine administration of a lower dose (1 mg/kg) with butorphanol (0.2 mg/kg) im.

6. Pethidine (3–5 mg/kg im or sc) will make some cats more tractable and provides some analgesia, although the sedative effects in certain individuals appear minimal.

Atropine (0.05 mg/kg im) or glycopyrrolate (0.01 mg/kg iv, 0.05 mg/kg im) can be administered prior to induction of anaesthesia to reduce salivation and protect the heart from vagally mediated bradycardia.

The dose rates of anaesthetic drugs listed below and in Table 6.15 can be reduced by 30%–50% if one of the drugs (1–6) listed above has been administered.

General anaesthesia

Injectable agents

Propofol (5–8 mg/kg iv) will provide about 10 min of surgical anaesthesia. Induction and recovery are smooth and rapid. Incremental doses can be used to prolong anaesthesia without unduly prolonging recovery times ((Glen, 1980); (Brearley et al., 1988), although there are reports of more prolonged recovery after extended periods of anaesthesia (150 min, (Pascoe et al., 2006).

Alphaxalone (5 mg/kg iv) provides about 10 min of surgical anaesthesia. Incremental injections of approximately 1–2 mg/kg can be given to prolong anaesthesia. Recovery can be associated with excitement and agitation, but this can be prevented by use of appropriate premedication, for example, with acepromazine.

Ketamine (20–30 mg/kg im) can be used to provide sufficient analgesia and restraint for minor surgical procedures. Improved muscle relaxation can be achieved by the concurrent administration of medetomidine or xylazine. The dosage of ketamine required can be reduced to 7 mg/kg im ketamine and medetomidine (80 μg/kg im or sc), or 22 mg/kg im for ketamine and xylazine (1.1 mg/kg im or sc). Addition of butorphanol enables further reduction of the ketamine dose. Partial reversal of anaesthesia can be achieved by administration of atipamezole (mg/kg) (Verstegen et al., 1990).

Ketamine (20 mg/kg) combined with acepromazine (0.11 mg/kg) provides light to moderate surgical anaesthesia (Ingwersen et al., 1988). The degree of analgesia may be improved by preanaesthetic administration of an opioid such as butorphanol (0.4 mg/kg sc) to increase the degree of intraoperative analgesia. As with other combinations, addition of a tranquillizer reduces the muscle rigidity associated with ketamine alone and appears to produce unconsciousness and a state more resembling conventional general anaesthesia, although the eyes remain open with a dilated pupil.

Pentobarbital (20–30 mg/kg iv) produces 30–90 min of light to moderate surgical anaesthesia. In order to avoid involuntary excitement during induction, half of the calculated dose should be administered rapidly, followed by the remainder more slowly, to effect. Pentobarbital has a relatively slow onset of action, so that administration of the remaining dose should generally take

TABLE 6.15 Anaesthetic dose rates in the cat.

Drug	Dose rate	Effect	Duration of anaesthesia (min)	Sleep time (min)
Alphaxalone	5 mg/kg iv	Surgical anaesthesia	10–15	30–60
Alpha-chloralose	70 mg/kg ip, 60 mg/kg iv	Light to medium anaesthesia	180–720	Nonrecovery only
Fentanyl + medetomidine	0.02 mg/kg im + 20 mg/kg im	Surgical anaesthesia	–	300
Ketamine/acepromazine	20 mg/kg im + 0.11 mg/kg im	Surgical anaesthesia	20–30	180–240
Ketamine/dexmedetomidine	7 mg/kg im + 40 µg/kg im	Surgical anaesthesia	30–40	180–240
Ketamine/medetomidine	7 mg/kg im + 80 µg/kg im	Surgical anaesthesia	30–40	180–240
Ketamine/medetomidine/butorphanol	5 mg/kg im + 80 µg/kg im + 0.4 mg/kg im	Surgical anaesthesia	30–40	180–240
Ketamine/midazolam	10 mg/kg im + 0.2 mg/kg im	Surgical anaesthesia	20–30	180–240
Ketamine/promazine	15 mg/kg im + 1.12 mg/kg im	Surgical anaesthesia	20–30	180–240
Ketamine/xylazine	22 mg/kg im + 1.1 mg/kg im	Surgical anaesthesia	20–30	180–240
Methohexital	4–8 mg/kg iv	Surgical anaesthesia	5–6	60–90
Pentobarbital	20–30 mg/kg iv	Surgical anaesthesia	60–90	240–480
Propanidid	8–16 mg/kg iv	Surgical anaesthesia	4–6	20–30
Propofol	5–8 mg/kg iv	Surgical anaesthesia	5–10	20
Thiamylal	12–18 mg/kg iv	Surgical anaesthesia	10–15	60–120
Thiopental	10–15 mg/kg iv	Surgical anaesthesia	5–10	60–120
Tiletamine/zolezepam	47.5 mg/kg im + 7.5 mg/kg im	Surgical anaesthesia	20–40	
Urethane	750 mg/kg iv, 1500 mg/kg ip	Surgical anaesthesia	360–480	Nonrecovery only

Duration of anaesthesia and sleep time (loss of righting reflex) are provided only as a general guide, since considerable between-animal variation occurs. For recommended techniques, see text.

around 5–6 min. Too rapid injection is frequently associated with apnoea and severe cardiovascular depression. Pentobarbital has a narrow safety margin in the cat, as in other species. Recovery can be very prolonged, especially if the animal is allowed to become hypothermic, and may be associated with excitement. Cats may remain ataxic and sedated for 8–24 h.

Inhalational agents

It is preferable to induce anaesthesia using an injectable agent and then maintain anaesthesia using an inhalational agent, since cats often resent the process of face mask induction. Prior administration of a sedative/tranquillizer coupled with expert handling may, however, enable smooth induction of anaesthesia by this method. Sevoflurane is better tolerated than the other inhalant agents, and the very rapid induction makes this a useful option when other agents are contraindicated, or when particularly rapid recovery is required (Tzannes et al., 2000). An alternative, which avoids the need for firm physical restraint, is to use an anaesthetic chamber.

Laryngospasm during induction with volatile anaesthetics may occur and the incidence of this problem may be reduced by increasing anaesthetic concentrations gradually.

Following induction of anaesthesia, with either an injectable or a volatile anaesthetic, the cat should be intubated using an uncuffed, 3–4 mm endotracheal tube. Endotracheal intubation in the cat can be carried out under direct vision using a paediatric laryngoscope blade. Care must be taken to spray the larynx with 2% lidocaine before attempting intubation, to help prevent the development of laryngospasm. In the United Kingdom, some formulations of lidocaine have been associated with the occurrence of laryngeal oedema; hence, it is advisable to check the suitability of any locally available product before use (see Chapter 1). In most instances, some spasm occurs immediately following spraying of the larynx, but this passes rapidly and intubation can then be successfully achieved. Alternatively, suxamethonium (1.0 mg/kg iv) can be administered following induction of anaesthesia and the animal can be ventilated for a short period following intubation. Under these circumstances ventilation can be carried out using a face mask if difficulties are experienced during intubation.

Following intubation, it is preferable to attach the animal to an Ayre's T-piece or Bain system since expiratory resistance and equipment dead space are minimal when using these systems.

Sevoflurane, isoflurane, halothane, and enflurane can all be used for maintenance of anaesthesia, but ether is best avoided because of its irritant nature.

Dogs

Preanaesthetic medication

Dogs respond positively to human contact, and if the animal's regular handler is present then restraint will rarely be a problem. It is often preferable, however, to administer preanaesthetic medication to dogs, to ease handling, to ensure a smooth and stress-free induction of anaesthesia and to provide a quiet and gradual recovery. Dogs should be fasted for 12 h prior to induction of anaesthesia. Intravenous injection for induction of anaesthesia is easy to carry out; particularly if the skin has been anaesthetized by prior application of EMLA cream (see Chapter 1) and a sedative or tranquillizer has been administered.

The following drugs can be used for preanaesthetic medication and are listed in order of preference (see also Table 6.16).

Medetomidine (10–80 µg/kg im, sc, or iv) or dexmedetomidine (5–40 µg/kg im, sc, or iv) produces light to deep sedation, and at higher dose rates, the dog is completely immobilized enabling minor procedures to be carried out. The degree of analgesia is insufficient for anything other than superficial surgical procedures. Sedation can be reversed completely and rapidly by administration of atipamezole (50–400 µg/kg im).

Buprenorphine (0.009 mg/kg im) and acepromazine (0.07 mg/kg im) produce moderate or deep sedation, enabling minor procedures such as radiography to be undertaken easily.

Acepromazine (0.2 mg/kg im) alone produces sedation, but has no analgesic action.

Fentanyl/fluanisone (Hypnorm, Janssen) (0.1–0.2 mL/kg) or fentanyl/droperidol (Innovar-Vet, Janssen) (0.1–0.15 mL/kg im) produces good analgesia, sufficient for minor surgical procedures, and heavy sedation. A moderate bradycardia is often produced, but this can be prevented by administration of atropine (see below). Partial reversal of these agents is possible using nalbuphine or other mixed agonist/antagonist opioids (Tables 5.1 and 5.2).

Xylazine (2.0 mg/kg im) produces good sedation and mild analgesia. Vomiting often occurs after administration and animals may be easily roused by loud noises. Other side-effects include production of bradycardia, occasional heart-block, and hyperglycaemia, although the cardiac effects can be prevented by pretreatment with atropine.

Atropine (0.05 mg/kg sc) or glycopyrrolate (0.01 mg/kg) should be administered prior to the use of fentanyl/fluanisone, fentanyl/droperidol, or xylazine. It may also be included as premedication prior to use of the anaesthetic regimens described below.

The dose rates of anaesthetic drugs listed below and in Table 6.17 can be reduced by 30%–50% if one of the drugs (1–6) listed above has been administered.

General anaesthesia

Injectable agents

Intravenous administration is easily carried out using the cephalic vein on the anterior surface of the forelimb, provided adequate restraint can be provided.

TABLE 6.16 Sedatives, tranquillizers, and other preanaesthetic medication for use in the dog.

Drug	Dose rate	Comments
Acepromazine	0.1–0.25 mg/kg im	Light to moderate sedation
Acepromazine/buprenorphine	0.07 mg/kg im + 0.009 mg/kg im	Heavy sedation, immobilization, some analgesia
Atropine	0.05 mg/kg sc or im	Anticholinergic
Dexmedetomidine	5–40 µg/kg im, sc, or iv	Light to heavy sedation, mild to moderate analgesia
Etorphine methotrime-prazine 'Immobilon SA'	0.5 mL/4 kg im	Immobilization/analgesia
Fentanyl/droperidol (Innovar-Vet)	0.1–0.15 mL/kg im	Immobilization/analgesia
Fentanyl/fluanisone (Hypnorm)	0.1–0.2 mL/kg im	Moderate to heavy sedation, moderate analgesia
Glycopyrrolate	0.01 mg/kg iv	Anticholinergic
Medetomidine	10–80 µg/kg im, sc, or iv	Light to heavy sedation, mild to moderate analgesia
Medetomidine + butorphanol	5–10 µg/kg im, sc + 0.1–0.5 mg.kg im	Light to heavy sedation, mild to moderate analgesia
Xylazine	1–2 mg/kg im	Light to moderate sedation, mild to moderate analgesia

TABLE 6.17 Anaesthetic dose rates in the dog.

Drug	Dose rate	Effect	Duration of anaesthesia (min)	Sleep time (min)
Alpha-chloralose	80 mg/kg iv	Light anaesthesia	360–600	Nonrecovery only
Alphaxalone	2 mg/kg iv	Surgical anaesthesia	10–15	15–20
Ketamine/dexmedetomidine	2.5–7.5 mg/kg im + 20 µg/kg im	Light to medium anaesthesia	30–45	60–120
Ketamine/medetomidine	2.5–7.5 mg/kg im + 40 µg/kg im	Light to medium anaesthesia	30–45	60–120
Ketamine/xylazine	5 mg/kg iv + 1–2 mg/kg iv or im	Light to medium anaesthesia	30–60	60–120
Methohexital	4–8 mg/kg iv	Surgical anaesthesia	4–5	10–20
Pentobarbital	20–30 mg/kg iv	Surgical anaesthesia	30–40	60–240
Propofol	5–7.5 mg/kg iv	Surgical anaesthesia	5–10	15–30
Thiamylal	10–15 mg/kg iv	Surgical anaesthesia	5–10	15–20
Thiopental	10–20 mg/kg iv	Surgical anaesthesia	5–10	20–30
Urethane	1000 mg/kg iv	Surgical anaesthesia	360–480	Nonrecovery only

Duration of anaesthesia and sleep time (loss of righting reflex) are provided only as a general guide, since considerable between-animal variation occurs. For recommended techniques, see text.

Propofol (5–7.5 mg/kg iv) produces a short period (5–10 min) of general anaesthesia, which can be prolonged by administration of incremental injections of 1–2 mg/kg every 10–15 min. To avoid apnoea during induction of anaesthesia, propofol should be administered slowly, over 60–90 s. Recovery is smooth and rapid, even after prolonged anaesthesia (Glen and Hunter, 1984; Hall and Chambers, 1987; Nolan and Reid, 1993a).

Alfaxalone (Alfaxan CD) (2 mg–4.5 mg/kg iv) produces smooth induction of anaesthesia, provided it is administered slowly (e.g. over 60–90 s) to avoid apnoea. Anaesthesia can be prolonged by repeated injections or as a continuous infusion (Herbert et al., 2013).

The barbiturates thiopental (10–20 mg/kg of a 1.25% or 2.5% solution) can be used to produce anaesthesia lasting 10–30 min, with recovery occurring within 15–20 min. Recovery can be associated with involuntary excitement and agitation unless a sedative or tranquillizer has been administered as preanaesthetic medication.

Pentobarbital is still used in research facilities, since it can provide 45–60 min of light anaesthesia following a single intravenous dose of the drug (20–30 mg/kg iv). It has the disadvantage of providing poor analgesia for major surgical procedures, unless high dosages are administered. At these higher doses, pentobarbital produces significant respiratory and cardiovascular system depression and it is preferable to ventilate the animal to maintain normal blood gas concentrations.

Ketamine is less widely used in the dog than in other species, primarily since it may cause behavioural disturbances. Despite these problems, ketamine (2.5–7.5 mg/kg im) and medetomidine (40 µg/kg im) can be used to produce surgical anaesthesia, as can ketamine (5 mg/kg iv) and xylazine (12 mg/kg iv or im).

Inhalational agents

Anaesthesia can be induced using a face mask in a co-operative animal, especially when using sevoflurane or following sedation with one of the drugs listed above in more apprehensive individuals. Even after sedation, some animals may resent this procedure. It is generally preferable to induce anaesthesia with an injectable anaesthetic agent (see above) followed by intubation and maintenance with a volatile anaesthetic. Intubation is a relatively straightforward procedure in the dog. The mouth can be opened widely to provide a clear view of the larynx, so that an endotracheal tube can be passed under direct vision. If difficulty is experienced in visualizing the larynx, a laryngoscope with a McGill or Soper blade can be used. Following intubation, the dog can be connected to an appropriate breathing system such as a Bain's or Magill system (see Chapter 1). Halothane (1%–2%), methoxyflurane (1.0%–1.5%), isoflurane (2%–3%), or enflurane (1%–2%) provides stable anaesthesia with good analgesia and muscle relaxation.

Ferrets

Preanaesthetic medication

If a ferret has become accustomed to being handled it can be easily restrained to enable injection of an anaesthetic agent. Some animals may resent physical restraint, and administration of drugs to sedate the animal may be required before induction of anaesthesia with intravenous or inhalational anaesthetic agents. Ferrets should be fasted for 12 h prior to induction of anaesthesia to minimize the risk of vomiting during induction of anaesthesia.

The following drugs can be used to produce sedation (see also Table 6.18):

1. Diazepam (2 mg/kg im) produces good sedation.
2. Acepromazine (0.2 mg/kg im) produces heavy sedation.
3. Ketamine (20–30 mg/kg im) produces deep sedation and light anaesthesia lasting about 30–40 min.
4. Fentanyl/fluanisone (Hypnorm, Janssen) (0.5 mL/kg im) or fentanyl/droperidol (Innovar-Vet) (0.15 mL/kg im) produces deep sedation and sufficient analgesia for minor surgical procedures.

TABLE 6.18 Sedatives, tranquillizers, and other preanaesthetic medication for use in the ferret.

Drug	Dose rate	Comments
Acepromazine	0.2 mg/kg im	Moderate sedation
Atropine	0.05 mg/kg sc or im	Anticholinergic
Dexmedetomidine	5–40 µg/kg sc or im	Light to heavy sedation, mild to moderate analgesia
Diazepam	2 mg/kg im	Light sedation
Fentanyl/fluanisone (Hypnorm)	0.5 mL/kg im	Immobilization, good analgesia
Ketamine	20–30 mg/kg	Immobilization, some analgesia
Medetomidine	10–80 µg/kg sc or im	Light to heavy sedation, mild to moderate analgesia
Medetomidine/butorphanol	80 µg/kg + 0.2 mg/kg sc or im	Light to heavy sedation, mild to moderate analgesia
Xylazine	0.1–0.5 mg/kg sc or im	Light to heavy sedation, mild to moderate analgesia

5. Medetomidine (0.1–0.5 mg/kg sc), dexmedetomidine (0.05–0.25 mg/kg im, sc, or iv), or xylazine (1–2 mg/kg im) produces light to heavy sedation in the ferret. Sedation can be reversed using atipamezole (1 mg/kg).

Atropine (0.05 mg/kg im) may be administered if necessary.

General anaesthesia

Injectable agents

The cephalic vein on the anterior aspect of the foreleg can be used for intravenous injection, although firm restraint is necessary. Intramuscular injections can easily be made into the hindlimb muscles. Anaesthetic dose rates are summarized in Table 6.19.

Ketamine (25 mg/kg im) and xylazine (1–2 mg/kg im), or ketamine (4–8 mg/kg im) and medetomidine (0.05–0.1 mg/kg im) (Plant and Lloyd, 2010) produces good surgical anaesthesia lasting 30–60 min. As in other species, administration of atipamezole will accelerate recovery. Ketamine combined with diazepam (2 mg/kg im) or acepromazine (0.25 mg/kg im) has effects to those of ketamine/xylazine.

Alphaxalone (5 mg/kg iv) produces surgical anaesthesia lasting 5–10 min. Additional doses of the drug can be administered to prolong the period of anaesthesia (Giral et al., 2014).

Pentobarbital (25–30 mg/kg iv, 36 mg/kg ip) can be used to provide 30–120 min of light to medium surgical anaesthesia.

Inhalational agents isoflurane, sevoflurane, and halothane can all be used to produce or maintain surgical anaesthesia in ferrets. Animals can be induced in an anaesthetic chamber, following which anaesthesia can be maintained using a face mask. Alternatively, the animal may be intubated.

Pigs

Preanaesthetic medication

Small pigs (<10 kg) are easily restrained humanely, but pigs of all sizes vocalize extremely loudly when restrained; hence, it may be useful to administer a sedative before induction of anaesthesia. Although it is possible to physically restrain larger pigs, use of preanaesthetic medication will considerably ease induction and reduce stress to the animal. Several of the preanaesthetic agents require administration of relatively large volumes of drug, and this appears to cause less distress if carried out slowly. A useful technique is to attach a 2 in. needle (or longer in animals >50 kg) to the syringe using an anaesthetic extension tube. The needle can be quickly placed in the pig's neck muscles, and the injection made slowly with the pig unrestrained.

Pigs are usually fasted for 12 h prior to induction of anaesthesia, although vomiting on induction is rare.

TABLE 6.19 Anaesthetic dose rates in the ferret.

Drug	Dose rate	Effect	Duration of anaesthesia (min)	Sleep time (min)
Alphaxalone	5 mg/kg iv	Surgical anaesthesia	10–15	20–30
Ketamine/acepromazine	25 mg/kg im + 0.25 mg/kg im	Surgical anaesthesia	20–30	60–120
Ketamine/dexmedetomidine	4–8 mg/kg im + 25–50 μg/kg im	Light-surgical anaesthesia	20–30	60–120
Ketamine/diazepam	25 mg/kg im + 2 mg/kg im	Surgical anaesthesia	20–30	60–120
Ketamine/medetomidine	4–8 mg/kg im + 50–100 μg/kg im	Light-surgical anaesthesia	20–30	60–120
Ketamine/medetomidine/butorphanol	8 mg/kg im + 80 μg/kg im + 0.2 mg/kg im	Surgical anaesthesia	20–30	60–120
Ketamine/xylazine	25 mg/kg im + 1–2 mg/kg im	Surgical anaesthesia	20–30	60–120
Pentobarbital	25–30 mg/kg iv, 36 mg/kg ip	Surgical anaesthesia	30–60	90–240
Urethane	1500 mg/kg ip	Surgical anaesthesia	360–480	Nonrecovery only

Duration of anaesthesia and sleep time (loss of righting reflex) are provided only as a general guide, since considerable between-animal variation occurs. For recommended techniques, see text.

The following drugs can be used for preanaesthetic medication (see also Table 6.20):

1. Diazepam (1–2.0 mg/kg im) provides rapid sedation, but is best followed by administration of ketamine (10–15 mg/kg im) to provide complete immobilization. Some preparations of diazepam can be mixed in the same syringe with ketamine; alternatively, midazolam (1–2 mg/kg) can be used. The large volume of injectate (6–8 mL) required for animals weighing over 15–20 kg limits the use of this combination for smaller pigs.

2. Ketamine (10 mg/kg im) used alone in juvenile and adult pigs immobilizes the animal, but spontaneous movements occur. In young animals, this drug appears less effective and higher dose rates (20 mg/kg) may be required. Even at higher doses considerable spontaneous movements may occur. Although this drug is useful in older animals, it is an expensive means of producing sedation.

3. Tiletamine and zolazepam (2–4 mg/kg of 'Zoletil', Virbac) combination produces heavy sedation and immobilization. An advantage of this combination is that the volume for injection can be reduced, making it particularly suitable for larger animals.

4. Alphaxalone (5 mg/kg im) produces good sedation in pigs but the volume of injection (10 mL for a 20 kg pig) limits the use of this drug to smaller animals (Santos et al., 2013). Deeper sedation can be produced by adding diazepam or midazolam (0.5 mg/kg im).

5. Azaperone (5 mg/kg im) produces sedation but has no analgesic effect.

TABLE 6.20 Sedatives, tranquillizers, and other preanaesthetic medication for use in the pig.

Drug	Dose rate	Comments
Acepromazine	0.2 mg/kg im	Moderate sedation
Alphaxalone/alphadolone	6 mg/kg im	Sedation
Atropine	0.05 mg/kg sc or im	Anticholinergic
Azaperone	5 mg/kg im	Moderate to deep sedation
Diazepam	1–2 mg/kg im	Light to moderate sedation
Ketamine	10–15 mg/kg im	Sedation, immobilization
Ketamine/acepromazine	22 mg/kg im + 1 mg/kg im	Immobilization
Ketamine/medetomidine	5 mg/kg + 30-80 g/kg im	Immobilization
Metomidate	2 mg/kg im	Moderate to deep sedation
Tiletamine/zolezepam	2–4 mg/kg im	Moderate to deep sedation

6. Acepromazine (0.2 mg/kg im) produces moderate sedation but has no analgesic action.
7. Medetomidine and xylazine are relatively ineffective in many strains of pigs,
   and the degree of sedation produced is highly variable, although these agents
   may potentiate the effects of other anaesthetics.

Atropine (0.05 mg/kg im) can be administered to reduce salivary and bronchial secretions.

General anaesthesia

Injectable agents

Following physical or chemical restraint, a number of different anaesthetic
agents can be administered by intravenous injection to produce surgical anaesthesia. The dose rates of anaesthetic drugs listed below and in Table 6.21 can be
reduced by 30%–50% if one of the drugs (1–7) listed above has been administered. The most convenient route is via the ear veins, and placement of an 'over-
the-needle' catheter to ensure reliable venous access is strongly recommended.

1. Propofol (2.5–3.5 mg/kg iv) produces surgical anaesthesia lasting 10 min. As
   with other species a short period of apnoea often occurs immediately after
   injection. Anaesthesia can be prolonged by administration of incremental
   injections (1–2 mg/kg every 10–15 min) or by continuous infusion (8–9 mg/
   kg/h). If propofol is used as the sole anaesthetic agent for major surgical
   procedures, significant respiratory depression may occur, and ventilation
   may need to be assisted. An alternative approach is to administer propofol
   at a lower rate (5–6 mg/kg/h) together with alfentanil (20–30 μg/kg iv followed by 2–5 μg/kg/min) to provide supplemental analgesia, although use
   of alfentanil will require assisted ventilation. Recovery following propofol
   is smooth and rapid, as with other species, and if necessary the alfentanil can
   be reversed by administration of nalbuphine (0.5 mg/kg iv).
2. Alphaxalone (1–2.0 mg/kg iv, to effect, after immobilization or sedation with
   one of the agents listed above) will produce surgical anaesthesia and good
   muscle relaxation with minimal respiratory depression. Prolonged anaesthesia can be achieved by continuous infusion of this drug (0.05–0.2 mg/kg
   per minute iv (Pfeiffer et al., 2013; Bigby et al., 2017).
3. Ketamine in combination with xylazine or medetomidine, alone, or together
   with other sedatives or analgesics (e.g. acepromazine or butorphanol) can all
   be used to produce light to moderate planes of surgical anaesthesia (Vainio
   et al., 1992; Sakaguchi et al., 1996; Linkenhoker et al., 2010). All of these
   combinations produce some degree of respiratory depression, so may require oxygen supplementation.
4. Thiopental (6–9 mg/kg iv) can be administered to produce 5–10 min of surgical anaesthesia. Recovery can be associated with excitement in some individuals unless a sedative or tranquillizer has been administered.

TABLE 6.21 Anaesthetic dose rates in the pig.

Drug	Dose rate	Effect	Duration of anaesthesia (min)	Sleep time (min)
Alphaxalone	5 mg/kg im then 1–2 mg/kg iv	Immobilization, surgical anaesthesia	–	10–20
			5–10	15–20
Ketamine	10–15 mg/kg im	Sedation, immobilization	20–30	60–120
Ketamine/acepromazine	22 mg/kg + 1.1 mg/kg im	Light anaesthesia	20–30	60–120
Ketamine/diazepam	10–15 mg/kg im + 0.5–2 mg/kg im	Immobilization/light anaesthesia	20–30	60–90
Ketamine/medetomidine	10 mg/kg im + 0.08 mg/kg im	Immobilization/light anaesthesia	40–90	120–240
Ketamine/midazolam	10–15 mg/kg im + 0.5–2 mg/kg im	Immobilization/light anaesthesia	20–30	60–90
Methohexital	5 mg/kg iv	Surgical anaesthesia	4–5	5–10
Pentobarbital	20–30 mg/kg iv	Light to surgical anaesthesia	15–60	60–120
Propofol	2.5–3.5 mg/kg iv (6–8 mg/kg if no premed given)	Surgical anaesthesia	5–10	10–20
Thiopental	6–9 mg/kg iv	Surgical anaesthesia	5–10	10–20
Tiletamine/zolezepam	2–4 mg/kg im	Immobilization	20–30	60–120
	6–8 mg/kg im	Light anaesthesia	20–30	90–180
Tiletamine/zolezepam + xylazine	2–7 mg/kg im + 0.2–1 mg/kg im	Light to medium anaesthesia	30–40	60–120

Duration of anaesthesia and sleep time (loss of righting reflex) are provided only as a general guide, since considerable between-animal variation occurs. For recommended techniques, see text.

5. Pentobarbital (20–30 mg/kg iv) produces light surgical anaesthesia in pigs. The high dose rates (30 mg/kg) needed to produce deep surgical anaesthesia may cause severe cardiovascular system depression. The duration of anaesthesia in pigs is shorter than in other species, surgical anaesthesia persisting for only 20–30 min. Full recovery can take 3–4 h, however.

Inhalational agents

It is possible to produce anaesthesia with volatile anaesthetics administered by means of a face mask, but providing the necessary degree of physical restraint can be a problem, even in small pigs. Considerable pollution of the environment with anaesthetic gases will occur and this should be avoided if possible. As in other species, sevoflurane provides rapid induction and this makes it a suitable alternative in smaller pigs (<10 kg) (Moeser et al., 2008). In larger animals, it is preferable to induce anaesthesia with an injectable anaesthetic, intubate the pig and maintain anaesthesia using an inhalational agent. Halothane, methoxyflurane, enflurane and isoflurane can all be used to maintain safe and effective anaesthesia. The potency of volatile anaesthetics appears lower in pigs than in other laboratory mammals, so slightly higher concentrations are required for induction and maintenance (Weiskopf and Bogetz, 1984; Heavner, 2001) A small number of pigs have been shown to develop malignant hyperthermia in response to volatile anaesthetics and, whenever possible, animals should be obtained from herds that have a low incidence of this problem (Jurkat-Rott et al., 2000).

Anaesthesia should be maintained in small pigs using a Bain or Magill breathing system, but large animals (>30 kg) may require closed-circuit anaesthesia in order to reduce the gas flow rates needed. As discussed in Chapter 1, closed-circuit anaesthesia requires considerable expertise and advice should be sought from a veterinary surgeon or medically qualified anaesthetist if this type of circuit is to be used.

Intubation of pigs is complicated by the difficulty of obtaining a clear view of the larynx and by the laryngeal anatomy that tends to obstruct passage of the tube. A brief description of the technique of intubation is given in Chapter 1. A more detailed description is given by Theisen et al. (2009).

Sheep and goats

Preanaesthetic medication

Opinion varies as to whether sheep and goats should be fasted before induction of general anaesthesia. Fasting has little effect on the volume of digesta present in the rumen, but may reduce the incidence of rumenal tympany (an accumulation of gas in the rumen caused by bacterial fermentation). This appears to be a greater problem in animals that are grazing. Unnecessary fasting should be avoided since it may cause distress to the animal, and the author has experienced few problems if food and water are provided up to an hour prior to induction of anaesthesia. If rumenal tympany develops it can be relieved by passage of a stomach tube (see Chapter 3). Should the condition occur repeatedly, preanaesthetic fasting may be introduced, although this may not resolve the problem.

Sheep and goats can generally be restrained easily for administration of anaesthetic agents. The stress associated with movement from its pen to the operating theatre can be reduced by use of sedatives and tranquillizers. High doses of sedatives and tranquillizers can also be used in conjunction with local anaesthetics to provide humane restraint and surgical anaesthesia. Useful reviews of anaesthetic techniques in sheep and goats is provided by Taylor (1991) and Galatos (2011).

The following drugs may be used for preanaesthetic medication (see also Table 6.22):

1. Diazepam (2 mg/kg im or 1 mg/kg iv) and midazolam (0.5 mg/kg iv) are particularly effective tranquillizers in sheep and goats (Stegmann and Bester, 2001). When combined with ketamine (4 mg/kg iv) moderate surgical anaesthesia is produced.
2. Xylazine (0.1 mg/kg im) will provide heavy sedation and good analgesia in sheep, lasting 30–35 min. It can be combined with ketamine (4 mg/kg iv) to produce light surgical anaesthesia. Goats appear more sensitive to xylazine, and lower doses (0.05 mg/kg im) are usually adequate.

TABLE 6.22 Sedatives, tranquillizers, and other preanaesthetic medication for use in the sheep and goat.

Drug	Dose rate	Comments
Acepromazine	0.05–0.1 mg/kg im	Moderate sedation
Dexmedetomidine	125 µg/kg im	Light to heavy sedation, some analgesia
Diazepam	1–2 mg/kg im, 1 mg/kg iv	Light to moderate sedation
Ketamine	20 mg/kg im	Moderate to heavy sedation, immobilization, some analgesia
Medetomidine	25 µg/kg im	Light to heavy sedation, some analgesia
Midazolam	0.5 mg/kg iv	Moderate sedation
Xylazine	0.1 mg/kg im or iv (sheep) 0.05 mg/kg im (goat)	Light to moderate sedation, some analgesia

3. Medetomidine (25 µg/kg im) is also effective in producing sedation and an-algesia. As with xylazine, this agent can be combined with ketamine to pro-duce surgical anaesthesia, but only a low dose of ketamine (1 mg/kg im) is required because of the potency of medetomidine in this species (Laitinen, 1990). Medetomidine, xylazine, and dexmedetomidine can produce hypoxia in sheep due to pulmonary effects (Celly et al., 1997; Kästner et al., 2007). Sedation, and any undesirable side-effects, can be reversed using atipa-mezole (100–200 µg/kg iv or im).
4. Acepromazine (0.05–0.1 mg/kg im) will sedate sheep but provides no analgesia.

The use of atropine in sheep is of limited value. Extremely high dose rates (0.5 mg/kg im) are needed to reduce salivary secretions and repeated doses of 0.2–0.3 mg/kg may be required every 15 min to maintain the effects.

General anaesthesia

Injectable agents

Intravenous injection is easily carried out using the marginal ear vein, anterior cephalic vein on the foreleg or jugular vein. Dose rates of injectable anaesthetics are summarized in Table 6.23.

1. Light to moderate surgical anaesthesia can be produced by use of ket-amine (4 mg/kg iv) + xylazine (1 mg/kg iv) or ketamine (10–5 mg/kg im or 4 mg/kg iv) + diazepam or midazolam (2 mg/kg im or 1 mg/kg iv) (Walsh et al., 2012) as described above. The combination of ketamine and diaz-epam appears to cause less cardiovascular and respiratory system depres-sion than does ketamine/xylazine.
2. Thiopental (10–15 mg/kg iv) provides 5–10 min of anaesthesia.
3. Alphaxalone (2–3 mg/kg iv in adults provides excellent stable anaesthesia in sheep. A previous report of using alphaxalone/alphadolone indicated that lambs required higher dose rates (x2) than adults and the dose of alphaxa-lone required may be similarly elevated in lambs (Eales and Small, 1982). Alphaxalone can be administered by continuous infusion to maintain anaes-thesia over prolonged periods (Andaluz et al., 2012; Granados et al., 2012).
4. Propofol can be used to induce anaesthesia in sheep (4–5 mg/kg iv) (Waterman, 1988; Vishwakarma et al., 2013) and goats (3 mg/kg iv, (Prassinos et al., 2005).
5. Pentobarbital (30 mg/kg iv) produces anaesthesia lasting 15–30 min. The dose required varies considerably in different animals, and the drug gener-ally produces marked respiratory depression.

Inhalational agents

Sheep may be restrained and anaesthesia induced using a face mask, but consid-erable pollution of the environment with inhalational anaesthetics will occur be-cause of the high fresh gas flows used when anaesthetizing these larger animals.

TABLE 6.23 Anaesthetic dose rates in the sheep and goat.

Drug	Dose rate	Effect	Duration of anaesthesia (min)	Sleep time (min)
Alphaxalone	2–3 mg/kg iv	Surgical anaesthesia	5–10	10–20
Etorphine/acepromazine (Immobilon LA)	0.5 mL per 50 kg im (>30 kg)	Immobilization, analgesia	Analgesia 30–40	60–90
Etorphine/methotrimeprazine (Immobilon SA)	0.5 mL per 4 kg im (>30 kg)	Immobilization, analgesia	Analgesia 30–40	60–90
Ketamine/diazepam	10–15 mg/kg + 1–2 mg/kg im or 4 mg/kg iv + 0.5–1 mg/kg iv	Light to medium anaesthesia Surgical anaesthesia	20–30 20–30	60–90 45–90
Ketamine/dexmedetomidine	1 mg/kg iv + 125 µg/kg iv	Surgical anaesthesia	30–60	60–90
Ketamine/medetomidine	1 mg/kg iv + 25 µg/kg iv	Surgical anaesthesia	30–60	60–90
Ketamine/xylazine	4 mg/kg + 0.2 mg/kg iv (sheep), 0.05 mg/kg iv (goat)	Surgical anaesthesia	15–20	30–90
Methohexital	4 mg/kg iv	Surgical anaesthesia	4–5	5–10
Pentobarbital	30 mg/kg iv	Immobilization, anaesthesia	15–30	30–60
Propofol	4–5 mg/kg iv	Light anaesthesia	5–10	10–15
Thiopental	10–15 mg/kg iv	Surgical anaesthesia	5–10	10–20
Urethane	1000 mg/kg iv	Surgical anaesthesia	360–480	Nonrecovery only

Duration of anaesthesia and sleep time (loss of righting reflex) are provided only as a general guide, since considerable between-animal variation occurs. For recommended techniques, see text.

It is generally preferable to induce anaesthesia with an injectable agent, intubate the animal, and maintain anaesthesia with an inhalational agent if required.

It is essential to intubate sheep immediately following induction of general anaesthesia since regurgitation of rumen contents invariably occurs and these may be inhaled, resulting in an inhalational pneumonia. Intubation is relatively straightforward, provided that a suitable laryngoscope blade (Table 1.2 and Chapter 1) is available. The vocal cords should be sprayed with lignocaine prior to passage of an endotracheal tube to prevent laryngospasm.

Halothane, methoxyflurane, enflurane, isoflurane, and sevoflurane can all be used to maintain effective anaesthesia in sheep. Anaesthesia should be maintained using a Bain or Magill breathing system. It may be advisable to use a circle system in large adult sheep to reduce the quantities of anaesthetic gases required.

Anaesthetic management

Following intubation it is advisable to pass a stomach tube to try to minimize the risk or the development of rumenal tympany. Sheep should, if possible, be positioned on their sides as when positioned in dorsal recumbency, the pressure of the rumen, and other viscera on the major abdominal blood vessels may interfere with venous return.

During the postoperative recovery period, sheep should be positioned on their sternum and observed carefully for signs of rumenal tympany.

Primates

Preanaesthetic medication

Small primates such as marmosets (*Callithrix jacchus*) can usually be restrained relatively easily to enable the intraperitoneal or intramuscular injection of an anaesthetic agent. Preanaesthetic medication to sedate these animals is generally only required prior to intravenous injection of induction agents or to enable administration of inhalational agents by means of a face mask. Larger primates such as baboons (*Papio* sp.) and macaque monkeys (*Macaca* sp.) can cause physical injury to their handler if inexpertly restrained and it is strongly recommended that chemical agents be used to produce deep sedation.

The following drugs may be used for preanaesthetic medication (see also Table 6.24):

1. Ketamine (5–25 mg/kg im) is probably the drug of choice in larger primates. At the lower dose rate, heavy sedation is produced; higher doses of ketamine produce light surgical anaesthesia (Banknieder et al., 1978).
2. Alphaxalone (8–12 mg/kg im) is the agent of choice for sedating marmosets and small primates. Heavy sedation is produced and additional doses of the drug can be administered intravenously to produce surgical anaesthesia (Bakker et al., 2013).

TABLE 6.24 Sedatives, tranquillizers, and preanaesthetic medication for use in the nonhuman primate.

Drug	Dose rate	Comments
Acepromazine	0.2 mg/kg im	Moderate sedation
Alphaxalone	8–12 mg/kg im	Heavy sedation
Atropine	0.05 mg/kg sc or im	Anticholinergic
Diazepam	1 mg/kg im	Light to moderate sedation
Fentanyl/dropiderol (Innovar-Vet)	0.3 mL/kg im	Heavy sedation, good analgesia
Fentanyl/fluanisone (Hypnorm)	0.3 mL/kg im	Heavy sedation, good analgesia
Ketamine	5–25 mg/kg im	Moderate sedation, immobilization, some analgesia
Medetomidine + midazolam + fentanyl	20 µg/kg + 0.5 mg/kg + 10 µg/kg im	Heavy sedation/immobilization (Rhesus monkey)
Xylazine	0.5 mg/kg im	Light to moderate sedation, some analgesia

3. Acepromazine (0.2 mg/kg im) produces sedation but will not immobilize the animal.
4. Diazepam (1 mg/kg im) sedates primates, but provides insufficient sedation for the safe handling of large primates.
5. Fentanyl/fluanisone (Hypnorm, Janssen) (0.3 mL/kg im) or fentanyl/droperidol (Innovar-Vet) (0.3 mL/kg im) produces heavy sedation and good analgesia (Field et al., 1966).
6. Medetomidine can be used to provide sedation, but animals may arouse in response to external stimuli (Miyabe et al., 2001) and this can present a significant hazard to the staff.
7. In Rhesus monkeys, a combination of medetomidine (20 µg/kg), midazolam (0.5 mg/kg), and fentanyl (10 µg/kg) im produces profound sedation or light anaesthesia. Animals should be monitored as there is a risk of hypoxia occurring, but this combination can be reversed using atipamezole and butorphanol (Bertrand et al., 2016). Recovery is rapid with no signs of residual sedation from the midazolam.

Atropine (0.05 mg/kg im) should be administered to minimize the bradycardia produced by neuroleptanalgesic combinations and to reduce the amount of salivary secretions. Primates should be fasted for 12–16 h prior to induction of anaesthesia.

General anaesthesia

Injectable agents

The cephalic vein on the anterior aspect of the forelimb of large primates or the lateral tail vein in marmosets can be used for intravenous injection. Dose rates of injectable anaesthetics are summarized in Table 6.25.

1. The combination of ketamine (10 mg/kg im) and xylazine (0.5 mg/kg im) or ketamine (5 mg/kg im) and medetomidine (50 μg/kg) or dexmedetomidine (25 μg/kg) produces surgical anaesthesia with good muscle relaxation, lasting 30–40 min. Ketamine (15 mg/kg im) and diazepam (1 mg/kg im) combination has similar effects. As in other species, reversal of the alpha2 agonist with atipamezole speeds recovery.
2. Alphaxalone (5–10 mg/kg iv) produces good surgical anaesthesia in both Old and New World primates, and prolonged periods of anaesthesia can be provided by administration of additional doses (2–5 mg/kg iv) every 10–15 min or by continuous infusion (0.1–0.2 mg/kg/min).
3. Propofol (7–8 mg/kg iv) can be used to induce and maintain anaesthesia in both marmosets and larger primates. Good surgical anaesthesia is produced with rapid and smooth recoveries (Glen, 1980; Fowler et al., 2001).

Thiopental (15–20 mg/kg iv) can be administered to produce 5–10 min of surgical anaesthesia. The dosage can be reduced by at least 50% if the animal has received ketamine as preanaesthetic medication.

Pentobarbital (25–35 mg/kg iv) will provide 30–60 min of light surgical anaesthesia, but severe respiratory depression often occurs at higher dose rates and recovery can be prolonged, especially if incremental doses are administered. It is usually better replaced with other anaesthetic agents. If it is necessary to use pentobarbital, the dose should be reduced by at least 50% if ketamine or other sedatives have been administered as preanaesthetic medication.

Inhalational agents

All the commonly available inhalational anaesthetics can be administered to primates. It is usually most convenient to induce anaesthesia using injectable agents. Small primates can then be maintained using an inhalational agent delivered by means of a face mask, or intubated (Thomas et al., 2012). With larger primates, it is usually preferable to intubate the animal. Endotracheal intubation is relatively straightforward in larger primates using a Magill laryngoscope blade. The larynx should be sprayed with lignocaine before attempting to pass an endotracheal tube. Following intubation, a T-piece or Bain breathing system should be used for administration of oxygen and the inhalational anaesthetic. As in other species, the concentration of inhalational agent can be reduced by administration of a continuous infusion of short-acting opioids (Table 6.25).

TABLE 6.25 Anaesthetic dose rates in the nonhuman primate.

Drug	Dose rate	Effect	Duration of anaesthesia (min)	Sleep time (min)
Alphaxalone	5–10 mg/kg iv	Surgical anaesthesia	5–10	10–20
Ketamine/diazepam	15 mg/kg im + 1 mg/kg im	Surgical anaesthesia	30–40	60–90
Ketamine/dexmedetomidine	5 mg/kg im + 25 µg/kg im	Surgical anaesthesia	30–40	60–120
Ketamine/medetomidine	5 mg/kg im + 50 µg/kg im	Surgical anaesthesia	30–40	60–120
Ketamine/xylazine	10 mg/kg im + 0.5 mg/kg im	Surgical anaesthesia	30–40	60–120
Methohexital	10 mg/kg iv	Surgical anaesthesia	4–5	5–10
Pentobarbital	25–35 mg/kg iv	Surgical anaesthesia	30–60	60–120
Propofol	7–8 mg/kg iv	Surgical anaesthesia	5–10	10–15
Thiopental	15–20 mg/kg iv	Surgical anaesthesia	5–10	10–15

Duration of anaesthesia and sleep time (loss of righting reflex) are provided only as a general guide, since considerable between-animal variation occurs. For recommended techniques, see text.

Other species

A full description of all of the available anaesthetic techniques for fish, reptiles, amphibia, and birds is beyond the scope of this book, but the following section gives initial guidance on anaesthesia of these species. Further information is available in a number of reviews and textbooks (Machin, 2004; Gunkel and Lafortune, 2005; Longley, 2008; Ross and Ross, 2009; Raftery, 2013).

Birds

A number of unique aspects of avian physiology influence the selection of anaesthetic agents and the overall management of anaesthesia. Birds, particularly smaller species, have higher metabolic rates relative to mammals of comparable size and have higher body temperatures (39–42°C). The higher body temperature results in an increased temperature gradient between core temperature and the external environmental temperature, and so cooling during anaesthesia is rapid. In small birds, as with mammals, the high surface area to body weight ratio also increases heat loss. It is therefore particularly important to adopt measures to minimize heat loss. In addition to those described in Chapter 3, avoid removing large numbers of feathers. Because of their high metabolic rate, small birds do not tolerate fasting and may develop hypoglycaemia, so only individuals weighing more than 1 kg should undergo preanaesthetic fasting.

The respiratory system in birds differs from that of mammals, having a series of air sacs that connect with the lungs. The presence of air sacs may allow a build-up of anaesthetic vapour in dependent areas of the respiratory system, and consequent overdosage. Induction of anaesthesia with volatile agents is rapid in birds. This is not a problem provided that the anaesthetist appreciates the shorter time frame within which induction may occur. Endotracheal intubation is easily accomplished, as the glottis is easily seen at the back of the pharynx. Use an uncuffed endotracheal tube, and do not insert the tube too far down the trachea, which narrows distally in some species.

When positioning the bird for surgery, avoid taping the wings and legs in full extension as this can inhibit both respiratory movements and venous return. Birds should be handled gently at all times, taking particular care to avoid obstructing respiratory movements, since even short periods of apnoea can result in hypoxia. As with small mammals, care must be taken to avoid laying instruments across the chest or resting the operator's hands on the bird, since this can easily impede respiration in small species.

In the postanaesthetic period, continued attention to maintaining body temperature is essential. Birds should recover in a heated incubator or cage (40°C for small birds, 35°C for larger, 0>250 g, species). The recovery area should be quiet, with subdued lighting. Prolonged recovery can be associated with episodes of wing flapping, and if not restrained, the bird may injure itself. Placing a temporary bandage or cloth around the wings can help to control this problem. Such difficulties can be largely avoided, however, by using isoflurane or sevoflurane for anaesthesia, since recovery from these agents is extremely rapid. Very little information is available concerning the use of analgesics for postoperative pain relief in birds. No clinical trials of their efficacy have been undertaken, and only very limited data are available from analgesiometry (Machin, 2005). Pharmacokinetic data are available for aspirin, flunixin, and meloxicam (Baert and De Backer, 2003). Suggestions based on clinical impression and an articular pain model include buprenorphine (0.05 mg/kg im), butorphanol (2–4 mg/kg im), or the NSAIDs flunixin (3 mg/kg), ketoprofen (12 mg/kg) (Hawkins and Paul-Murphy, 2011; Hocking et al., 2005), or meloxicam (2 mg/kg) (Desmarchelier et al., 2012). However, care should be taken when using NSAIDs in birds, since toxicity of this class of analgesic appears higher in some species (Cuthbert et al., 2007). Surveys of analgesic use by veterinarians suggest that meloxicam may be the NSAID of choice in terms of safety profile (Cuthbert et al., 2014). Dose rates of anaesthetics and analgesics are summarized in Table 6.26.

Preanaesthetic medication

Ketamine

Ketamine can be administered to a wide range of avian species, but its effects can vary considerably. In the domestic fowl, 15–20 mg/kg im produces immobilization and some individuals may be lightly anaesthetized (Lierz and Korbel, 2012). Following initial chemical restraint with ketamine, anaesthesia can be deepened using isoflurane. When using ketamine in small birds (e.g. small finches, body weight, 20–49 g), the required dose (30–40 mg/kg) is best administered by diluting the commercial veterinary preparation with saline to provide a 10 mg/mL solution. A volume of 0.1 mL/bird im will then provide heavy sedation and 0.2 mL/bird will produce light anaesthesia.

General anaesthesia

Injectable agents

Ketamine combinations: Ketamine in combination with xylazine or medetomidine or dexmedetomidine will produce light to moderate surgical anaesthesia in birds. As with ketamine alone, the effects vary between species, and it may be necessary to carry out a pilot study to assess the response of the species that are to be anaesthetized. Allometric scaling of ketamine/xylazine doses appears to provide a reasonable guide to an appropriate dose rate, with doses ranging from 10 to 30 mg/kg ketamine and 2 to 6 mg/kg xylazine, smaller birds requiring higher dose rates per kilogram.

Ketamine (20–40 mg/kg) and diazepam (1–1.5 mg/kg) or midazolam (4 mg/kg), given by intramuscular injection, produce light to medium surgical anaesthesia in birds, but as with other ketamine combinations, dose rates vary with the body weight and species involved.

TABLE 6.26 Anaesthetic, sedative, and analgesic drugs for use in birds.

Drug	Dose rate	Effect	Duration of anaesthesia (min)	Sleep time (min)
Alphaxalone	6–10 mg/kg iv	Light anaesthesia	10–15	20–60
Buprenorphine	0.01–0.05 mg/kg im	Analgesia		
Butorphanol	2–4 mg/kg im	Analgesia		
Equithesin[a]	2.5 mL/kg im	Light to medium anaesthesia	20–30	60–120
Flunixin	1–10 mg/kg im	Analgesia		
Ketamine >1 kg	15–20 mg/kg im	Immobilization, some analgesia	20–30	30–90
Ketamine <1 kg	30–40 mg/kg im			
Ketamine/diazepam	20–40 mg/kg im + 1–1.5 mg/kg im	Medium surgical anaesthesia	20–30	30–90
Ketamine/ dexmedetomidine	5–10 mg/kg im + 25–50 µg/kg im	Light to medium surgical anaesthesia	10–30	30–60
Ketamine/medetomidine	5–10 mg/kg im + 50–100 µg/kg im	Light to medium surgical anaesthesia	10–30	30–60
Ketamine/midazolam	20–40 mg/kg im + 4 mg/kg im	Medium surgical anaesthesia	20–30	30–90
Ketamine/xylazine	5–30 mg/kg im + 0.2–5 mg/kg im	Light to medium surgical anaesthesia	10–30	30–60
Ketoprofen	2 mg/kg sc	Analgesia		
Propofol	5–10 mg/kg iv	Medium surgical anaesthesia	10	20

Duration of anaesthesia and sleep time (loss of righting reflex) are provided only as a general guide, since considerable species variation occurs. For recommended techniques, see text.
[a] See Appendix 3.

Alphaxalone has unpredictable effects when given intramuscularly, but it can be administered by the intravenous route (6–10 mg/kg) in some larger species to produce light surgical anaesthesia.

Propofol: Propofol produces smooth and rapid induction of anaesthesia if administered intravenously (up to 10 mg/kg). As in mammalian species, it should be administered slowly as rapid injection can cause apnoea (Machin, 2004). Further doses or a continuous infusion can be administered to prolong anaesthesia.

'Equithesin' (pentobarbital, chloral hydrate, and magnesium sulphate, see Appendix 3): Equithesin (2.5 mL/kg im) produces medium planes of surgical anaesthesia in pigeons and domestic fowl. It provides effective anaesthesia in domestic fowl chicks (0.15 mL/40 g chick ip), although occasional postanaesthetic mortality may occur.

Inhalational agents

Inhalational agents can be administered via a face mask or endotracheal tube, but in birds use can also be made of the caudal air sac; this can be of particular value if birds are placed in a stereotaxic frame for surgical procedures (Nilson et al., 2005).

Isoflurane: Isoflurane is widely regarded as the anaesthetic agent of choice for birds. It provides smooth and rapid induction of anaesthesia (4%–5%), and anaesthesia may be maintained with concentrations of 2%–3%. The depth of anaesthesia can be changed very rapidly by changing the inspired concentration, allowing birds to be maintained at an anaesthetic plane appropriate to the degree of surgical stimulus. This feature probably contributes to this agent's reputation for providing 'safe' anaesthesia, since unnecessarily deep planes of anaesthesia can be avoided. Induction can be achieved using a face mask or by placing the bird in an anaesthetic chamber. Recovery is rapid, and usually free from involuntary excitement.

Sevoflurane: Sevoflurane appears nonirritant in many species of birds, and face mask induction is smooth and rapid. Recovery also seems smoother and more rapid than with other agents. Induction and maintenance concentrations are similar to those in mammals (7%–8% and 3%–4%).

Halothane: Halothane can be used to provide surgical anaesthesia in birds, but the margin of safety appears to be considerably less than that provided by isoflurane. In addition, recovery is more prolonged, and birds may be inappetent. Provided the bird is observed carefully, however, induction with 3%–4% halothane and maintenance with 1.5%–2% provides reasonably safe and effective anaesthesia.

Reptiles

Anaesthesia of many species of reptiles can be complicated due to their ability to hold their breath for several minutes. This can slow the speed of induction when using volatile anaesthetics, or make their use impracticable, and can cause alarm when breath holding occurs after administration of injectable agents. Breath holding is commonly seen in snakes and chelonians and some species of lizards. Once anaesthesia has been induced, intubation is relatively simple as the larynx is easily visualized. This should be undertaken as a routine procedure, since in many reptiles the glottis may close as anaesthesia is deepened. Ventilation can be assisted if required, but only low inflation pressures are needed (usually less than 10 cm water; Longley, 2008).

Recovery from anaesthesia in these species is particularly influenced by environmental temperature; however, it is not advisable to try to accelerate recovery by placing the animals in a very warm environment. Animals are best recovered in their preferred optimum temperature range, and this varies with different species of reptiles. Small snakes should be fasted for 24 h before anaesthesia, and larger species should be deprived of food for 7 days. Chelonians and lizards do not require preanaesthetic fasting.

General anaesthesia

Injectable agents

Ketamine: Ketamine is the most widely used injectable anaesthetic for reptiles, producing light to moderate anaesthesia in most species. In snakes, doses of 50 mg/kg im produce sedation and 50–80 mg/kg im results in light to moderate anaesthesia. The effects of ketamine may persist for 1–2 days. Chelonians are usually lightly anaesthetized at dose rates of 60 mg/kg im, although once again recovery can take up to 24 h. Lizards are generally lightly anaesthetized at dose rates of 25–50 mg/kg im, and recovery may take up to 6 h. In all species, anaesthesia may be deepened by administration of volatile anaesthetics. It has also been recommended that better results are obtained by using lower dose rates (5–20 mg/kg) in combination with benzodiazepines or alpha$_2$ agonists (Mosley, 2005; Sladky and Mans, 2012).

Alphaxalone and propofol: Alphaxalone (5–9 mg/kg iv, 10–20 mg/kg im) can be used to produce surgical anaesthesia and is particularly effective in chelonians (Sladky and Mans, 2012). Propofol is now considered the anaesthetic of choice in reptiles (Longley, 2008), provided that it can be administered by the intravenous or intraosseous route (12–15 mg/kg iv, chelonians; 5–10 mg/kg, other reptiles).

Inhalational agents

Sevoflurane, isoflurane, halothane, and methoxyflurane can all be used to produce safe and effective anaesthesia. Use of an anaesthetic chamber is convenient for most smaller species of reptiles. Anaesthesia can then be maintained using a face mask or, preferably, the animal can be intubated and maintained on an appropriate anaesthetic breathing system.

Amphibia

Anaesthesia of amphibia can be achieved either by injection of anaesthetic or administration by inhalation. Alternatively, the animal can be placed in water or a moist environment and liquid anaesthetic or anaesthetic vapour added. Absorption occurs through the skin, resulting in induction of anaesthesia. During anaesthesia and recovery, the skin must be kept moist in frogs and newts, but complete immersion in water must be avoided until the animal has regained consciousness, otherwise it might drown. Preanaesthetic fasting is not necessary.

Hypothermia has been suggested as a suitable means of immobilizing amphibia for surgery, but this technique is not considered humane since the degree of analgesia produced is unknown.

General anaesthesia

Injectable agents

Immersion in tricaine methanesulphonate (MS 222) rapidly induces anaesthesia. The concentration of agent required ranges from 0.2 to 0.5 g/L for larvae and newts, 1 to 2 g/L for adult frogs and salamanders, and is 3 g/L for toads. The animal can then be removed from the anaesthetic solution. Anaesthesia generally lasts for 18–30 min, and can be prolonged by applying anaesthetic solution to the skin. During anaesthesia and recovery, the skin should be kept moist. Recovery usually occurs within 30–90 min and this can be reduced by washing the animal with water to remove surplus anaesthetic. The solution should be buffered to a pH of 7–7.4 before use, and this is easily achieved by addition of sodium bicarbonate.

Inhalational agents

Methoxyflurane can be used to provide safe and effective anaesthesia in amphibia, by exposure to the vapour in an anaesthetic chamber. During induction, the base of the chamber should be lined with moist cotton wool to prevent drying of the skin.

Fish

Fish are most easily anaesthetized by immersion in anaesthetic solution. Since these animals may be sensitive to sudden changes in pH and temperature, it may be advisable to use some of the water from their normal tank to fill the anaesthetic chamber (Sneddon, 2012). The induction tank should be aerated using a standard aquarium pump and airstone. Following induction of anaesthesia, the fish can be removed from the solution of anaesthetic and wrapped in moist gauze to prevent desiccation, and any procedure should be undertaken rapidly. For some procedures, it is possible to position the fish so that its gills remain submerged in anaesthetic solution. Alternatively, a more complex system, in which oxygenated anaesthetic solution is passed over the gills, can be constructed. A simpler recirculating system has been described (Longley, 2008). It is important to minimize handling of the fish during anaesthesia, since the skin is easily damaged, resulting in infections postoperatively. Fish should be fasted for 24–48 h prior to anaesthesia, as they may vomit and this can interfere with gill function.

The signs of onset of anaesthesia in fish have been described in detail (Sneddon, 2012) and differ significantly from mammals. Briefly, after loss of equilibrium and muscle tone, and onset of very shallow opercular movements, the response to pressure on the muscles at the tail base is reduced, but not abolished. At this stage, the fish can be removed from the anaesthetic solution and surgery or other manipulations carried out. If surgical stimuli cause muscle spasms, then either the fish can be returned to the anaesthetic solution, or additional solution can be dripped or sprayed over the gills, for example, by placing a drip in the buccal cavity. Overdosage is indicated by loss of regular opercular movements and occasional exaggerated respiratory movements. Cardiac arrest follows in 1–2 min unless the fish is resuscitated. This can be achieved either by flushing the mouth, and hence the gills, with fresh water, or by placing the fish in a tank of fresh water and moving it back and forth with its mouth open.

General anaesthesia

Injectable agents

Tricaine methanesulphonate (MS222): Tricaine is used for induction and maintenance of anaesthesia of a wide range of fish species (Carter et al., 2011; Topic Popovic et al., 2012). It is administered as a 25–300 mg/L solution, by immersion; the concentration used determines the depth of anaesthesia. Most small to medium-sized fish (e.g. goldfish, trout) require 100 mg/L for surgical anaesthesia. Anaesthesia is induced in around 2 min, and recovery occurs about 5 min after removal from the anaesthetic solution. The anaesthetic solution should be buffered before use, using sodium bicarbonate. The effects of MS222 have been evaluated in zebra fish embryos for both short- and long-term (24 h) immobilization (Rombough, 2007). MS222, in common with several other anaesthetics has been shown to be aversive in fish, and etomidate has been recommended as an alternative (Readman et al., 2013).

Etomidate: Etomidate has been shown to be nonaversive in fish (Readman et al., 2013) and to produce safe and effective anaesthesia (Kazuń and Siwicki, 2012). Dose rates vary between species, but are generally 2.0–4.0 mg/L (Amend et al., 1982).

Benzocaine: Benzocaine should be administered as a freshly prepared solution of 200 mg benzocaine in 5 mL acetone, which when added to 8 L of water provides a solution of 25 ppm (25 mg/L). This concentration is sedative, enabling minor manipulations to be undertaken. Higher concentrations (50 ppm, 50 mg/L) induce surgical anaesthesia.

Appendix 1

Physiological data

	Rat	Mouse	Gerbil	Hamster	Guinea pig	Rabbit	Dog
Adult body weight	250–350 g	30–40 g	90–100 g	100–150 g	500–1000 g	3–6 kg	15–20 kg
Body temperature	38°C	37.4°C	39°C	37.4°C	38–39°C	38–39°C	38.3°C
Respiration rate	80 min^{-1}	180 min^{-1}	90 min^{-1}	80 min^{-1}	120 min^{-1}	55 min^{-1}	25 min^{-1}
Resting heart rate	350 min^{-1}	570 min^{-1}	260–300 min^{-1}	350 min^{-1}	155 min^{-1}	220 min^{-1}	100 min^{-1}

	Cat	Ferret	Pig	Sheep	Goat	Primate (marmoset)	Primate (rhesus)
Adult body weight	3–5 kg	500–1000 g	40–200 kg	60–80 kg	40–100 kg	500 g	8–12 kg
Body temperature	38.6°C	39°C	39°C	39.1°C	39.4°C	38.5–40°C	37–39°C
Respiration rate	26 min^{-1}	33–36 min^{-1}	12–18 min^{-1}	20 min^{-1}	20 min^{-1}	min^{-1}	35 min^{-1}
Resting heart rate	150 min^{-1}	250 min^{-1}	220 min^{-1}	75 min^{-1}	80 min^{-1}	225 min^{-1}	150 min^{-1}

Appendix 2

Estimation of required quantities of volatile anaesthetics and anaesthetic gases

Oxygen: Oxygen cylinders are coloured black with a white top segment in the United Kingdom and green in the United States. A size E cylinder, when full contains approximately 680 L of oxygen, sufficient for 340 h use at 2 L/min. The quantity of gas remaining (in litres) in a size E cylinder can be estimated from the pressure, in psi, multiplied by 0.3.

Nitrous oxide cylinders (coloured blue in the United Kingdom and in the United States) contain liquid N_2O, and the pressure reading on the pressure reducing valve does not indicate whether the cylinder is full or almost empty. When the pressure does fall, it will do so very rapidly as the cylinder empties. A full size E cylinder of nitrous oxide can deliver approximately 1800 L of gas (at room temperature), in other words 900 h at 2 L/min.

Volatile anaesthetics: The quantity of volatile anaesthetic required can be calculated from the molecular weight (1 g mole of anaesthetic produces 22.4 L of vapour at standard temperature and pressure) and the density of the liquid anaesthetic. For the most commonly used anaesthetics, at a temperature of 21°C:

Agent	Liquid density (g/mL)	Molecular weight	Volume from 1 mL (L)	Concentration for maintenance of anaesthesia	Quantity of agent (mL/min) for maintenance at 4 L/min fresh gas flow
Desflurane	1.47	168	0.210	9%	1.7
Enflurane	1.52	184.5	0.198	3%	0.6
Halothane	1.87	197	0.228	1.5%	0.26
Isoflurane	1.5	184.5	0.195	2%	0.41
Methoxyflurane	1.43	146	0.235	0.4%	0.07
Sevoflurane	1.52	200.1	0.183	4%	0.87

From this, and a knowledge of the price/bottle, the relative costs of the anaesthetics can be calculated. At the time of publication, typical costs of the agents available in the United Kingdom were

Agent	Cost per unit	Cost/mL	Cost/min with 4L/min flow (see above table)
Desflurane	£76/240 mL	£0.32/mL	£0.54
Halothane	£25/250 mL	£0.10/mL	£0.26
Isoflurane	£25/250 mL	£0.10/mL	£0.41
Sevoflurane	£150/250 mL	£0.60/mL	£0.52

Appendix 3

Examples of dilutions of some commonly used anaesthetic mixtures for small rodents

- Look up dose of each drug in mg kg^{-1}.
- Convert to mL/kg according to concentration of stock solution.
- Convert to mL/100 g (rats), mL/10 g (mice).
- Add diluent (water for injection, WFI) to make an appropriate volume per animal (e.g. 0.2 mL/100 g ip for rats, 0.1 mL/10 g ip for mice).

Before making up these mixtures, check that the strengths of the stock solutions you are using are the same as those used here (ketamine, 100 mg/mL, xylazine, 20 mg/mL, medetomidine, 1 mg/mL, dexmedetomidine, 0.5 mg/mL, midazolam, 5 mg/mL, acepromazine, 2 mg/mL or 10 mg/mL, fentanyl, 50 μg/mL, atipamezole 5 mg/mL and butorphanol 10 mg/mL).

Rat

Except for fentanyl/medetomidine and fentanyl/fluanisone/midazolam and the reversal agents, the volumes listed below make up sufficient mixture for animals with a total bodyweight of 1 kg (i.e. 4–5 young adults). The dilutions are adjusted to provide a volume for injection of 0.2 mL/100 g.

Ketamine/xylazine

Dose (mg kg^{-1}): 75 mg kg^{-1} ketamine + 10 mg kg^{-1} xylazine i/p.
Dose (mL/kg): 0.75 mL (75 mg) ketamine + 0.5 mL (10 mg) xylazine + 0.75 mL WFI provides approximately 4–5 doses of 0.2 mL/100 g of this mixture.

Ketamine/medetomidine

75 mg kg^{-1} ketamine + 0.5 mg kg^{-1} medetomidine i/p.
0.75 mL (75 mg) ketamine + 0.5 mL (0.5 mg) medetomidine + 0.75 mL WFI gives provides approximately 4–5 doses of 0.2 mL/100 g of this mixture.

Ketamine/dexmedetomidine

$75\,mg\,kg^{-1}$ ketamine $+0.25\,mg\,kg^{-1}$ dexmedetomidine i/p.
$0.75\,mL$ ($75\,mg$) ketamine $+0.5\,mL$ ($0.25\,mg$) dexmedetomidine $+0.75\,mL$ WFI provides approximately 4–5 doses of $0.2\,mL/100\,g$ of this mixture.

Ketamine/midazolam

$75\,mg\,kg^{-1}$ ketamine $+5\,mg\,kg^{-1}$ midazolam i/p.
$0.75\,mL$ ($75\,mg$) ketamine $+1\,mL$ ($5\,mg$) midazolam $+0.25\,mL$ WFI provides approximately 4–5 doses of $0.2\,mL/100\,g$ of this mixture.

Ketamine/acepromazine

$75\,mg\,kg^{-1}$ ketamine $+2.5\,mg\,kg^{-1}$ acepromazine i/p.
$0.75\,mL$ ($75\,mg$) ketamine $+0.25\,mL$ ($2.5\,mg$) acepromazine $+1\,mL$ WFI provides approximately 4–5 doses of $0.2\,mL/100\,g$ of this mixture.

Fentanyl/fluanisone ("Hypnorm")/midazolam

mL "Hypnorm" ($0.315\,mg$ fentanyl/mL; $10\,mg$ fluanisone/mL) $+1\,mL$ midazolam ($5\,mg$) $+2\,mL$ WFI provides approximately 4–5 doses of $0.33\,mL/100\,g$ i/p of this mixture. (Add water for injection to "Hypnorm" *before* adding midazolam.)

Fentanyl/medetomidine

$300\,\mu g\,kg^{-1}$ fentanyl $+300\,\mu g\,kg^{-1}$ medetomidine i/p.
$2\,mL$ ($100\,\mu g$) fentanyl $+0.1\,mL$ ($100\,\mu g$) medetomidine gives 1 dose of $0.63\,mL/100\,g$.

Fentanyl/dexmedetomidine

$300\,\mu g\,kg^{-1}$ fentanyl $+150\,\mu g\,kg^{-1}$ dexmedetomidine i/p.
$2\,mL$ ($100\,\mu g$) fentanyl $+0.1\,mL$ ($50\,\mu g$) medetomidine gives 1 dose of $0.63\,mL/100\,g$.

Reversal for fentanyl/medetomidine or fentanyl/ dexmedetomidine

Butorphanol

$2\,mg\,kg^{-1}$ sc.
$0.2\,mL$ ($2\,mg$) $+0.8\,mL$ WFI provides approximately 4–5 doses of $0.1\,mL/100\,g$.

Atipamezole

1 mg kg^{-1} sc.
0.2 mL (1 mg) + 0.8 mL WFI provides approximately 4–5 doses of 0.1 mL/100 g.

Mouse

The quantities listed below make up sufficient material for animals with a total body weight of 500 g (i.e. 15–20 young adults). Except for "Hypnorm"/midazolam, the dilution is adjusted to provide a volume of injectate of 0.1 mL/10 g.

Ketamine/xylazine

100 mg kg^{-1} ketamine + 10 mg kg^{-1} xylazine i/p.
0.5 mL (75 mg) ketamine + 0.25 mL (5 mg) xylazine + 4.25 mL WFI gives approximately 17 doses of 0.1 mL/10 g.

Ketamine/midazolam

100 mg kg^{-1} ketamine + 5 mg kg^{-1} midazolam i/p.
0.5 mL (50 mg) ketamine + 0.5 mL (2.5 mg) midazolam + 3.75 mL WFI gives approximately 17 doses of 0.1 mL/10 g.

Ketamine/acepromazine

100 mg kg^{-1} ketamine + 5 mg kg^{-1} acepromazine i/p.
0.5 mL (50 mg) ketamine + 1.25 mL (2.5 mg) acepromazine + 3 mL WFI provides approximately 17 doses of 0.1 mL/10 g of this mixture.

Fentanyl/fluanisone ("Hypnorm")/midazolam

mL "Hypnorm" (0.315 mg fentanyl/mL; 10 mg fluanisone/mL) + 1 mL midazolam (5 mg) + 2 mL WFI provides approximately 4–5 doses of 0.1 mL/10 g i/p of this mixture.

Ketamine/medetomidine

75 mg kg^{-1} ketamine + 1 mg kg^{-1} medetomidine.
0.38 mL (38 mg) ketamine + 0.5 mL (0.5 mg) medetomidine + 4.22 mL provides approximately 17 doses of 0.1 mL/10 g of this mixture.

Ketamine/dexmedetomidine

75 mg kg^{-1} ketamine + 0.5 mg kg^{-1} dexmedetomidine.
0.38 mL (38 mg) ketamine + 0.5 mL (0.25 mg) dexmedetomidine + 4.22 mL provides approximately 17 doses of 0.1 mL/10 g of this mixture.

Guinea-pig

The quantities listed below make up sufficient material for animals with a total body weight of 1 kg (i.e. 2 young adults). Except for ketamine/acepromazine and "Hypnorm"/midazolam, the dilution is adjusted to provide a volume of injectate of $2\,mL\,kg^{-1}$.

Ketamine/xylazine

$40\,mg\,kg^{-1}$ ketamine + $5\,mg\,kg^{-1}$ xylazine i/p.
0.4 mL (40 mg) ketamine + 0.25 mL (5 mg) xylazine + 1.35 mL WFI provides enough mixture for 1 kg at $2.0\,mL\,kg^{-1}$.

Ketamine/acepromazine

$125\,mg\,kg^{-1}$ Ketamine + $5\,mg\,kg^{-1}$ Acepromazine i/p.
1.25 mL (125 mg) ketamine + 2.5 mL (5 mg) acepromazine + 0.25 mL WFI provides enough mixture for 1 kg at $4.0\,mL\,kg^{-1}$.

Fentanyl/fluanisone ("Hypnorm")/midazolam

2 mL "Hypnorm" (0.315 mg fentanyl/mL; 10 mg fluanisone/mL) + 2 mL midazolam (5 mg) + 4 mL WFI provides enough mixture for 1 kg at $8\,mL\,kg^{-1}$ i/p.

Ketamine/medetomidine

$40\,mg\,kg^{-1}$ ketamine + $0.5\,mg\,kg^{-1}$ medetomidine.
0.4 mL (40 mg) ketamine + 0.5 mL (0.5 mg) medetomidine + 1.1 mL WFI provides enough mixture for 1 kg at $2.0\,mL\,kg^{-1}$.

Ketamine/dexmedetomidine

$40\,mg\,kg^{-1}$ ketamine + $0.25\,mg\,kg^{-1}$ dexmedetomidine.
0.4 mL (40 mg) ketamine + 0.5 mL (0.25 mg) dexmedetomidine + 1.1 mL WFI provides enough mixture for 1 kg at $2.0\,mL\,kg^{-1}$.

Birds

Equithesin

5.25 g chloral hydrate + 12.5 mL absolute alcohol.
20.25 mL pentobarbital (60 mg/mL).
49.5 mL propylene glycol.
2.65 g magnesium sulphate + 25 mL sterile water for injection.

Mix all of the above and make up total volume to 125 mL with sterile water for injection. Dose rate of mixture is $2.5\,mL\,kg^{-1}$ i/m.

Appendix 4

Manufacturers of equipment and other items illustrated or cited in the text. If not listed, products are marketed via third party distribution companies.

3M (www.3M.com)
(Micropore tape)

3M Bair Hugger (www.bairhugger.com)
(Bair Hugger forced air warming blankets)

AAS (Advanced Anaesthesia Services) and Darvall Vet
(www.aasmedical.com, www.darvallvet.com)
info@aasmedical.com.au
Anaesthetic equipment, warming devices, vaporisers

Columbus Instruments (www.colinst.com)
(Low sample volume capnograph)
950 N. Hague Ave., Columbus, OH 43204, United States

Hallowell EMC (www.hallowell.com)
(Rodent intubation systems, ventilators)
239 West St., Pittsfield, MA 01201, United States

Harvard Apparatus (www.harvardapparatus.com)
(Infusion pumps, heating blankets, anaesthetic equipment)
22 Cambridge Science Park, Milton Road, Cambridge CB4 0FJ, United Kingdom

Kent Scientific Corporation (www.kentscientific.com)
(Anaesthetic and monitoring equipment)
1116 Litchfield Street, Torrington, CT 06790, United States

Nonin Medical, Inc. (www.nonin.com)
(Pulse oximeter)
13700 1st Avenue North, Plymouth, MN 55441-5443, United States

Penlon Limited (www.penlon.com)
(Anaesthetic circuits, vaporizers)
Abingdon Science Park, Barton Lane, Abingdon OX14 3PH, United Kingdom

Petlife International Ltd. (www.petlifeonline.co.uk)
(Veterinary bedding)
Unit 2
Cavendish Road, Bury St Edmunds, Suffolk IP33 3TE, United Kingdom

SA Instruments Inc. (www.i4sa.com)
(MRI compatible monitors)
PO Box 740, Stony Brook, NY 11790, United States

Sigma-Aldrich Company Ltd. (www.sigmaaldrich.com)
(Anaesthetic drugs—e.g. inactin)
The Old Brickyard
New Road, Gillingham, Dorset SP8 4XT, United Kingdom

Starr Life Sciences Corporation (www.starrlifesciences.com)
(Mouseox pulse oximeter)
333 Alleheny Avenue, Suite 300, Oakmont, PA 15139, United States

Smiths Medical (www.smiths-medical.com)
5200 Upper Metro Place, Suite 200, Dublin, OH 43017, United States

Smiths Medical International (UK) (www.smiths-medical.com)
(Portex low-dead space connectors, endotracheal tubes)
500 Eureka Park, Lower Pemberton, Ashford, Kent TN25 4BF, United Kingdom

Thames Medical (www.thamesmedical.com)
Anaesthetic monitoring equipment

VetEquip, Inc. (http://www.vetequip.com)
(Rat nose cone, anaesthetic equipment)
1452 N Vasco Rd. #303, Livermore, CA 94551, United States

VetaPharma (www.vetapharma.co.uk)
('Hypnorm')
Sherburn Enterprise Park, Sherburn-in-Elmet, Leeds LS25 6NB, United Kingdom

VetTech Solutions (www.vet-tech.co.uk, info@vet-tech.co.uk)
(Waste anaesthetic gas scavenging systems, ventilators, anaesthetic chambers)

Vetronic Services (www.vetronic.co.uk, enquiries@vetronic.co.uk)
(Merlin ventilator, capnography)

Vygon Ltd. (www.vygon.com)
(Connectors, catheters)

References

Abdelkhalek, A.S., et al., 2021. Anesthetic protocols for urodynamic studies of the lower urinary tract in small rodents—a systematic review. PLoS ONE 16 (6), e0253192.

Abelson, K.S., et al., 2012. Voluntary ingestion of nut paste for administration of buprenorphine in rats and mice. Lab. Anim. 46 (4), 349–351.

Abrão, J., et al., 2014. Effect of local anaesthetic infiltration with bupivacaine and ropivacaine on wound healing: a placebo-controlled study. Int. Wound J. 11 (4), 379–385.

Acierno, M.J., et al., 2010. Agreement between directly measured blood pressure and pressures obtained with three veterinary-specific oscillometric units in cats. J. Am. Vet. Med. Assoc. 237 (4), 402–406.

Adam, H.K., et al., 1980. Pharmacokinetics in laboratory animals of ICI 35 868, a new iv anaesthetic agent. Br. J. Anaesth. 52 (8), 743–746.

Adetunji, A., et al., 2009. Evaluation of diazepam-ketamine-pentazocine anaesthesia in rabbits. Afr. J. Biomed. Res. 12 (3), 237–240.

Aeschbacher, G., Webb, A.I., 1993. Propofol in rabbits. 2. Long-term anesthesia. Lab. Anim. Sci. 43 (4), 328–335.

Affaitati, G., et al., 2002. Effects of tramadol on behavioural indicators of colic pain in a rat model of ureteral calculosis. Fundam. Clin. Pharmacol. 16 (1), 23–30.

Ailiani, A.C., et al., 2014. Quantifying the effects of inactin vs isoflurane anesthesia on gastrointestinal motility in rats using dynamic magnetic resonance imaging and spatio-temporal maps. Neurogastroenterol. Motil. 26 (10), 1477–1486.

Albrecht, M., et al., 2014. Effects of isoflurane, ketamine-xylazine and a combination of medetomidine, midazolam and fentanyl on physiological variables continuously measured by telemetry in Wistar rats. BMC Vet. Res. 10 (1), 198.

Allen, D.G., et al., 1986. Evaluation of a xylazine-ketamine hydrochloride combination in the cat. Can. J. Vet. Res. 50 (1), 23–26.

Allison, S.O., et al., 2007. Assessment of buprenorphine, carprofen, and their combination for postoperative analgesia in olive baboons (*Papio anubis*). J. Am. Assoc. Lab. Anim. Sci. 46 (3), 24.

Allweiler, S., et al., 2010. The use of propofol and sevoflurane for surgical anaesthesia in New Zealand White rabbits. Lab. Anim. 44 (2), 113–117.

Al-Shaikh, B., Stacey, S.G., 2018. Essentials of Equipment in Anaesthesia, Critical Care, and Peri-Operative Medicine, fifth ed. Elsevier Health Sciences.

Alstrup, A.K.O., Smith, D.F., 2013. Anaesthesia for positron emission tomography scanning of animal brains. Lab. Anim. 47 (1), 12–18.

Alves, H.C., et al., 2007. Intraperitoneal propofol and propofol fentanyl, sufentanil and remifentanil combinations for mouse anaesthesia. Lab. Anim. 41 (3), 329–336.

Alves, H.C., et al., 2009. Intraperitoneal anaesthesia with propofol, medetomidine and fentanyl in mice. Lab. Anim. 43 (1), 27–33.

Alves, H.N.C., et al., 2010. Anesthesia with intraperitoneal propofol, medetomidine, and fentanyl in rats. J. Am. Assoc. Lab. Anim. Sci. 49 (4), 454–459.

Amarpal, X., et al., 2010. Evaluation of xylazine, acepromazine and medetomidine with ketamine for general anaesthesia in rabbits. Scand. J. Lab. Anim. Sci. 37 (3), 223–229.

Amend, D.F., et al., 1982. Etomidate: effective dosages for a new fish anesthetic. Trans. Am. Fish. Soc. 111 (3), 337–341.

Amornyotin, S., 2014. Ketamine: pharmacology revisited. Int. J. Anesthesiol. Res. 2, 42–44.

Andaluz, A., et al., 2012. The effects on cardio-respiratory and acid-base variables of the anaesthetic alfaxalone in a 2-hydroxypropyl-β-cyclodextrin (HPCD) formulation in sheep. Vet. J. 191 (3), 389–392.

Andreoni, V., Giorgi, M., 2009. Transdermal lidocaine patch 5% and lidocaine cream 5%: a PK/PD approach in the horse. Med. Weter. 65 (9), 612–616.

Andrews, N., et al., 2012. Spontaneous burrowing behaviour in the rat is reduced by peripheral nerve injury or inflammation associated pain. Eur. J. Pain 16 (4), 485–495.

Andrews, D.D., et al., 2020. A comparison of buprenorphine, sustained release buprenorphine, and high concentration buprenorphine in male New Zealand white rabbits. J. Am. Assoc. Lab. Anim. Sci. 59 (5), 546–556.

Antognini, J.F., et al., 2005. Movement as an index of anesthetic depth in humans and experimental animals. Comp. Med. 55, 413–418.

Appadu, B., Vaidya, A., 2008. Monitoring techniques: neuromuscular blockade and depth of anaesthesia. Anaesth. Intensive Care Med. 9 (6), 247–250.

Arenillas, M., Gomez de Segura, I.A., 2018. Anaesthetic effects of alfaxalone administered intraperitoneally alone or combined with dexmedetomidine and fentanyl in the rat. Lab. Anim. 52 (6), 588-598.

Arras, M., et al., 2001. Optimization of intraperitoneal injection anesthesia in mice: drugs, dosages, adverse effects, and anesthesia depth. Comp. Med. 51 (5), 443–456.

Arras, M., et al., 2007. Assessment of post-laparotomy pain in laboratory mice by telemetric recording of heart rate and heart rate variability. BMC Vet. Res. 3 (1), 16.

Aung, H.H., et al., 2004. Methylnaltrexone prevents morphine-induced kaolin intake in the rat. Life Sci. 74 (22), 2685–2691.

Austin, V.C., et al., 2005. Confounding effects of anesthesia on functional activation in rodent brain: a study of halothane and α-chloralose anesthesia. Neuroimage 24 (1), 92–100.

Ayre, P., 1937. Anaesthesia for hare-lip and cleft palate operations on babies. Br. J. Surg. 25 (97), 131–132.

Bachmanov, A.A., et al., 2002. Food intake, water intake, and drinking spout side preference of 28 mouse strains. Behav. Genet. 32 (6), 435–443.

Baert, K., De Backer, P., 2003. Comparative pharmacokinetics of three non-steroidal anti-inflammatory drugs in five bird species. Comp. Biochem. Physiol. C Toxicol. Pharmacol. 134 (1), 25–33.

Bagis, H., et al., 2004. Exposure to warmer postoperative temperatures reduces hypothermia caused by anaesthesia and significantly increases the implantation rate of transferred embryos in the mouse. Lab. Anim. 38 (1), 50–54.

Bailey, J.M., 1997. Context-sensitive half-times and other decrement times of inhaled anesthetics. Anesth. Analg. 85 (3), 681–686.

Bain, J.A., Spoerel, W.E., 1972. A streamlined anaesthetic system. Can. Anaesth. Soc. J. 19 (4), 426–435.

Bainbridge, D., et al., 2012. Perioperative and anaesthetic-related mortality in developed and developing countries: a systematic review and meta-analysis. Lancet 380 (9847), 1075–1081.

Bakker, J., et al., 2013. Comparison of three different sedative-anaesthetic protocols (ketamine, ketamine-medetomidine and alphaxalone) in common marmosets (*Callithrix jacchus*). BMC Vet. Res. 9 (1), 113.

Banchi, P., et al., 2020. Reliability and construct validity of a composite pain scale for rabbit (CAN-CRS) in a clinical environment. PLoS ONE 15 (4), e0221377.

Banchi, P., et al., 2022. A composite scale to recognize abdominal pain and its variation over time in response to analgesia in rabbits. Vet. Anaesth. Analg. 49 (3), 323–328.

Banknieder, A.R., et al., 1978. Comparison of ketmine with the combination of ketamine and xylazine for effective anesthesia in the rhesus monkey (*Macaca mulatta*). Lab. Anim. Sci. 28 (6), 742–745.

Baral, P., et al., 2019. Pain and immunity: implications for host defence. Nat. Rev. Immunol. 19 (7), 433–447.

Bar-Ilan, A., Marder, J., 1980. Acid base status in unanesthetized, unrestrained guinea pigs. Pflugers Arch. 384 (1), 93–97.

Barletta, M., et al., 2016. Determination of the minimum alveolar concentration of isoflurane that blunts adrenergic responses in sheep and evaluation of the effects of fentanyl. Am. J. Vet. Res. 77 (2), 119–126.

Barter, L.S., Hopper, K., 2011. Transcutaneous monitor approximates PaCO2 but not PaO2 in anesthetized rabbits. Vet. Anaesth. Analg. 38 (6), 568–575.

Barter, L.S., et al., 2004. Animal dependence of inhaled anaesthetic requirements in cats. Br. J. Anaesth. 92 (2), 275–277.

Bartocci, M., et al., 2006. Response to David Bowsher's comment: the jump from cerebral neurovascular events to the subjective feeling of pain in neonates. Pain 126 (1–3), 321–322. Available at: http://linkinghub.elsevier.com/retrieve/pii/S0304395906003848.

Barzago, M.M., et al., 1994. Respiratory and hemodynamic functions, blood-gas parameters, and acid-base balance of ketamine-xylazine anesthetized guinea pigs. Lab. Anim. Sci. 44 (6), 648–650.

Bass, L.M., et al., 2009. Comparison of femoral and auricular arterial blood pressure monitoring in pigs. Vet. Anaesth. Analg. 36 (5), 457–463.

Bateman, S.W., et al., 2008. Comparison of the analgesic efficacy of hydromorphone and oxymorphone in dogs and cats: a randomized blinded study. Vet. Anaesth. Analg. 35 (4), 341–347.

Bauer, D.J., et al., 2003. Acetaminophen as a postsurgical analgesic in rats: a practical solution to neophobia. Contemp. Top. Lab. Anim. Sci. 42 (2), 20–25.

Baumgartner, C., et al., 2010. Effects of medetomidine-midazolam-fentanyl IV bolus injections and its reversal by specific antagonists on cardiovascular function in rabbits. Can. J. Vet. Res. 74 (4), 286–298.

Baumgartner, C., et al., 2011. Comparison of dipyrone/propofol versus fentanyl/propofol anaesthesia during surgery in rabbits. Lab. Anim. 45 (1), 38–44.

Baysinger, A., et al., 2021. Proposed multidimensional pain outcome methodology to demonstrate analgesic drug efficacy and facilitate future drug approval for piglet castration. Anim. Health Res. Rev., 1–14.

Beck, C., et al., 2013. Evaluation of a new side-stream, low dead space, end-tidal carbon dioxide monitoring system in rats. Lab. Anim., 0023677213501657.

Bednarski, R.M., Muir, W., 2011. Capnography in veterinary medicine. Capnography, 272.

Beier, H., et al., 2007. Peritoneal microdialysis in freely moving rodents: an alternative to blood sampling for pharmacokinetic studies in the rat and the mouse. Eur. J. Pharm. Sci. 30 (1), 75–83.

Bellieni, C.V., 2021. Analgesia for fetal pain during prenatal surgery: 10 years of progress. Pediatr. Res. 89 (7), 1612–1618.

Bellieni, C.V., 2022. Foetal pain and anaesthesia during prenatal surgery. Clin. Exp. Obstet. Gynecol. 49 (4), 79.

Bellini, L., et al., 2014. Evaluation of three medetomidine-based protocols for chemical restraint and sedation for non-painful procedures in companion rats (*Rattus norvegicus*). Vet. J. 200 (3), 456–458.

Benato, L., et al., 2021. Development of the Bristol Rabbit Pain Scale (BRPS): a multidimensional composite pain scale specific to rabbits (*Oryctolagus cuniculus*). PLoS ONE 16 (6), e0252417.

Beninson, J.A., et al., 2018. Analgesic efficacy and hematologic effects of robenacoxib in mice. J. Am. Assoc. Lab. Anim. Sci. 57 (3), 258–267.

Bertrand, H.G., et al., 2016. Comparison of the effects of ketamine and fentanyl-midazolam-medetomidine for sedation of rhesus macaques (*Macaca mulatta*). BMC Vet. Res. 12 (1), 1–9.

Bertrand, H.G., et al., 2017a. Comparison of emergence times and quality between isoflurane and sevoflurane in rhesus macaque (*Macaca mulatta*) undergoing neurosurgical procedure. Lab. Anim. 51 (5), 518–525.

Bertrand, H.G., et al., 2017b. A combination of alfaxalone, medetomidine and midazolam for the chemical immobilization of Rhesus macaque (*Macaca mulatta*): preliminary results. J. Med. Primatol. 46 (6), 332–336.

Bertrand, H.G., et al., 2018. The use of desflurane for neurosurgical procedures in rhesus macaque (*Macaca mulatta*). Lab. Anim. 52 (3), 292–299.

Beyers, T.M., et al., 1991. Axonal degeneration and self-mutilation as a complication of the intramuscular use of ketamine and xylazine in rabbits. Lab. Anim. Sci. 41 (5), 519–520.

Beynen, A.C., et al., 1987. Assessment of discomfort in gallstone-bearing mice: a practical example of the problems encountered in an attempt to recognize discomfort in laboratory animals. Lab. Anim. 21 (1), 35–42.

Bigby, S.E., et al., 2017. The use of alfaxalone for premedication, induction and maintenance of anaesthesia in pigs: a pilot study. Vet. Anaesth. Analg. 44 (4), 905–909.

Bigeleisen, P.E., Wempe, M., 2001. Identification of the precipitate in alkalinized solutions of mepivacaine and bupivacaine at 37 °C. J. Clin. Pharm. Ther. 26 (3), 171–173.

Birch, J., et al., 2020. Dimensions of animal consciousness. Trends Cogn. Sci. 24 (10), 789–801.

Blaha, M.D., Leon, L.R., 2008. Effects of indomethacin and buprenorphine analgesia on the postoperative recovery of mice. J. Am. Assoc. Lab. Anim. Sci. 47 (4), 8–19.

Blake, D.W., et al., 1988. Haemodynamic and heart rate reflex responses to propofol in the rabbit comparison with Althesin. Br. J. Anaesth. 61 (2), 194–199.

Blevins, C.E., et al., 2021. Effects of oxygen supplementation on injectable and inhalant anesthesia in C57BL/6 mice. J. Am. Assoc. Lab. Anim. Sci. 60 (3), 289–297.

Blouin, A., Cormier, Y., 1987. Endotracheal intubation in guinea pigs by direct laryngoscopy. Lab. Anim. Sci. 37 (2), 244–245.

Bo, P., et al., 2003. Quantified EEG analysis monitoring in a novel model of general anaesthesia in rats. Brain Res. Protocol. 11 (3), 155–161.

Bongiovanni, T., et al., 2021. Systematic review and meta-analysis of the association between non-steroidal anti-inflammatory drugs and operative bleeding in the perioperative period. J. Am. Coll. Surg. 232 (5), 765–790.

Bonnet, F., Marret, E., 2007. Postoperative pain management and outcome after surgery. Best Pract. Res. Clin. Anaesthesiol. 21, 99–107.

Booij, L.H.D.J., et al., 2009. In vivo animal studies with sugammadex. Anaesthesia 64 (Suppl. 1(s1)), 38–44.

Borges, L.P., et al., 2016. Behavioral and cardiopulmonary effects of dexmedetomidine alone and in combination with butorphanol, methadone, morphine or tramadol in conscious sheep. Vet. Anaesth. Analg. 43 (5), 549–560.

Bosgraaf, C.A., et al., 2004. What's your diagnosis? Respiratory distress in rats. Lab. Anim. 33 (3), 21–22.

Bosiack, A.P., et al., 2010. Comparison of ultrasonic Doppler flow monitor, oscillometric, and direct arterial blood pressure measurements in ill dogs. J. Vet. Emerg. Crit. Care 20 (2), 207–215.

Botting, R., Ayoub, S.S., 2005. COX-3 and the mechanism of action of paracetamol/acetaminophen. Prostaglandins Leukot. Essent. Fatty Acids 72 (2), 85–87.

Bowdle, D.T.A., 1998. Adverse effects of opioid agonists and agonist-antagonists in anaesthesia. Drug Saf. 19 (3), 173–189.

Bowman, W.C., 2006. Neuromuscular block. Br. J. Pharmacol. 147 (Suppl. 1(S1)), S277–S286.

Bowsher, D., 2006. Pain activates cortical areas in the preterm newborn brain. Pain 126 (1–3), 320–321.

Box, P.G., Ellis, K.R., 1973. Use of CT1341 anaesthetic ("Saffan") in monkeys. Lab. Anim. 7 (2), 161–170.

Bradbury, A.G., Eddleston, M., Clutton, R.E., 2016. Pain management in pigs undergoing experimental surgery; a literature review (2012–4). Br. J. Anaesth. 116 (1), 37–45.

Bradfield, J.F., et al., 1992. Behavioral and physiologic effects of inapparent wound infection in rats. Lab. Anim. Sci. 42 (6), 572–578.

Bradley, M.P., et al., 2022. Evaluation of alfaxalone total intravenous anesthesia in rabbits (*Oryctolagus cuniculus*) premedicated with dexmedetomidine or dexmedetomidine and buprenorphine. Vet. Anaesth. Analg. 49 (3), 308–312.

Brammer, A., et al., 1993. A comparison of propofol with other injectable anaesthetics in a rat model for measuring cardiovascular parameters. Lab. Anim. 27 (3), 250–257.

Brattwall, M., et al., 2012. Brief review: theory and practice of minimal fresh gas flow anesthesia. Can. J. Anaesth. 59 (8), 785–797.

Brearley, J.C., et al., 1988. Propofol anaesthesia in cats. J. Small Anim. Pract. 29 (5), 315–322.

Breivik, H., 1994. Pain management. Baillieres Clin. Anaesthesiol. 8, 775–795.

Brioni, J.D., et al., 2017. A clinical review of inhalation anesthesia with sevoflurane: from early research to emerging topics. J. Anesth. 31 (5), 764–778.

Briscoe, J.A., Syring, R., 2004. Techniques for emergency airway and vascular access in special species. Semin. Avian Exot. Pet Med. 13 (3), 118–131.

Brodbelt, D.C., et al., 2008. The risk of death: the confidential enquiry into perioperative small animal fatalities. Vet. Anaesth. Analg. 35 (5), 365–373.

Brody, S., 1945. Metabolism and pulmonary ventilation in relation to body weight during growth. In: Bioenergetics and Growth: With Special Reference to the Efficiency Complex in Domestic Animals. Reinhold, New York, pp. 404–469.

Brosnan, R.J., et al., 2007. Anesthetic properties of carbon dioxide in the rat. Anesth. Analg. 105 (1), 103–106.

Brouwer, G.J., Snowdon, S.L., 1986. Breathing systems in current canine anaesthetic practice: a review. Vet. Anaesth. Analg. 14 (1), 152–168.

Brown, B.R., et al., 1974. Mechanisms of acute hepatic toxicity: chloroform, halothane, and glutathione. Anesthesiology 41 (6), 554–561.

Brown, J.N., et al., 1989. Blood pressure and other physiological responses in awake and anesthetized guinea pigs. Lab. Anim. Sci. 39 (2), 142–148.

Brunell, M.K., 2012. Comparison of noncontact infrared thermometry and 3 commercial subcutaneous temperature transponding microchips with rectal thermometry in rhesus macaques (*Macaca mulatta*). J. Am. Assoc. Lab. Anim. Sci. 51 (4), 479–484.

Bruniges, N., Yates, D., 2020. Effects of atipamezole dosage and timing of administration on recovery time and quality in cats following injectable anaesthesia incorporating ketamine. J. Feline Med. Surg. 22 (6), 589–597.

Brun-Pascaud, M., et al., 1982. Arterial blood gases and acid-base status in awake rats. Respir. Physiol. 48 (1), 45–57.

Brydges, N.M., et al., 2011. Environmental enrichment induces optimistic cognitive bias in rats. Anim. Behav. 81 (1), 169–175.

Buelke-Sam, J., et al., 1978. Comparative stability of physiological parameters during sustained anesthesia in rats. Lab. Anim. Sci. 28 (2), 157–162.

Bugnon, P., et al., 2016. What the literature tells us about score sheet design. Lab. Anim. 50 (6), 414–417.

Buitrago, S., et al., 2008. Safety and efficacy of various combinations of injectable anesthetics in BALB/c mice. J. Am. Assoc. Lab. Anim. Sci. 47 (1), 11–17.

Burnside, W.M., et al., 2013. A comparison of medetomidine and its active enantiomer dexmedetomidine when administered with ketamine in mice. BMC Vet. Res. 9 (1), 48.

Burwell, R.D., et al., 1992. Effects of aging on the diurnal pattern of water intake in rats. Behav. Neural Biol. 58 (3), 196–203.

Buscail, E., Deraison, C., 2022. Postoperative ileus: a pharmacological perspective. Br. J. Pharmacol. https://doi.org/10.1111/bph.15800.

Busch, U., et al., 1998. Pharmacokinetics of meloxicam in animals and the relevance to humans. Drug Metab. Dispos. 26 (6), 576–584.

Bushnell, M.C., Čeko, M., Low, L.A., 2013. Cognitive and emotional control of pain and its disruption in chronic pain. Nat. Rev. Neurosci. 14 (7), 502–511.

Byrd, C.J., et al., 2019. Assessment of disbudding pain in dairy calves using nonlinear measures of heart rate variability. J. Dairy Sci. 102 (9), 8410–8416.

Cagle, L.A., et al., 2017. Injectable anesthesia for mice: combined effects of dexmedetomidine, tiletamine-zolazepam, and butorphanol. Anesthesiol. Res. Pract. 2017. https://doi.org/10.1155/2017/9161040.

Calderone, L., et al., 1986. Acute reversible cataract induced by xylazine and by ketamine-xylazine anesthesia in rats and mice. Exp. Eye Res. 42 (4), 331–337.

Caldwell, J.E., 1994. Desflurane clinical pharmacokinetics and pharmacodynamics. Clin. Pharmacokinet. 27 (1), 6–18.

Callahan, L.M., et al., 2014. Mortality associated with using medetomidine and ketamine for general anesthesia in pregnant and nonpregnant Wistar rats. Lab. Anim. 43 (6), 208–214.

Callaway, J.K., et al., 2012. Isoflurane induces cognitive deficits in the Morris water maze task in rats. Eur. J. Anaesthesiol. 29 (5), 239–245.

Camu, F., Vanlersberghe, C., 2002. Pharmacology of systemic analgesics. Best Pract. Res. Clin. Anaesthesiol. 16 (4), 475–488.

Cappon, G.D., et al., 2003. Relationship between cyclooxygenase 1 and 2 selective inhibitors and fetal development when administered to rats and rabbits during the sensitive periods for heart development and midline closure. Birth Defects Res. B Dev. Reprod. Toxicol. 68 (1), 47–56.

Carbone, L., 2019. Ethical and IACUC considerations regarding analgesia and pain management in laboratory rodents. Comp. Med. 69 (6), 443–450.

Carbone, L., Austin, J., 2016. Pain and laboratory animals: publication practices for better data reproducibility and better animal welfare. PLoS ONE 11 (5), e0155001.

Carbone, E.T., et al., 2012. Duration of action of sustained-release buprenorphine in 2 strains of mice. J. Am. Assoc. Lab. Anim. Sci. 51 (6), 815–819.

Cardoso, C.G., et al., 2020. A comparative study of the cardiopulmonary and sedative effects of a single intramuscular dose of ketamine anesthetic combinations in rabbits. Res. Vet. Sci. 128, 177–182.

Carli, F., Asenjo, J.F., 2003. Is multimodal analgesia necessary to facilitate postoperative recovery? Tech. Reg. Anesth. Pain Manag. 7 (3), 133–139.

Caro, A.C., et al., 2013. Comparison of thermoregulatory devices used during anesthesia of C57BL/6 mice and correlations between body temperature and physiologic parameters. J. Am. Assoc. Lab. Anim. Sci. 52 (5), 577–583.

Carpenter, K.C., et al., 2019. The influence of pain and analgesia in rodent models of sepsis. Comp. Med. 69 (6), 546–554.

Carroll, G.L., et al., 2005. Analgesic efficacy of preoperative administration of meloxicam or butorphanol in onychectomized cats. J. Am. Vet. Med. Assoc. 226 (6), 913–919.

Carruba, M.O., et al., 1987. Effects of diethyl ether, halothane, ketamine and urethane on sympathetic activity in the rat. Eur. J. Pharmacol. 134 (1), 15–24.

Carter, K.M., et al., 2011. A review of tricaine methanesulfonate for anesthesia of fish. Rev. Fish Biol. Fish. 21 (1), 51–59.

Celeste, N.A., et al., 2021. Effects of cling film draping material on body temperature of mice during surgery. J. Am. Assoc. Lab. Anim. Sci. 60 (2), 195–200.

Celly, C.S., et al., 1997. The comparative hypoxaemic effect of four $\alpha2$ adrenoceptor agonists (xylazine, romifidine, detomidine and medetomidine) in sheep. J. Vet. Pharmacol. Ther. 20 (6), 464–471.

Chambers, D.J., 2019. Principles of intravenous drug infusion. Anaesth. Intensive Care Med. 20 (1), 61–64.

Chan, E.D., et al., 2013. Pulse oximetry: understanding its basic principles facilitates appreciation of its limitations. Respir. Med. 107 (6), 789–799.

Chandrasekharan, N.V., et al., 2002. COX-3, a cyclooxygenase-1 variant inhibited by acetaminophen and other analgesic/antipyretic drugs: cloning, structure, and expression. Proc. Natl. Acad. Sci. 99 (21), 13926–13931.

Chatigny, F., et al., 2017. Uses and doses of local anesthetics in fish, amphibians, and reptiles. J. Am. Assoc. Lab. Anim. Sci. 56 (3), 244–253.

Child, K.J., et al., 1971. The pharmacological properties in animals of CT1341—a new steroid anaesthetic agent. Br. J. Anaesth. 43 (1), 2–13.

Child, K.J., et al., 1972a. Anaesthetic, cardiovascular and respiratory effects of a new steroidal agent CT 1341: a comparison with other intravenous anaesthetic drugs in the unrestrained cat. Br. J. Pharmacol. 46 (2), 189–200.

Child, K.J., et al., 1972b. An endocrinological evaluation of CT1341 (Althesin) with special reference to reproduction. Postgrad. Med. J. 48, 51–55.

Christy, A.C., et al., 2014. Evaluation of medicated gel as a supplement to providing acetaminophen in the drinking water of C57BL/6 mice after surgery. J. Am. Assoc. Lab. Anim. Sci. 53 (2), 180–184.

Chu, E.R., et al., 2014. Intraocular pressure measurement in acepromazine-sedated mice. Clin. Experiment. Ophthalmol. 42 (4), 395–397.

Chuang, S.M., et al., 2013. Dual involvements of cyclooxygenase and nitric oxide synthase expressions in ketamine-induced ulcerative cystitis in rat bladder. Neurourol.Urodyn. 32 (8), 1137–1143.

Chum, H.H., et al., 2014. Antinociceptive effects of sustained-release buprenorphine in a model of incisional pain in rats (*Rattus norvegicus*). J. Am. Assoc. Lab. Anim. Sci. 53 (2), 193–197.

Ciccone, G.K., Holdcroft, A., 1999. Drugs and sex differences: a review of drugs relating to anaesthesia. Surv. Anesthesiol. 43 (5), 293–294.

Clark, J.A., et al., 1997. Pica behavior associated with buprenorphine administration in the rat. Lab. Anim. Sci. 47 (3), 300–303.

Clowry, G.J., Flecknell, P.A., 2000. The successful use of fentanyl/fluanisone ("Hypnorm") as an anaesthetic for intracranial surgery in neonatal rats. Lab. Anim. 34 (3), 260–264.

Clutton, R.E., et al., 2011. Reducing the oxygen concentration of gases delivered from anaesthetic machines unadapted for medical air. Vet. Rec. 169 (17), 440.

Coble, D.J., et al., 2011. Analgesic effects of meloxicam, morphine sulfate, flunixin meglumine, and xylazine hydrochloride in African-clawed frogs (*Xenopus laevis*). J. Am. Assoc. Lab. Anim. Sci. 50 (3), 355–360.

Cockshott, I.D., et al., 1992. The pharmacokinetics of propofol in laboratory animals. Xenobiotica 22 (3), 369–375.

Coderre, T.J., et al., 1993. Contribution of central neuroplasticity to pathological pain: review of clinical and experimental evidence. Pain 52 (3), 259–285.

Columbano, N., et al., 2018a. Determination of the minimum alveolar concentration (MAC) and cardiopulmonary effects of sevoflurane in sheep. Vet. Anaesth. Analg. 45 (4), 487–495.

Columbano, N., et al., 2018b. Determination of minimum alveolar concentration and cardiovascular effects of desflurane in positive-pressure ventilated sheep. Am. J. Vet. Res. 79 (7), 727–732.

Conour, L.A., et al., 2006. Preparation of animals for research—issues to consider for rodents and rabbits. ILAR J. 47 (4), 283–293.

Constant, C., et al., 2022. Peri-anesthetic hypothermia in rodents: a factor to consider for accurate and reproducible outcomes in orthopedic device-related infection studies. J. Orthop. Res. https://doi.org/10.1002/jor.25397.

Conzemius, M.G., et al., 1997. Correlation between subjective and objective measures used to determine severity of postoperative pain in dogs. J. Am. Vet. Med. Assoc. 210 (11), 1619–1622.

Cook, C.D., et al., 2000. Sex-related differences in the antinociceptive effects of opioids: importance of rat genotype, nociceptive stimulus intensity, and efficacy at the mu opioid receptor. Psychopharmacology (Berl) 150 (4), 430–442.

Cook, J.C., et al., 2003. Analysis of the nonsteroidal anti-inflammatory drug literature for potential developmental toxicity in rats and rabbits. Birth Defects Res. B Dev. Reprod. Toxicol. 68 (1), 5–26.

Cookson, J.H., Mills, F.J., 1983. Continuous infusion anaesthesia in baboons with alphaxolone-alphadolone. Lab. Anim. 17 (3), 196–197.

Cooper, D.M., et al., 2005. Duration of effects on clinical parameters and referred hyperalgesia in rats after abdominal surgery and multiple doses of analgesic. Comp. Med. 55 (4), 344–353.

Corder, G., Ahanonu, B., Grewe, B.F., Wang, D., Schnitzer, M.J., Scherrer, G., 2019. An amygdalar neural ensemble that encodes the unpleasantness of pain. Science 363 (6424), 276–281.

Costa, D.L., et al., 1986. Transoral tracheal intubation of rodents using a fiberoptic laryngoscope. Lab. Anim. Sci. 36 (3), 256–261.

Costa, E.D., et al., 2014. Development of the horse grimace scale (HGS) as a pain assessment tool in horses undergoing routine castration. PLoS ONE 9 (3), e92281.

Costello, M.F., 2004. Principles of cardiopulmonary cerebral resuscitation in special species. Semin. Avian Exot. Pet Med. 13 (3), 132–141.

Cotran, R.S., et al., 1968. Resistance of Wistar/Furth rats to the mast cell-damaging effect of horseradish peroxidase. J. Histochem. Cytochem. 16 (5), 382–383.

Coulter, C.A., et al., 2009. Reported analgesic administration to rabbits, pigs, sheep, dogs and non-human primates undergoing experimental surgical procedures. Lab. Anim. 43 (3), 232–238.

Cousins, M.J., et al., 2000. 1996 Labat lecture: pain—a persistent problem. Reg. Anesth. Pain Med. 25, 6–21.

Cowan, A., et al., 1977a. The animal pharmacology of buprenorphine, an oripavine analgesic agent. Br. J. Pharmacol. 60 (4), 547–554.

Cowan, A., et al., 1977b. Agonist and antagonist properties of buprenorphine, a new antinociceptive agent. Br. J. Pharmacol. 60 (4), 537–545.

Cox, A.K., et al., 1994. Evaluation of detomidine and ketamine-detomidine for anesthesia in laboratory rats. Contemp. Top. Lab. Anim. Sci. 33 (2), 52–55.

Craft, R.M., McNiel, D.M., 2003. Agonist/antagonist properties of nalbuphine, butorphanol and (−)-pentazocine in male vs. female rats. Pharmacol. Biochem. Behav. 75 (1), 235–245.

Craig, K.D., et al., 1993. Pain in the preterm neonate: behavioural and physiological indices. Pain 52 (3), 287–299.

Criado, A.B., et al., 2003. Reduction of isoflurane MAC by fentanyl or remifentanil in rats. Vet. Anaesth. Analg. 30 (4), 250–256.

Crile, G., 1913. The kinetic theory of shock and its prevention through anoci-association (shockless operation). Lancet 182 (4688), 7–16.

Crook, R.J., 2021. Behavioral and neurophysiological evidence suggests affective pain experience in octopus. Iscience 24 (3), 102229.

Crook, R.J., et al., 2013. Squid have nociceptors that display widespread long-term sensitization and spontaneous activity after bodily injury. J. Neurosci. 33 (24), 10021–10026.

Cruz, J.I., et al., 1998. Observations on the use of medetomidine/ketamine and its reversal with atipamezole for chemical restraint in the mouse. Lab. Anim. 32 (1), 18–22.

Curl, J.L., Peters, L.L., 1983. Ketamine hydrochloride and xylazine hydrochloride anaesthesia in the golden hamster (*Mesocricetus auratus*). Lab. Anim. 17 (4), 290–293.

Cuthbert, R., et al., 2007. Comparative toxicity studies of NSAIDs in birds: a criticism of Reddy et al. Environ. Toxicol. Pharmacol. 23 (2), 254–255.

Cuthbert, R.J., et al., 2014. Avian scavengers and the threat from veterinary pharmaceuticals. Philos. Trans. R. Soc. Lond. B Biol. Sci. 369 (1656), 20130574.

D'Alleinne, C.P., Mann, D.D., 1982. Evaluation of ketamine/xylazine anesthesia in the guinea pig: toxicological parameters. Vet. Hum. Toxicol. 24 (6), 410–412.

Danneman, P.J., Mandrell, T.D., 1997. Evaluation of five agents/methods for anesthesia of neonatal rats. Lab. Anim. Sci. 47 (4), 386–395.

Das, R.G., North, D., 2007. Implications of experimental technique for analysis and interpretation of data from animal experiments: outliers and increased variability resulting from failure of intraperitoneal injection procedures. Lab. Anim. 41 (3), 312–320.

Davey, A.J., Diba, A., 2011. Ward's Anaesthetic Equipment, sixth ed. Elsevier.

Davidson, C.D., et al., 2004. Plasma fentanyl concentrations and analgesic effects during full or partial exposure to transdermal fentanyl patches in cats. J. Am. Vet. Med. Assoc. 224 (5), 700–705.

Davis, J., Musk, G.C., 2014. Pressure and volume controlled mechanical ventilation in anaesthetized pregnant sheep. Lab. Anim. 48 (4), 321–327.

de Boer, H.D., et al., 2006. Reversal of profound rocuronium neuromuscular blockade by sugammadex in anesthetized rhesus monkeys. Anesthesiology 104 (4), 718–723.

de Segura, I.A.G., de la Víbora, J.B., Criado, A., 2009. Determination of the minimum alveolar concentration for halothane, isoflurane and sevoflurane in the gerbil. Lab. Anim. 43 (3), 239–242.

De Sousa, A.B., et al., 2008. Pharmacokinetics of tramadol and o-desmethyltramadol in goats after intravenous and oral administration. J. Vet. Pharmacol. Ther. 31 (1), 45–51. Available at: http://onlinelibrary.wiley.com/doi/10.1111/j.1365-2885.2007.00916.x/full.

De Wolf, A.M., et al., 2012. Theoretical effect of hyperventilation on speed of recovery and risk of rehypnotization following recovery—a GasMan® simulation. BMC Anesthesiol. 12 (1), 1–6.

Deacon, R.M.J., 2006. Burrowing in rodents: a sensitive method for detecting behavioral dysfunction. Nat. Protoc. 1 (1), 118–121.

Deacon, R., 2009. Burrowing: a sensitive behavioural assay, tested in five species of laboratory rodents. Behav. Brain Res. 200 (1), 128–133.

Deacon, R., 2012. Assessing burrowing, nest construction, and hoarding in mice. J. Vis. Exp. 59, e2607.

Deacon, R.M.J., Rawlins, J.N.P., 1996. Equithesin without chloral hydrate as an anaesthetic for rats. Psychopharmacology (Berl) 124 (3), 288–290.

Deacon, R., et al., 2007. A comparison of the behavior of C57BL/6 and C57BL/10 mice. Behav. Brain Res. 179 (2), 239–247.

de Jong, R.H., Bonin, J.D., 1980. Deaths from local anesthetic-induced convulsions in mice. Anesth. Analg. 59 (6), 401–405.

del Portillo, I.P., et al., 2014. Oxygen therapy in critical care: a double edged sword. Health 2014 (15), 2035–2046.

Delk, K.W., et al., 2014. Pharmacokinetics of meloxicam administered orally to rabbits (*Oryctolagus cuniculus*) for 29 days. Am. J. Vet. Res. 75 (2), 195–199.

DeMarco, G.J., Nunamaker, E.A., 2019. A review of the effects of pain and analgesia on immune system function and inflammation: relevance for preclinical studies. Comp. Med. 69 (6), 520–534.

Desborough, J.P., 2000. The stress response to trauma and surgery. Br. J. Anaesth. 85 (1), 109–117.

Descovich, K.A., et al., 2019. Opportunities for refinement in neuroscience: indicators of wellness and post-operative pain in laboratory macaques. ALTEX 36 (4), 535–554.

Desjardins, C., 1981. Endocrine signaling and male reproduction. Biol. Reprod. 24 (1), 1–21.

Desmarchelier, M., et al., 2012. Analgesic effects of meloxicam administration on postoperative orthopedic pain in domestic pigeons (*Columba livia*). Am. J. Vet. Res. 73 (3), 361–367.

Dholakia, U., et al., 2017. Anesthetic effects and body weight changes associated with ketamine-xylazine-lidocaine administered to CD-1 mice. PLoS One 12 (9), e0184911.

Dickinson, A.L., et al., 2009. The analgesic effects of oral paracetamol in two strains of mice undergoing vasectomy. Lab. Anim. 43 (4), 357–361.

Difilippo, S.M., et al., 2004. A comparison of xylazine and medetomidine in an anesthetic combination in New Zealand white rabbits. Contemp. Top. Lab. Anim. Sci. 43 (1), 32–34.

Divers, S.J., Stahl, S.J. (Eds.), 2018. Mader's Reptile and Amphibian Medicine and Surgery-e-Book. Elsevier Health Sciences.

Dix, G.M., et al., 2006. Methods used in veterinary practice to maintain the temperature of intravenous fluids. Vet. Rec. 159 (14), 451–455.

Dobromylskyj, P., 1993. Assessment of methadone as an anaesthetic premedicant in cats. J. Small Anim. Pract. 34 (12), 604–608.

Doerning, C.M., et al., 2018. Effects of subcutaneous alfaxalone alone and in combination with dexmedetomidine and buprenorphine in guinea pigs (*Cavia porcellus*). Vet. Anaesth. Analg. 45 (5), 658–666.

Douglas, B.G., Dagirmanjian, R., 1975. The effects of magnesium deficiency on ketamine sleeping times in the rat. Br. J. Anaesth. 47 (3), 336–340.

Drummond, J.C., 1985. MAC for halothane, enflurane, and isoflurane in the New Zealand white rabbit: and a test for the validity of MAC determinations. Anesthesiology 62 (3), 336–338.

Drummond, J.C., et al., 1996. Use of neuromuscular blocking drugs in scientific investigations involving animal subjects. The benefit of the doubt goes to the animal. Anesthesiology 85 (4), 697–699.

Dugdale, A., 2007. The ins and outs of ventilation 2. Mechanical ventilators. In Pract. 29 (5), 272–282.

Dugdale, A.H., et al., 2020. Veterinary Anaesthesia: Principles to Practice. John Wiley & Sons.

Duke, T., 2000. Local and regional anesthetic and analgesic techniques in the dog and cat: part II, infiltration and nerve blocks. Can. Vet. J. 41 (12), 949–952.

Dum, J.E., Herz, A., 1981. In vivo receptor binding of the opiate partial agonist, buprenorphine, correlated with its agonistic and antagonistic actions. Br. J. Pharmacol. 74 (3), 627–633.

Duncan, I.J.H., 1996. Animal welfare defined in terms of feelings. Acta. Agric. Scand. A: Anim. Sci. 27 (suppl.), 29–35.

Dupras, J., et al., 2001. Anesthesia of the New Zealand rabbit using the the combination of tiletamine-zolazepam and ketamine-midazolam with or without xylazine. Can. Vet. J. 42 (6), 455–460.

Dürsteler, C., et al., 2007. Synergistic interaction between dexamethasone and tramadol in a murine model of acute visceral pain. Fundam. Clin. Pharmacol. 21 (5), 515–520.

Dyson, D.H., et al., 1987. Effects of saffan on cardiopulmonary function in healthy cats. Can. J. Vet. Res. 51 (2), 236–239.

Eales, F.A., Small, J., 1982. Alphaxalone/alphadolone anaesthesia in the lamb. Vet. Rec. 110 (12), 273–275.

Eatwell, K., et al., 2013. Use of arterial blood gas analysis as a superior method for evaluating respiratory function in pet rabbits (*Oryctolagus cuniculus*). Vet. Rec. 173 (7), 166.

Edmunson, A.M., et al., 2021. Indicators of postoperative pain in Syrian hamsters (*Mesocricetus auratus*). Comp. Med. 71 (1), 76–85.

Eger, E.I., 1981. Isoflurane: a review. Anesthesiology 55 (5), 559–576.

Eger, E.I., 1992. Desflurane animal and human pharmacology: aspects of kinetics, safety, and MAC. Anesth. Analg. 75 (4 Suppl), S3–S7 (discussion S8–9).

Eger II, E.I., Shafer, S.L., 2005. Tutorial: context-sensitive decrement times for inhaled anesthetics. Anesth. Analg. 101 (3), 688–696.

Eger, E.I.I., Johnson, B.H., 1987. Rates of awakening from anesthesia with I-653, halothane, isoflurane, and sevoflurane: a test of the effect of anesthetic concentration and duration in rats. Anesth. Analg. 66 (10), 977.

Eger, E.I., et al., 2003. Women appear to have the same minimum alveolar concentration as men: a retrospective study. Anesthesiologists 99 (5), 1059–1061.

Egger, C.M., et al., 2007. Efficacy and cost-effectiveness of transdermal fentanyl patches for the relief of post-operative pain in dogs after anterior cruciate ligament and pelvic limb repair. Vet. Anaesth. Analg. 34 (3), 200–208.

Ellen, Y., et al., 2016. Evaluation of using behavioural changes to assess post-operative pain in the guinea pig (*Cavia porcellus*). PLoS ONE 11 (9), e0161941.

Elmer, G.I., et al., 1998. Genetic variance in nociception and its relationship to the potency of morphine-induced analgesia in thermal and chemical tests. Pain 75, 129–140.

Erhardt, W., et al., 1984. A comparative study with various anesthetics in mice (pentobarbitone, ketamine-xylazine, carfentanyl-etomidate). Res. Exp. Med. 184 (3), 159–169.

Erhardt, W., et al., 2001. Comparison of the anaesthesia combinations racemic-ketamine/medetomidine and S-Ketamine/medetomidine in syrian golden hamsters (*Mesocricetus auratus*). Vet. Anaesth. Analg. 28 (4), 212–213.

Erickson, R.L., et al., 2019. Alfaxalone–xylazine anesthesia in laboratory mice (*Mus musculus*). J. Am. Assoc. Lab. Anim. Sci. 58 (1), 30–39.

Evangelista, M.C., et al., 2022. Measurement properties of grimace scales for pain assessment in nonhuman mammals: a systematic review. Pain 163 (6), e697–e714.

Evangelista-Vaz, R., et al., 2018. Analgesic efficacy of subcutaneous–oral dosage of tramadol after surgery in C57BL/6J mice. J. Am. Assoc. Lab. Anim. Sci. 57 (4), 368–375.

Fabian, N.J., et al., 2021. Pharmacokinetics of single-dose intramuscular and subcutaneous injections of buprenorphine in common marmosets (*Callithrix jacchus*). J. Am. Assoc. Lab. Anim. Sci. 60 (5), 568–575.

Fagin, K.D., Shinsako, J., 1983. Effects of housing and chronic cannulation on plasma ACTH and corticosterone in the rat. Am. J. Physiol. Endocrinol. Metab. 245, E515–E520.

Fairbanks, C.A., 2003. Spinal delivery of analgesics in experimental models of pain and analgesia. Adv. Drug Deliv. Rev. 55 (8), 1007–1041.

Faller, K.M.E., et al., 2015. Refinement of analgesia following thoracotomy and experimental myocardial infarction using the mouse grimace scale. Exp. Physiol. 100 (2), 164–172.

Fanton, J.W., et al., 2000. Cardiovascular responses to propofol and etomidate in long-term instrumented rhesus monkeys (*Macaca mulatta*). Comp. Med. 50 (3), 303–308.

Farraj, A.K., et al., 2011. The utility of the small rodent electrocardiogram in toxicology. Toxicol. Sci. 121 (1), 11–30.

Fechner, J., et al., 2009. Fospropofol disodium, a water-soluble prodrug of the intravenous anesthetic propofol (2,6-diisopropylphenol). Expert Opin. Investig. Drugs 18 (10), 1565–1571.

Feldman, E.R., et al., 2021. Effects of cisapride, buprenorphine, and their combination on gastrointestinal transit in New Zealand white rabbits. J. Am. Assoc. Lab. Anim. Sci. 60 (2), 221–228.

Fellows, I.W., et al., 1983. Adrenocortical suppression with etomidate. Lancet 2 (8340), 54–55.

Ferre, P.J., et al., 2006. Plasma pharmacokinetics of alfaxalone in dogs after an intravenous bolus of Alfaxan-CD RTU. Vet. Anaesth. Analg. 33 (4), 229–236.

Ferrini, E., et al., 2020. Alfaxalone and dexmedetomidine as an alternative to gas anesthesia for micro-CT lung imaging in a bleomycin-induced pulmonary fibrosis murine model. Front. Vet. Sci. 7, 588592.

Festing, M.F., 2002. The design and statistical analysis of animal experiments. ILAR J. 43 (4), 191–193.

Field, K.J., Lang, C.M., 1988. Hazards of urethane (ethyl carbamate): a review of the literature. Lab. Anim. 22 (3), 255–262.

Field, W.E., et al., 1966. Use of droperidol and fentanyl for analgesia and sedation in primates. J. Am. Vet. Med. Assoc. 149 (7), 896–901.

Field, K.J., et al., 1993. Anaesthetic effects of chloral hydrate, pentobarbitone and urethane in adult male rats. Lab. Anim. 27 (3), 258–269.

Fiorito, G., et al., 2015. Guidelines for the care and welfare of cephalopods in research—a consensus based on an initiative by CephRes, FELASA and the Boyd Group. Lab. Anim. 49 (2_suppl), 1–90.

Fiorucci, S., Distrutti, E., 2011. COXIBs, CINODs and H2S-releasing NSAIDs: current perspectives in the development of safer non steroidal anti-inflammatory drugs. Curr. Med. Chem. 18 (23), 3494–3505.

Fitz, C.B., Goodroe, A.E., Moody, D.E., Fang, W.B., Capuano III, S.V., 2021. Pharmacokinetics of buprenorphine and sustained-release buprenorphine in common marmosets (*Callithrix jacchus*). J. Am. Assoc. Lab. Anim. Sci. 60 (2), 188–194.

Fitzgerald, M., 2005. The development of nociceptive circuits. Nat. Rev. Neurosci. 6 (7), 507–520.

Flecknell, P.A., 1983. Injectable anaesthetic techniques in 2 species of gerbil (*Meriones libycus* and *Meriones unguiculatus*). Lab. Anim. 17 (2), 118–122.

Flecknell, P.A., 1984. The relief of pain in laboratory animals. Lab. Anim. 18 (2), 147–160.

Flecknell, P.A., 1994. Refinement of animal use-assessment and alleviation of pain and distress. Lab. Anim. 28 (3), 222–231.

Flecknell, P.A., Liles, J.H., 1990. Assessment of the analgesic action of opioid agonist-antagonists in the rabbit. Vet. Anaesth. Analg. 17 (1), 24–29.

Flecknell, P.A., Liles, J.H., 1991. The effects of surgical procedures, halothane anaesthesia and nalbuphine on locomotor activity and food and water consumption in rats. Lab. Anim. 25 (1), 50–60.

Flecknell, P.A., Liles, J.H., 1996. Halothane anaesthesia in the rabbit: a comparison of the effects of medetomidine, acepromazine and midazolam on breath-holding during induction. Vet. Anaesth. Analg. 23 (1), 11–14.

Flecknell, P.A., Mitchell, M., 1984. Midazolam and fentanyl-fluanisone: assessment of anaesthetic effects in laboratory rodents and rabbits. Lab. Anim. 18 (2), 143–146.

Flecknell, P.A., et al., 1983. Neuroleptanalgesia in the rabbit. Lab. Anim. 17 (2), 104–109.

Flecknell, P.A., et al., 1989a. Long-term anaesthesia with alfentanil and midazolam for lung transplantation in the dog. Lab. Anim. 23 (3), 278–284.

Flecknell, P.A., et al., 1989b. Reversal of fentanyl/fluanisone neuroleptanalgesia in the rabbit using mixed agonist/antagonist opioids. Lab. Anim. 23 (2), 147–155.

Flecknell, P.A., et al., 1990a. Long-term anaesthesia with propofol and alfentanil in the dog and its partial reversal with nalbuphine. Vet. Anaesth. Analg. 17 (1), 11–16.

Flecknell, P.A., et al., 1990b. The use of lignocaine-prilocaine local anaesthetic cream for pain-free venepuncture in laboratory animals. Lab. Anim. 24 (2), 142–146.

Flecknell, P.A., et al., 1991. Post-operative analgesia following thoracotomy in the evaluation of the effects of bupivacaine intercostal block and nalbuphine on respiratory function. Lab. Anim. 25, 319–324.

Flecknell, P.A., et al., 1999a. Induction of anaesthesia with sevoflurane and isoflurane in the rabbit. Lab. Anim. 33 (1), 41–46.

Flecknell, P.A., et al., 1999b. Use of oral buprenorphine ("buprenorphine jello") for postoperative analgesia in rats-a clinical trial. Lab. Anim. 33 (2), 169–174.

Fleischman, R.W., et al., 1977. Adynamic ileus in the rat induced by chloral hydrate. Lab. Anim. Sci. 27 (2), 238–243.

Fleischmann, T., et al., 2016. Injection anaesthesia with fentanyl–midazolam–medetomidine in adult female mice: importance of antagonization and perioperative care. Lab. Anim. 50 (4), 264–274.

Foley, P.L., et al., 2011. Evaluation of a sustained-release formulation of buprenorphine for analgesia in rats. J. Am. Assoc. Lab. Anim. Sci. 50 (2), 198–204.

Fowler, K.A., et al., 2001. Anesthetic protocol: propofol use in Rhesus macaques (*Macaca mulatta*) during magnetic resonance imaging with stereotactic head frame application. Brain Res. Protocol. 7 (2), 87–93.

Franken, N.D., et al., 2008. Evaluation of analgesic and sedative effects of continuous infusion of dexmedetomidine by measuring somatosensory- and auditory-evoked potentials in the rat. Vet. Anaesth. Analg. 35 (5), 424–431.

Franks, N.P., Lieb, W.R., 1996. Temperature dependence of the potency of volatile general anesthetics: implications for in vitro experiments. J. Am. Soc. Anesthesiol. 84 (3), 716–720.

Fraser, D., 2009. Animal behaviour, animal welfare and the scientific study of affect. Appl. Anim. Behav. Sci. 118 (3–4), 108–117.

Frommel, E., Joye, E., 1964. On the analgesic power of morphine in relation to age and sex of guinea pigs. Pharmacology 11 (1), 43–46.

Fudickar, A., Bein, B., 2009. Propofol infusion syndrome: update of clinical manifestation and pathophysiology. Minerva Anestesiol. 75 (5), 339.

Fulkerson, P.J., Gustafson, S.B., 2007. Use of laryngeal mask airway compared to endotracheal tube with positive-pressure ventilation in anesthetized swine. Vet. Anaesth. Analg. 34 (4), 284–288.

Gaarde, L., et al., 2021. The effects of post-operative oxygen supply on blood oxygenation and acid-base status in rats anaesthetized with fentanyl/fluanisone and midazolam. PLoS ONE 16 (8), e0255829.

Gades, N.M., et al., 2000. The magnitude and duration of the analgesic effect of morphine, butorphanol, and buprenorphine in rats and mice. Contemp. Top. Lab. Anim. Sci. 39 (2), 8–13.

Galatos, A.D., 2011. Anesthesia and analgesia in sheep and goats. Vet. Clin. North Am. Food Anim. Pract. 27 (1), 47–59.

Gan, T.J., Habib, A.S., Miller, T.E., White, W., Apfelbaum, J.L., 2014. Incidence, patient satisfaction, and perceptions of post-surgical pain: results from a US national survey. Curr. Med. Res. Opin. 30 (1), 149–160.

Garrido, M.J., et al., 2003. Pharmacokinetic/pharmacodynamic modeling of the antinociceptive effects of (+)-tramadol in the rat: role of cytochrome P450 2D activity. J. Pharmacol. Exp. Ther. 305 (2), 710–718.

Gaynor, J.S., Muir, W.W., 2014. Handbook of Veterinary Pain Management, third ed. Elsevier Health Sciences.

Ge, R., et al., 2013. Adrenocortical suppression and recovery after continuous hypnotic infusion: etomidate versus its soft analogue cyclopropyl-methoxycarbonyl metomidate. Crit. Care 17 (1), R20.

Gebhart, G.F., et al., 2009. Recognition and Alleviation of Pain in Laboratory Animals. National Academy of Sciences. https://nap.nationalacademies.org/catalog/12526/recognition-and-alleviation-of-pain-in-laboratory-animals.

Giannoudis, P.V., et al., 2006. Surgical stress response. Injury 37, S3–S9.

Gibney, B.C., et al., 2011. Dynamic determination of oxygenation and lung compliance in murine pneumonectomy. Exp. Lung Res. 37 (5), 301–309.

Giorgi, M., 2008. Pharmacokinetic differences of tramadol in several animal species and human beings. J. Vet. Res. 178 (2), 272–277.

Giorgi, M., 2012. Tramadol vs tapentadol: anew horizon in pain treatment? Am. J. Anim. Vet. Sci. 7 (1), 7–11.

Giorgi, M., et al., 2012. Pharmacokinetics of the novel atypical opioid tapentadol following oral and intravenous administration in dogs. Vet. J. 194 (3), 309–313.

Giorgi, M., et al., 2013. Plasma concentrations of tapentadol and clinical evaluations of a combination of tapentadol plus sevoflurane for surgical anaesthesia and analgesia in rabbits (*Oryctolagus cuniculus*) undergoing orchiectomy. Isr. J. Vet. Med. 68, 141–148.

Giral, M., et al., 2014. Anaesthetic effects in the ferret of alfaxalone alone and in combination with medetomidine or tramadol: a pilot study. Lab. Anim. 48 (4), 313–320.

Glaab, T., et al., 2001. Tidal midexpiratory flow as a measure of airway hyperresponsiveness in allergic mice. Am. J. Physiol. Lung Cell. Mol. Physiol. 280 (3), L565–L573.

Glaab, T., et al., 2007. Invasive and noninvasive methods for studying pulmonary function in mice. Resp. Res. 8 (1), 1–10.

Gleerup, K.B., et al., 2015. Pain evaluation in dairy cattle. Appl. Anim. Behav. Sci. 171, 25–32.

Glen, J.B., 1980. Animal studies of the anaesthetic activity of ici 35 868. Br. J. Anaesth. 52 (8), 731–742.

Glen, J.B., Hunter, S.C., 1984. "Diprivan": an update. Vet. Anaesth. Analg. 12 (1), 40–47.

Glynn, C.J., 1987. Intrathecal and epidural administration of opiates. Baillieres Clin. Anaesthesiol. 1 (4), 915–933.

Godlkuhl, R., et al., 2010. Effects of voluntarily-ingested buprenorphine on plasma corticosterone levels, body weight, water intake, and behaviour in permanently catheterised rats. In Vivo 24 (2), 131–135.

Goecke, J.C., et al., 2005. Evaluating postoperative analgesics in mice using telemetry. Comp. Med. 55, 37–44.

Gong, D., et al., 1998. Rat strain minimally influences anesthetic and convulsant requirements of inhaled compounds in rats. Anesth. Analg. 87 (4), 963–966.

Gonsowski, C.T., Eger, E.I., 1994. Nitrous oxide minimum alveolar anesthetic concentration in rats is greater than previously reported. Anesth. Analg. 79 (4), 710–712.

Goodchild, C.S., et al., 2015. Alphaxalone reformulated: a water-soluble intravenous anesthetic preparation in sulfobutyl-ether-β-cyclodextrin. Anesth. Analg. 120 (5), 1025–1031.

Goutchtat, R., et al., 2021. Long-term analgesia following a single application of fentanyl transdermal solution in pigs. Eur. Surg. Res. 62 (2), 115–120.

Granados, M.M., et al., 2012. Anaesthetic and cardiorespiratory effects of a constant-rate infusion of alfaxalone in desflurane-anaesthetised sheep. Vet. Rec. 171 (5), 125.

Grandjean, J., et al., 2014. Optimization of anesthesia protocol for resting-state fMRI in mice based on differential effects of anesthetics on functional connectivity patterns. NeuroImage 102 (P2), 838–847.

Granholm, M., et al., 2006. Evaluation of the clinical efficacy and safety of dexmedetomidine or medetomidine in cats and their reversal with atipamezole. Vet. Anaesth. Analg. 33 (4), 214–223. https://doi.org/10.1111/j.1467-2995.2005.00259.x.

Grant, C., Upton, R.N., 2004. Comparison of the analgesic effects of xylazine in sheep via three different administration routes. Aust. Vet. J. 82 (5), 304–307.

Grant, G.J., et al., 2000. An in vivo method for the quantitative evaluation of local anesthetics. J. Pharmacol. Toxicol. Methods 43 (1), 69–72.

Grape, S., Tramèr, M.R., 2007. Do we need preemptive analgesia for the treatment of postoperative pain? Best Pract. Res. Clin. Anaesthesiol. 21 (1), 51–63. Available at: http://linkinghub.elsevier.com/retrieve/pii/S1521689606000784.

Green, C.J., 1975. Neuroleptanalgesic drug combinations in the anaesthetic management of small laboratory animals. Lab. Anim. 9 (3), 161–178.

Green, C.J., et al., 1978. Alphaxolone-alphadolone anaesthesia in laboratory animals. Lab. Anim. 12 (2), 85–89.

Green, C.J., et al., 1981a. Ketamine alone and combined with diazepam or xylazine in laboratory animals: a 10 year experience. Lab. Anim. 15 (2), 163–170.

Green, C.J., et al., 1981b. Metomidate, etomidate and fentanyl as injectable anaesthetic agents in mice. Lab. Anim. 15 (2), 171–175.

Greene, S.A., Thurmon, J.C., 1988. Xylazine—a review of its pharmacology and use in veterinary medicine. J. Vet. Pharmacol. Ther. 11 (4), 295–313.

Gregory, P., Edsell, M., 2014. Fatigue and the anaesthetist. Contin. Educ. Anaesth. Crit. Care Pain 14 (1), 18–22.

Grimm, K.A., et al. (Eds.), 2015. Veterinary Anesthesia and Analgesia. John Wiley & Sons.

Grint, N.J., Murison, P.J., 2008. A comparison of ketamine-midazolam and ketamine-medetomidine combinations for induction of anaesthesia in rabbits. Vet. Anaesth. Analg. 35 (2), 113–121.

Grint, N.J., et al., 2008. Clinical evaluation of alfaxalone in cyclodextrin for the induction of anaesthesia in rabbits. Vet. Rec. 163 (13), 395–396.

Groeben, H., 2003. Heritable differences in respiratory drive and breathing pattern in mice during anaesthesia and emergence. Br. J. Anaesth. 91 (4), 541–545.

Grunau, R.E., et al., 1998. Bedside application of the neonatal facial coding system in pain assessment of premature infants. Pain 76 (3), 277–286.

Guedel, A.E., 1920. Signs of Inhalational Anesthesia. A fundamental guide. MacMillan Co., New York.

Guedes, S.R., et al., 2017. Mice aversion to sevoflurane, isoflurane and carbon dioxide using an approach-avoidance task. Appl. Anim. Behav. Sci. 189, 91–97.

Gumbleton, M., et al., 1990. Differential influence of laboratory anaesthetic regimens upon renal and hepatosplanchnic haemodynamics in the rat. J. Pharm. Pharmacol. 42 (10), 693–697.

Guneli, E., et al., 2007. Analysis of the antinociceptive effect of systemic administration of tramadol and dexmedetomidine combination on rat models of acute and neuropathic pain. Pharmacol. Biochem. Behav. 88 (1), 9–17.

Gunkel, C., Lafortune, M., 2005. Current techniques in avian anesthesia. In: Seminars in Avian and Exotic Pet Medicine, vol. 14, no. 4. WB Saunders, pp. 263–276.

Hacker, S.O., et al., 2005. A comparison of target-controlled infusion versus volatile inhalant anesthesia for heart rate, respiratory rate, and recovery time in a rat model. Contemp. Top. Lab. Anim. Sci. 44 (5), 7–12.

Häger, C., et al., 2017. The sheep grimace scale as an indicator of post-operative distress and pain in laboratory sheep. PLoS ONE 12 (4), e0175839.

Häger, C., et al., 2018. Running in the wheel: defining individual severity levels in mice. PLoS Biol. 16 (10), e2006159.

Hall, L.W., Chambers, J.P., 1987. A clinical trial of propofol infusion anaesthesia in dogs. J. Small Anim. Pract. 28 (7), 623–637.

Hamacher, J., et al., 2008. Microscopic wire guide-based orotracheal mouse intubation: description, evaluation and comparison with transillumination. Lab. Anim. 42 (2), 222–230.

Hanneman, S.K., et al., 2004. Comparison of methods of temperature measurement in swine. Lab. Anim. 38 (3), 297–306.

Hara, K., Harris, R.A., 2002. The anesthetic mechanism of urethane: the effects on neurotransmitter-gated ion channels. Anesth. Analg. 94 (2), 313–318.

Hardman, J.G., Aitkenhead, A.R., 2005. Awareness during anaesthesia. Contin. Educ. Anaesth. Crit. Care Pain 5 (6), 183–186.

Harrison, P.K., et al., 2006. The presence of atropinesterase activity in animal plasma. Naunyn Schmiedebergs Arch. Pharmacol. 373 (3), 230–236.

Hart, M.V., et al., 1984. Hemodynamics in the guinea pig after anesthetization with ketamine/xylazine. Am. J. Vet. Res. 45 (11), 2328–2330.

Hartrick, C.T., Rodríguez Hernandez, J.R., 2012. Tapentadol for pain: a treatment evaluation. Expert Opin. Pharmacother. 13 (2), 283–286.

Harvey-Clark, C.J., et al., 2000. Transdermal fentanyl compared with parenteral buprenorphine in post-surgical pain in swine: a case study. Lab. Anim. 34 (4), 386–398.

Hasiuk, M.M.M., et al., 2014. A comparison of alfaxalone and propofol on intraocular pressure in healthy dogs. Vet. Ophthalmol. 17 (6), 411–416.

Hawkins, M.G., Paul-Murphy, J., 2011. Avian analgesia. Vet. Clin. North Am. Exot. Anim. Pract. 14 (1), 61–80.

Hawkins, M., et al., 2016. Recognition, assessment and management of pain in birds. In: Speer, B. (Ed.), Current Therapy in Avian Medicine and Surgery. Elsevier.

Hayes, K.E., et al., 2000. An evaluation of analgesic regimens for abdominal surgery in mice. Contemp. Top. Lab. Anim. Sci. 39 (6), 18–23.

Heavner, J.E., 2001. Anesthesia update: agents, definitions, and strategies. Comp. Med. 51 (6), 500–503.

Hedenqvist, P., et al., 2000. Sufentanil and medetomidine anaesthesia in the rat and its reversal with atipamezole and butorphanol. Lab. Anim. 34 (3), 244–251.

Hedenqvist, P., et al., 2001. Assessment of ketamine/medetomidine anaesthesia in the New Zealand White rabbit. Vet. Anaesth. Analg. 28 (1), 18–25.

Hedenqvist, P., et al., 2002. Anaesthesia with ketamine/medetomidine in the rabbit: influence of route of administration and the effect of combination with butorphanol. Vet. Anaesth. Analg. 29 (1), 14–19.

Hedenqvist, P., et al., 2014. Anaesthesia in medetomidine premedicated New Zealand White rabbits: a comparison between intravenous sufentanil-midazolam and isoflurane anaesthesia for orthopaedic surgery. Lab. Anim. 48 (2), 155–163.

Hedlund, L.W., et al., 2000. MR-compatible ventilator for small animals: computer-controlled ventilation for proton and noble gas imaging. Magn. Reson. Imaging 18 (6), 753–759.

Heikkinen, E.M., et al., 2015. Fentanyl pharmacokinetics in pregnant sheep after intravenous and transdermal administration to the ewe. Basic Clin. Pharmacol. Toxicol. 117 (3), 156–163.

Henke, J., et al., 1996. Clinical investigations of an i.m. combination anesthesia with fentanyl/climazolam/xylazine and postoperative i.v. antagonism with naloxone/sarmazenil/yohimbine in guinea pigs. Tierarztl. Prax. 24 (1), 85–87.

Henke, J., et al., 2004. Clinical comparison of isoflurane and sevoflurane anaesthesia in the gerbil (*Meriones unguiculatus*). Berl. Munch. Tierarztl. Wochenschr. 117 (7–8), 296–303.

Henke, J., et al., 2005. Comparative study of three intramuscular anaesthetic combinations (medetomidine/ketamine, medetomidine/fentanyl/midazolam and xylazine/ketamine) in rabbits. Vet. Anaesth. Analg. 32 (5), 261–270.

Herbert, G.L., et al., 2013. Alfaxalone for total intravenous anaesthesia in dogs undergoing ovariohysterectomy: a comparison of premedication with acepromazine or dexmedetomidine. Vet. Anaesth. Analg. 40 (2), 124–133.

Hermansen, K., et al., 1986. The analgesic effect of buprenorphine, etorphine and pethidine in the pig: a randomized double blind cross-over study. Acta Pharmacol. Toxicol. 59 (1), 27–35.

Hernandez-Avalos, I., et al., 2019. Review of different methods used for clinical recognition and assessment of pain in dogs and cats. Int. J. Vet. Sci. Med. 7 (1), 43–54.

Herrmann, K., Flecknell, P., 2019. Retrospective review of anesthetic and analgesic regimens used in animal research proposals. ALTEX 36, 65–80.

Hildebrandt, I.J., et al., 2008. Anesthesia and other considerations for in vivo imaging of small animals. ILAR J. 49 (1), 17–26.

Hill, W.A., et al., 2013. Repeated administration of tribromoethanol in C57BL/6NHsd mice. J. Am. Assoc. Lab. Anim. Sci. 52 (2), 176–179.

Hinchcliffe, J.K., et al., 2022. The use of ball pits and playpens in laboratory Lister hooded male rats induces ultrasonic vocalisations indicating a more positive affective state and can reduce the welfare impacts of aversive procedures. Lab. Anim., 00236772211065920.

Hinz, B., et al., 2007. Drug insight: cyclo-oxygenase-2 inhibitors—a critical appraisal. Nat. Clin. Pract. Rheumatol. 3 (10), 552–560 (quiz 1 p following 589).

Hird, J.F.R., Carlucci, F., 1977. The use of the coaxial circuit to control the degree of rebreathing in the anaesthetised dog. Vet. Anaesth. Analg. 7 (1), i–xii.

Ho, H., et al., 2020. An inhalation anaesthesia approach for neonatal mice allowing streamlined stereotactic injection in the brain. J. Neurosci. Methods 342, 108824.

Hocking, P.M., et al., 2005. Effects of non-steroidal anti-inflammatory drugs on pain-related behaviour in a model of articular pain in the domestic fowl. Res. Vet. Sci. 78 (1), 69–75.

Hodgson, D.S., 2007. Anesthetic concentrations in enclosed chambers using an innovative delivery device. Vet. Anaesth. Analg. 34 (2), 99–106.

Hofstetter, C., et al., 2007. Anti-inflammatory effects of sevoflurane and mild hypothermia in endotoxemic rats. Acta Anaesthesiol. Scand. 51 (7), 893–899.

Hollmann, M.W., Sear, J.W., 2015. Another steroid hypnotic: more of the same or something different? Anesth. Analg. 120 (5), 980–982.

Holstein-Rathlou, N.H., et al., 1982. Effects of halothane-nitrous oxide inhalation anesthesia and Inactin on overall renal and tubular function in Sprague-Dawley and Wistar rats. Acta Physiol. Scand. 114 (2), 193–201.

Morgan, D.W., Legge, K., 1989. Clinical evaluation of propofol as an intravenous anaesthetic agent in cats and dogs. Vet. Rec. 124 (2), 31–33.

Holtman Jr., J.R., Wala, E.P., 2007. Characterization of the antinociceptive and pronociceptive effects of methadone in rats. Anesthesiology 106 (3), 563–571.

Holzgrefe, H.H., et al., 1987. Alpha-chloralose as a canine anesthetic. Lab. Anim. Sci. 37 (5), 587–595.

Horncastle, E., Lumb, A.B., 2019. Hyperoxia in anaesthesia and intensive care. BJA Educ. 19 (6), 176.

Hotz-Behofsits, C., et al., 2010. Role of COX-2 in nonsteroidal anti-inflammatory drug enteropathy in rodents. 45 (7–8), 822–827.

Hovard, A., et al., 2014. The applicability of a gel delivery system for self-administration of buprenorphine to laboratory mice. Lab. Anim. 49 (1), 40–45.

Hsu, W.H., et al., 1986. Xylazine-ketamine-induced anesthesia in rats and its antagonism by yohimbine. J. Am. Vet. Med. Assoc. 189 (9), 1040–1043.

Hu, C., et al., 1992. Fentanyl and medetomidine anaesthesia in the rat and its reversal using atipamazole and either nalbuphine or butorphanol. Lab. Anim. 26 (1), 15–22.

Huang, Q., Riviere, J.E., 2014. The application of allometric scaling principles to predict pharmacokinetic parameters across species. Expert Opin. Drug Metab. Toxicol. 10 (9), 1241–1253.

Hudson, C., et al., 2008. Recognition and management of pain in cattle. In Pract. 30 (3), 126–134.

Hughes, E.W., et al., 1982. Effects of urethane-chloralose anaesthesia on respiration in the rat. Clin. Exp. Pharmacol. Physiol. 9 (2), 119–127.

Hughes, M.A., et al., 1992. Context-sensitive half-time in multicompartment pharmacokinetic models for intravenous anesthetic drugs. Anesthesiology 76 (3), 334–341.

Hughes, P.J., et al., 1993. A rabbit model for the evaluation of epidurally administered local anaesthetic agents. Anaesth. Intensive Care 21 (3), 298–303.

Hunt, J.R., et al., 2013. Comparison of premedication with buprenorphine or methadone with meloxicam for postoperative analgesia in dogs undergoing orthopaedic surgery. J. Small Anim. Pract. 54 (8), 418–424.

Hunter, S.C., et al., 1984. A modified anaesthetic vapour extraction system. Lab. Anim. 18 (1), 42–44.

Hurst, J.L., et al., 1998. Housing and welfare in laboratory rats: the welfare implications of social isolation and social contact among females. Anim. Welf. 7, 121–136.

Huss, M.K., et al., 2019. Influence of pain and analgesia on orthopedic and wound-healing models in rats and mice. Comp. Med. 69 (6), 535–545.

Ikeda, K., et al., 1991. Indirect systolic and mean blood pressure determination by a new tail cuff method in spontaneously hypertensive rats. Lab. Anim. 25 (1), 26–29.

Imbe, H., et al., 2006. Stress-induced hyperalgesia: animal models and putative mechanisms. Front. Biosci. 11 (3), 2179–2192.

Ingrao, J.C., et al., 2013. Aqueous stability and oral pharmacokinetics of meloxicam and carprofen in male C57BL/6 mice. J. Am. Assoc. Lab. Anim. Sci. 52 (5), 553–559.

Ingvast Larsson, C., et al., 2010. Clinical pharmacology of methadone in dogs. Vet. Anaesth. Analg. 37 (1), 48–56.

Ingwersen, W., et al., 1988. Cardiopulmonary effects of a ketamine hydrochloride/acepromazine combination in healthy cats. Can. J. Vet. Res. 52 (1), 1–4.

Ison, S.H., et al., 2016. A review of pain assessment in pigs. Front. Vet. Sci. 3, 108.

Itah, R., et al., 2004. A replacement for methoxyflurane (Metofane) in open-circuit anaesthesia. Lab. Anim. 38 (3), 280–285.

Iversen, N.K., et al., 2012. The normal acid–base status of mice. Respir. Physiol. Neurobiol. 180 (2–3), 252–257.

Izer, J.M., et al., 2018. Development of a pain scoring system for use in sheep surgically implanted with ventricular assist devices. J. Invest. Surg. 32 (8), 706–715.

Jablonski, P., Howden, B.O., 2002. Oral buprenorphine and aspirin analgesia in rats undergoing liver transplantation. Lab. Anim. 36 (2), 134–143.

Jackson, T., et al., 2014. Associations between pain appraisals and pain outcomes: meta-analyses of laboratory pain and chronic pain literatures. J. Pain 15 (6), 586–601.

Jacobsen, K.R., et al., 2012. Postsurgical food and water consumption, fecal corticosterone metabolites, and behavior assessment as noninvasive measures of pain in vasectomized BALB/c mice. J. Am. Assoc. Lab. Anim. Sci. 51 (1), 69–75.

Jang, H.S., et al., 2009. Evaluation of the anaesthetic effects of medetomidine and ketamine in rats and their reversal with atipamezole. Vet. Anaesth. Analg. 36 (4), 319–327.

Janssen, B.J.A., 2004. Effects of anesthetics on systemic hemodynamics in mice. Am. J. Physiol. Heart Circ. Physiol. 287 (4), H1618–H1624.

Janssen, P.A., et al., 1975. Etomidate, a potent non-barbiturate hypnotic. Intravenous etomidate in mice, rats, guinea-pigs, rabbits and dogs. Arch. Int. Pharmacodyn. Ther. 214 (1), 92–132.

Janssen, C.F., et al., 2017. Comparison of atipamezole with yohimbine for antagonism of xylazine in mice anesthetized with ketamine and xylazine. J. Am. Assoc. Lab. Anim. Sci. 56 (2), 142–147.

Jirkof, P., et al., 2013. Assessment of postsurgical distress and pain in laboratory mice by nest complexity scoring. Lab. Anim. 47 (3), 0023677213475603–161.

Jirkof, P., et al., 2014. Buprenorphine for pain relief in mice: repeated injections vs sustained-release depot formulation. Lab. Anim., 0023677214562849.

Jirkof, P., et al., 2010. Burrowing behavior as an indicator of post-laparotomy pain in mice. Front. Behav. Neurosci. 4, 165. https://doi.org/10.3389/fnbeh.2010.00165.

Jirkof, P., et al., 2019. Assessing affective state in laboratory rodents to promote animal welfare—what is the progress in applied refinement research? Animals 9 (12), 1026. https://doi.org/10.3390/ani9121026.

Jirkof, P., 2017. Side effects of pain and analgesia in animal experimentation. Lab. Anim. 46 (4), 123–128.

Johnson-Delaney, C.A., 2016. Analgesia and anaesthesia. In: Ferret Medicine and Surgery. CRC Press, pp. 407–418.

Jonckers, E., et al., 2014. Different anesthesia regimes modulate the functional connectivity outcome in mice. Magn. Reson. Med. 72 (4), 1103–1112.

Joshi, G.P., Ogunnaike, B.O., 2005. Consequences of inadequate postoperative pain relief and chronic persistent postoperative pain. Anesthesiol. Clin. North America 23 (1), 21–36.

Jurkat-Rott, K., et al., 2000. Genetics and pathogenesis of malignant hyperthermia. Muscle Nerve 23 (1), 4–17.

Kallet, R.H., Matthay, M.A., 2013. Hyperoxic acute lung injury. Respir. Care 58 (1), 123–141.

Kalliokoski, O., et al., 2011. Serum concentrations of buprenorphine after oral and parenteral administration in male mice. Vet. J. 187 (2), 251–254.

Kandasamy, R., Morgan, M.M., 2021. "Reinventing the wheel" to advance the development of pain therapeutics. Behav. Pharmacol. 32 (2-# x000263), 142.

Kapoor, A., Matthews, S.G., 2005. Short periods of prenatal stress affect growth, behaviour and hypothalamo–pituitary–adrenal axis activity in male guinea pig offspring. J. Physiol. 566 (3), 967–977.

Kashimoto, S., et al., 1997. The minimum alveolar concentration of sevoflurane in rats. Eur. J. Anaesthesiol. 14 (4), 359–361.

Katz, J., Clarke, H., Seltzer, Z., 2011. Preventive Analgesia: Quo Vadimus? Anesth. Analg. 113 (5), 1242–1253.

Kazuń, K., Siwicki, A.K., 2012. Propiscin—a safe new anaesthetic for fish. Arch. Pol. Fish. 20 (3), 1–5.

Kästner, S.B., 2006. A2-agonists in sheep: a review. Vet. Anaesth. Analg. 33 (2), 79–96.

Kästner, S.B.R., et al., 2006. Comparative pharmacokinetics of medetomidine enantiomers in goats and sheep during sevoflurane anaesthesia. J. Vet. Pharmacol. Ther. 29 (1), 63–66.

Kästner, S.B.R., et al., 2007. Dexmedetomidine-induced pulmonary alterations in sheep. Res. Vet. Sci. 83 (2), 217–226.

Kain, M.L., Nunn, J.F., 1967. Fresh gas flow and rebreathing in the Magill Circuit with spontaneous respiration. Proc. R. Soc. Med. 60 (8), 749–750.

Kawakami, Y., et al., 2018. Mouse body temperature measurement using infrared thermometer during passive systemic anaphylaxis and food allergy evaluation. J. Vis. Exp. (139), 58391.

Keates, H., 2003. Induction of anaesthesia in pigs using a new alphaxalone formulation. Vet. Rec. 153 (20), 627–628.

Keating, S.C.J., et al., 2012. Evaluation of EMLA cream for preventing pain during tattooing of rabbits: changes in physiological, behavioural and facial expression responses. PLoS ONE. https://doi.org/10.1371/journal.pone.0044437.

Kehlet, H., Dahl, J.B., 2003. Anaesthesia, surgery, and challenges in postoperative recovery. Lancet 362 (9399), 1921–1928.

Keilholz, S.D., et al., 2004. Functional MRI of the rodent somatosensory pathway using multislice echo planar imaging. Magn. Reson. Med. 52 (1), 89–99.

Kelly, K.R., et al., 2011. Pharmacokinetics of oxymorphone in titi monkeys (Callicebus spp.) and rhesus macaques (*Macaca mulatta*). J. Am. Assoc. Lab. Anim. Sci. 50 (2), 212–220.

Kero, P., Thomasson, B., Soppi, A.-M., 1981. Spinal anaesthesia in the rabbit. Lab. Anim. 15 (4), 347–348.

Kest, B., Palmese, C., Hopkins, E., 2000. A comparison of morphine analgesic tolerance in male and female mice. Brain Res. 879 (1–2), 17–22.

Kessler, M., et al., 2018. Activation in the auditory pathway of the gerbil studied with 18F-FDG PET: effects of anesthesia. Brain Struct. Funct. 223 (9), 4293–4305.

Khosravi, H., et al., 2021. Pain-induced aggression and changes in social behavior in mice. Aggress. Behav. 47 (1), 89–98.

Kiefer, D., et al., 2022. Intravenous propofol, ketamine (ketofol) and rocuronium after sevoflurane induction provides long lasting anesthesia in ventilated rats. Exp. Anim. 71 (2), 231–239.

Kilic, N., Henke, J., 2004. Comparative studies on the effect of S (+)-ketamine-medetomidine and racemic ketamine-medetomidine in mouse. YYÜ Vet Fak Derg 15 (2004), 15–17.

Kilic, N., et al., 2004. Ketamine/medetomidine-anaesthesia in the hamster: a clinical comparison between the subcutaneous and intraperitoneal way of application. Tierärztliche Praxis Kleintiere 32 (6), 384–388.

Kilpatrick, G.J., 2021. Remimazolam: non-clinical and clinical profile of a new sedative/anesthetic agent. Front. Pharmacol., 1850.

Kim, T.-W., Giorgi, M., 2013. A brief overview of the coxib drugs in the veterinary field. Am. J. Anim. Vet. Sci. 8 (2), 89–97.

Kimura, L.F., et al., 2022. How environmental enrichment balances out neuroinflammation in chronic pain and comorbid depression and anxiety disorders. Br. J. Pharmacol. 179 (8), 1640–1660.

Kissin, I., et al., 1983. Inotropic and anesthetic potencies of etomidate and thiopental in dogs. Anesth. Analg. 62 (11), 961–965.

Kissin, I., 2000. Preemptive analgesia. Anesthesiology 93 (4), 1138–1143.

Kittleson, M.D., 1983. Measurement of systemic arterial blood pressure. Vet. Clin. North Am. Small Anim. Pract. 13, 321–336.

Knaevelsrud, T., Framstad, T., 1992. Measurement of arterial blood pressure in the sow. A comparison between an invasive and an automatic oscillometric method. Vet. Anaesth. Analg. 19 (1), 10–12.

Ko, J.C., et al., 1992. A comparison of medetomidine-propofol and medetomidine-midazolam-propofol anesthesia in rabbits. Lab. Anim. Sci. 42 (5), 503–507.

Ko, J., et al., 2007. Plasma concentrations of lidocaine in dogs following lidocaine patch application. J. Am. Anim. Hosp. Assoc. 43 (5), 280–283.

Ko, J.C., et al., 2008. Pharmacokinetics of lidocaine following the application of 5% lidocaine patches to cats. J. Vet. Pharmacol. Ther. 31 (4), 359–367.

Koblin, D.D., 1992. Characteristics and implications of desflurane metabolism and toxicity. Anesth. Analg. 75 (4 Suppl), S10–S16.

Koehn, D., et al., 2015. Ketamine/xylazine-induced corneal damage in mice. PLoS ONE 10 (7), e0132804.

Kohn, D.F., et al., 2007. Guidelines for the assessment and management of pain in rodents and rabbits. J. Am. Assoc. Lab. Anim. Sci. 46, 97–108.

Kolb, B., Cioe, J., 2001. Cryoanethesia on postnatal day 1, but not day 10, affects adult behavior and cortical morphology in rats. Brain Res. Dev. Brain Res. 130 (1), 9–14.

Komatsu, R., et al., 2007. Remifentanil for general anaesthesia: a systematic review. Anaesthesia 62 (12), 1266–1280.

Korner, P.I., et al., 1968. The effects of chloralose-urethane and sodium pentobarbitone anaesthesia on the local and autonomic components of the circulatory response to arterial hypoxia. J. Physiol. 199 (2), 283–302.

Kounensis, G., et al., 1992. Comparative study of the H2-receptor antagonists cimetidine, ranitidine, famotidine and Nizatidine on the rabbit stomach fundus and sigmoid colon. J. Pharmacobiodyn. 15 (10), 561–565.

Kögel, B., et al., 2005. Interaction of μ-opioid receptor agonists and antagonists with the analgesic effect of buprenorphine in mice. Eur. J. Pain 9 (5), 599–611.

Krall, C., et al., 2019. Behavioural anxiety predisposes rabbits to intra-operative apnoea and cardio-respiratory instability. Appl. Anim. Behav. Sci. 221, 104875.

Krugner-Higby, L., et al., 2003. Liposome-encapsulated oxymorphone hydrochloride provides prolonged relief of postsurgical visceral pain in rats. Comp. Med. 53 (3), 270–279.

Krugner-Higby, L., et al., 2009. Pharmacokinetics and behavioral effects of an extended-release, liposome-encapsulated preparation of oxymorphone in rhesus macaques. J. Pharmacol. Exp. Ther. 330 (1), 135–141.

Kruse-Elliott, K.T., et al., 1990. Duration of etomidate-induced adrenocortical supression in canine surgical patients. Vet. Surg. 18, 250.

Krutrök, N., et al., 2022. Ventilation via nose cone results in similar hemodynamic parameters and blood gas levels as endotracheal intubation during open chest surgery in rats. Lab. Anim. 56 (2), 157–164.

Kukanich, B., Papich, M.G., 2004. Pharmacokinetics of tramadol and the metabolite O-desmethyl-tramadol in dogs. J. Vet. Pharmacol. Ther. 27 (4), 239–246.

KuKanich, B., Spade, J., 2013. Pharmacokinetics of hydrocodone and hydromorphone after oral hydrocodone in healthy Greyhound dogs. Vet. J. 196 (2), 266–268.

KuKanich, B., et al., 2012. Clinical pharmacology of nonsteroidal anti-inflammatory drugs in dogs. Vet. Anaesth. Analg. 39 (1), 69–90.

Kumar, S., et al., 2005. Effects of perioperative hypothermia and warming in surgical practice. Int. Wound J. 2 (3), 193–204.

Kurtz, T.W., et al., 2005. Recommendations for blood pressure measurement in humans and experimental animals. Part 2: blood pressure measurement in experimental animals: a statement for professionals from the subcommittee of professional and public education of the American Heart Association council on high blood pressure research. Hypertension 45 (2), 299–310.

Kuwahara, M., et al., 1996. Non-invasive measurement of systemic arterial pressure in guinea pigs by an automatic oscillometric device. Blood Press. Monit. 1 (5), 433–437.

Laferriere, C.A., Pang, D.S., 2020. Review of intraperitoneal injection of sodium pentobarbital as a method of euthanasia in laboratory rodents. J. Am. Assoc. Lab. Anim. Sci. 59 (3), 254–263.

LaFollette, M.R., et al., 2018. Practical rat tickling: determining an efficient and effective dosage of heterospecific play. Appl. Anim. Behav. Sci. 208, 82–91.

Laitinen, O.M., 1990. Clinical observations on medetomidine/ketamine anaesthesia in sheep and its reversal by atipamezole. Vet. Anaesth. Analg. 17 (1), 17–19.

Lambert, H., et al., 2019. Given the cold shoulder: a review of the scientific literature for evidence of reptile sentience. Animals 9 (10), 821.

Lamon, T.K., et al., 2008. Adverse effects of incorporating ketoprofen into established rodent studies. J. Am. Assoc. Lab. Anim. Sci. 47 (4), 20–24.

Lamont, L.A., et al., 2004. Relationship of bispectral index to minimum alveolar concentration multiples of sevoflurane in cats. Am. J. Vet. Res. 65 (1), 93–98.

Langford, D.J., et al., 2010. Coding of facial expressions of pain in the laboratory mouse. Nat. Methods 7 (6), 447–449.

Larson, C.M., et al., 2019. Defining and managing pain in stroke and traumatic brain injury research. Comp. Med. 69 (6), 510–519.

Lascelles, B.D.X., et al., 1995. Central sensitization as a result of surgical pain: investigation of the pre-emptive value of pethidine for ovariohysterectomy in the rat. Pain 62 (2), 201–212.

Lascelles, B.D.X., et al., 2007. Nonsteroidal anti-inflammatory drugs in cats: a review. Vet. Anaesth. Analg. 34 (4), 228–250.

Lascelles, X.B.D., et al., 1997. Post-operative central hypersensitivity and pain: the pre-emptive value of pethidine for ovariohysterectomy. Pain 73 (3), 461–471.

Lau, C., et al., 2013. Plasma pharmacokinetics of alfaxalone after a single intraperitoneal or intravenous injection of Alfaxan® in rats. J. Vet. Pharmacol. Ther. 36 (5), 516–520.

Lavy, E., et al., 2014. Use of the novel atypical opioid tapentadol in goats (*Capra hircus*): pharmacokinetics after intravenous, and intramuscular administration. J. Vet. Pharmacol. Ther. 37 (5), 518–521.

Le Bars, D., et al., 2001. Animal models of nociception. Pharmacol. Rev. 53 (4), 597–652.

Leach, M.C., et al., 2010a. Influence of preferred foodstuffs on the antinociceptive effects of orally administered buprenorphine in laboratory rats. Lab. Anim. 44 (1), 54–58.

Leach, M.C., et al., 2010b. A preliminary investigation into the practicality of use and duration of action of slow-release preparations of morphine and hydromorphone in laboratory rats. Lab. Anim. 44 (1), 59–65.

Leach, M.C., et al., 2009. Behavioural effects of ovariohysterectomy and oral administration of meloxicam in laboratory housed rabbits. Res. Vet. Sci. 87 (2), 336–347.

Leach, M.C., et al., 2012. The assessment of post-vasectomy pain in mice using behaviour and the Mouse Grimace Scale. PLoS ONE 7 (4), e35656.

Ledowski, T., et al., 2012. Effects of acute postoperative pain on catecholamine plasma levels, hemodynamic parameters, and cardiac autonomic control. Pain 153 (4), 759–764.

Lee, E.J., et al., 2009. Dynamic arterial blood gas analysis in conscious, unrestrained C57BL/6J mice during exposure to intermittent hypoxia. J. Appl. Physiol. 107 (1), 290–294.

Lee, H.K., et al., 2013. Pharmacokinetics of the novel atypical opioid tapentadol after intravenous, intramuscular and subcutaneous administration in cats. Vet. J. 198 (3), 620–624.

Lee, J.I., et al., 2012. Reference values of hematology, chemistry, electrolytes, blood gas, coagulation time, and urinalysis in the Chinese rhesus macaques (*Macaca mulatta*). Xenotransplantation 19 (4), 244–248.

Lees, P., et al., 2004. Pharmacodynamics and pharmacokinetics of nonsteroidal anti-inflammatory drugs in species of veterinary interest. J. Vet. Pharmacol. Ther. 27 (6), 479–490.

Lees, P., et al., 1991. Pharmacology and therapeutics of nonsteroidal antiinflammatory drugs in the dog and cat: 1 general pharmacology. J. Small Anim. Pract. 32 (4), 183–193.

Lees, P., et al., 2022. Pharmacology, safety, efficacy and clinical uses of the COX-2 inhibitor robenacoxib. J. Vet. Pharmacol. Ther. https://doi.org/10.1111/jvp.13052.

Lemberg, K., et al., 2006. Morphine, oxycodone, methadone and its enantiomers in different models of nociception in the rat. Anesth. Analg. 102, 1768–1774.

Levin-Arama, M., et al., 2016. Subcutaneous compared with intraperitoneal ketamine–xylazine for anesthesia of mice. J. Am. Assoc. Lab. Anim. Sci. 55 (6), 794–800.

Levinson, B.L., et al., 2021. Pharmacokinetic and histopathologic study of an extended-release, injectable formulation of buprenorphine in sprague–dawley rats. J. Am. Assoc. Lab. Anim. Sci. 60 (4), 462–469.

Lewis, S.R., et al., 2013. Nonsteroidal anti-inflammatory drugs and perioperative bleeding in paediatric tonsillectomy. Cochrane Database Syst. Rev. 2013 (7), CD003591.

Li, R., et al., 2012. Minimum infusion rates and recovery times from different durations of continuous infusion of fospropofol, a prodrug of propofol, in rabbits: a comparison with propofol emulsion. Vet. Anaesth. Analg. 39 (4), 373–384.

Liao, L., et al., 2014. Evaluation of pain in rats through facial expression following experimental tooth movement. Eur. J. Oral Sci. 122 (2), 121–124.

Lidster, K., et al., 2016. Opportunities for improving animal welfare in rodent models of epilepsy and seizures. J. Neurosci. Methods 260, 2–25.

Lieggi, C.C., et al., 2005. An evaluation of preparation methods and storage conditions of tribromoethanol. J. Am. Assoc. Lab. Anim. Sci. 44 (1), 11–16.

Lierz, M., Korbel, R., 2012. Anesthesia and analgesia in birds. J. Exot. Pet Med. 21 (1), 44–58.

Liles, J.H., Flecknell, P.A., 1993. The effects of surgical stimulus on the rat and the influence of analgesic treatment. Br. Vet. J. 149 (6), 515–525.

Liles, J.H., Flecknell, P.A., 1992. The use of non-steroidal anti-inflammatory drugs for the relief of pain in laboratory rodents and rabbits. Lab. Anim. 26 (4), 241–255.

Lin, H., Passler, T., Clark-Price, S. (Eds.), 2022. Farm Animal Anesthesia: Cattle, Small Ruminants, Camelids, and Pigs. John Wiley & Sons.

Linde, H.W., Berman, M.L., 1971. Nonspecific stimulation of drug-metabolizing enzymes by inhalation anesthetic agents. Anesth. Analg. 50 (4), 656–667.

Linkenhoker, J.R., et al., 2010. Effective and safe anesthesia for Yorkshire and Yucatan swine with and without cardiovascular injury and intervention. J. Am. Assoc. Lab. Anim. Sci. 49 (3), 344–351.

Lipman, N.S., et al., 1990. A comparison of ketamine/xylazine and ketamine/xylazine/acepromazine anesthesia in the rabbit. Lab. Anim. Sci. 40 (4), 395–398.

Lipman, N.S., et al., 1987. Reversal of ketamine/xylazine anesthesia in the rabbit with yohimbine. Lab. Anim. Sci. 37 (4), 474–477.

Loepke, A.W., et al., 2006. The physiologic effects of isoflurane anesthesia in neonatal mice. Anesth. Analg. 102 (1), 75–80.

Longley, L., 2008. Anaesthesia of Exotic Pets. Elsevier Saunders.

Lovell, D.P., 1986a. Variation in pentobarbitone sleeping time in mice 2. Variables affecting test results. Lab. Anim. 20 (2), 91–96.

Lovell, D.P., 1986b. Variation in pentobarbitone sleeping time in mice. 1. Strain and sex differences. Lab. Anim. 20 (2), 85–90.

Luckl, J., et al., 2008. Alpha-chloralose is a suitable anesthetic for chronic focal cerebral ischemia studies in the rat: a comparative study. Brain Res. 1191, 157–167.

Ludders, J.W., 2015. Comparative anesthesia and analgesia of birds. In: Veterinary Anesthesia and Analgesia: The Fifth Edition of Lumb and Jones. Wiley, pp. 800–816.

Lukasik, V.M., et al., 1998a. Minimal alveolar concentration and cardiovascular effects of desflurane in sheep. Vet. Surg. 27, 167.

Lukasik, V.M., et al., 1998b. Minimal alveolar concentration and cardiovascular effects of sevoflurane in sheep. Vet. Surg. 27, 168.

Lunam, C.A., et al., 1985. Guinea-pig model of halothane-associated hepatotoxicity in the absence of enzyme induction and hypoxia. J. Pharmacol. Exp. Ther. 232 (3), 802–809.

Luna, S.P.L., et al., 2020. Validation of the UNESP-Botucatu pig composite acute pain scale (UPAPS). PLoS ONE 15 (6), e0233552.

Mach, W.J., et al., 2011. Consequences of hyperoxia and the toxicity of oxygen in the lung. Nurs. Res. Pract. 2011, 260482.

Machin, K., 2004. Waterfowl anesthesia. Semin. Avian Exot. Pet Med. 13 (4), 206–212.

Machin, K.L., 2005. Avian analgesia. Semin. Avian Exot. Pet Med. 14 (4), 236–242.

Mackiewicz, A.L., et al., 2019. Pharmacokinetics of a long-lasting, highly concentrated buprenorphine solution after subcutaneous administration in rhesus macaques (*Macaca mulatta*). J. Am. Assoc. Lab. Anim. Sci. 58 (4), 501–509.

Maggi, C.A., Meli, A., 1986a. Suitability of urethane anesthesia for physiopharmacological investigations in various systems part 1: general considerations. Experientia 42 (2), 109–114.

Maggi, C.A., Meli, A., 1986b. Suitability of urethane anesthesia for physiopharmacological investigations in various systems. Part 2: cardiovascular system. Experientia 42 (3), 292–297.

Maggi, C.A., Meli, A., 1986c. Suitability of urethane anesthesia for physiopharmacological investigations. Part 3: other systems and conclusions. Experientia 42 (5), 531–537.

Mahmoudi, N.W., et al., 1989. Insufficient anesthetic potency of nitrous oxide in the rat. Anesthesiology 70 (2), 345–349.

Malavasi, L.M., et al., 2006. Effects of epidural morphine and transdermal fentanyl analgesia on physiology and behaviour after abdominal surgery in pigs. Lab. Anim. 40 (1), 16–27.

Malik, A., Valentine, A., 2018. Pain in birds: a review for veterinary nurses. Vet. Nurs. J. 33 (1), 11–25.

Manley, S.V., McDonell, W.N., 1979. A new circuit for small animal anesthesia: the Bain coaxial circuit. J. Am. Anim. Hosp. Assoc. 15, 61–65.

Marini, R.P., et al., 1992. Ketamine/xylazine/butorphanol: a new anesthetic combination for rabbits. Lab. Anim. Sci. 42 (1), 57–62.

Marini, R.P., et al., 1993. An evaluation of three neuroleptanalgesic combinations in rabbits. Lab. Anim. Sci. 43 (4), 338–345.

Marini, R.P., Haupt, J., 2019. Anesthesia and select surgical procedures. In: The Common Marmoset in Captivity and Biomedical Research. Academic Press, pp. 177–194.

Marshall, M., 2004. Capnography in dogs. Compendium 26 (10).

Martenson, M., et al., 2005. A simple device for humidification of inspired gases during volatile anesthesia in rats. Contemp. Top. Lab. Anim. Sci. 44 (2), 46–48.

Martin, L., 1999. All you Really Need to Know to Interpret Arterial Blood Gases. Lippincott Williams & Wilkins.

Martin, L.B., et al., 2001. Analgesic efficacy of orally administered buprenorphine in rats. Comp. Med. 51 (1), 43–48.

Martin, T.J., et al., 2004. Effects of laparotomy on spontaneous exploratory activity and conditioned operant responding in the rat: a model for postoperative pain. Anesthesiology 101 (1), 191–203.

Martins, T.L., et al., 2010. Comparison of the effects of tramadol, codeine, and ketoprofen alone or in combination on postoperative pain and on concentrations of blood glucose, serum cortisol, and serum interleukin-6 in dogs undergoing maxillectomy or mandibulectomy. Am. J. Vet. Res. 71 (9), 1019–1026.

Martins, T., et al., 2019. Anaesthetics and analgesics used in adult fish for research: a review. Lab. Anim. 53 (4), 325–341.

Martín-Cancho, M.F., et al., 2006. Relationship of bispectral index values, haemodynamic changes and recovery times during sevoflurane or propofol anaesthesia in rabbits. Lab. Anim. 40 (1), 28–42.

Mason, G.J., Lavery, J.M., 2022. What is it like to be a bass? Red herrings, fish pain and the study of animal sentience. Front. Vet. Sci. 9.

Mather, L.E., 1983. Pharmacokinetic and pharmacodynamic factors influencing the choice, dose and route of administration of opiates for acute pain. Clin. Anesthesiol. 1 (1), 17–40.

Mathews, F., et al., 2002. Use of inhalation anaesthesia for wild mammals in the field. Vet. Rec. 150 (25), 785–787.

Mathews, K., et al., 1987. Renal-failure in dogs associated with flunixin meglumine and methoxy-flurane anesthesia. Vet. Surg. 16 (4), 323.

Mathews, K.A., 2000. Nonsteroidal anti-inflammatory analgesics: indications and contraindications for pain management in dogs and cats. Vet. Clin. North Am. Small Anim. Pract. 30 (4), 783–804.

Mathews, K.A., et al., 1996. A comparison of ketorolac with flunixin, butorphanol, and oxymor-phone in controlling postoperative pain in dogs. Can. Vet. J. 37 (9), 557–567.

Mathiesen, O., et al., 2014. Adverse effects of perioperative paracetamol, NSAIDs, glucocorticoids, gabapentinoids and their combinations: a topical review. Acta Anaesthesiol. Scand. 58 (10), 1182–1198.

Matsumiya, L.C., et al., 2012. Using the mouse grimace scale to reevaluate the efficacy of postoperative analgesics in laboratory mice. J. Am. Assoc. Lab. Anim. Sci. 51 (1), 42–49.

Maze, M., Fujinaga, M., 2000. Recent advances in understanding the actions and toxicity of nitrous oxide. Anaesthesia 55 (4), 311–314.

Mazze, R.I., et al., 1985. Halothane, isoflurane, and enflurane MAC in pregnant and nonpregnant female and male mice and rats. Anesthesiology 62 (3), 339–341.

McCann, M.E., et al., 2004. In vitro effects and in vivo efficacy of a novel cyclooxygenase-2 inhibitor in dogs with experimentally induced synovitis. Am. J. Vet. Res. 65 (4), 503–512.

McLennan, K.M., et al., 2016. Development of a facial expression scale using footrot and mastitis as models of pain in sheep. Appl. Anim. Behav. Sci. 176, 19–26.

McLennan, K.M., et al., 2019. Conceptual and methodological issues relating to pain assessment in mammals: the development and utilisation of pain facial expression scales. Appl. Anim. Behav. Sci. 217, 1–15.

McDowell, A., et al., 2014. A cyclodextrin formulation to improve use of the anesthetic tribromo-ethanol (Avertin®). J. Pharm. Bioallied Sci. 6 (1), 16–21.

McKeon, G.P., et al., 2011. Analgesic effects of tramadol, tramadol-gabapentin, and buprenorphine in an incisional model of pain in rats (*Rattus norvegicus*). J. Am. Assoc. Lab. Anim. Sci. 50 (2), 192–197.

McQuay, H.J., et al., 2012. Evidence for analgesic effect in acute pain—50years on. Pain 153 (7), 1364–1367.

Mellor, D.J., Diesch, T.J., 2006. Onset of sentience: the potential for suffering in fetal and newborn farm animals. Appl. Anim. Behav. Sci. 100 (1–2), 48–57.

Mellor, D.J., et al., 2005. The importance of "awareness" for understanding fetal pain. Brain Res. Brain Res. Rev. 49 (3), 455–471.

Mestre, C., et al., 1994. A method to perform direct transcutaneous intrathecal injection in rats. J. Pharmacol. Toxicol. Methods 32 (4), 197–200.

Michalot, G., et al., 1980. 24-hour althesin-fentanyl anaesthesia in dogs. Time course of haemodynamic changes. Br. J. Anaesth. 52 (1), 19–22.

Michou, J.N., et al., 2012. Comparison of pain on injection during induction of anaesthesia with alfaxalone and two formulations of propofol in dogs. Vet. Anaesth. Analg. 39 (3), 275–281.

Mickley, G.A., et al., 2006. Acetaminophen self-administered in the drinking water increases the pain threshold of rats (*Rattus norvegicus*). J. Am. Assoc. Lab. Anim. Sci. 45 (5), 48–54.

Middleton, D.J., et al., 1982. Physiological effects of thiopentone, ketamine and CT 1341 in cats. Res. Vet. Sci. 32 (2), 157–162.

Millar, T.J., et al., 1989. Urethane as a sole general anaesthetic in cats used for electroretinogram studies. Neurosci. Lett. 103 (1), 108–112.

Miller, A.L., et al., 2016. The influence of isoflurane anaesthesia on the rat grimace scale. PLoS ONE 11 (11), e0166652.

Miller, A., et al., 2015. The effect of isoflurane anaesthesia and buprenorphine on the mouse grimace scale and behaviour in CBA and DBA/2 mice. Appl. Anim. Behav. Sci. 172, 58–62.

Miller, A.L., Leach, M.C., 2016. The effect of handling method on the mouse grimace scale in two strains of laboratory mice. Lab. Anim. 50 (4), 305–307.

Miller, A., et al., 2022. Evaluating pain and analgesia effectiveness following routine castration in rabbits using behavior and facial expressions. Front. Vet. Sci. 9, 782486.

Mills, P.C., Cross, S.E., 2006. Transdermal drug delivery: basic principles for the veterinarian. Vet. J. 172 (2), 218–233.

Minville, V., et al., 2011. Ondansetron does not block paracetamol-induced analgesia in a mouse model of fracture pain. Br. J. Anaesth. 106 (1), 112–118.

Mion, G., Villevieille, T., 2013. Ketamine pharmacology: an update (pharmacodynamics and molecular aspects, recent findings). CNS Neurosci. Ther. 19 (6), 370–380.

Miranda, H.F., et al., 2008. Isobolographic analysis of multimodal analgesia in an animal model of visceral acute pain. Pharmacol. Biochem. Behav. 88 (4), 481–486.

Miranda, H.F., et al., 2013. Systemic synergism between codeine and morphine in three pain models in mice. Pharmacol. Rep. 65 (1), 80–88.

Mirra, A., et al., 2022. Usability of the SedLine® electroencephalographic monitor of depth of anaesthesia in pigs: a pilot study. J. Clin. Monit. Comput., 1–12.

Mitchell, A.Z., et al., 2010. Sensitivity of two noninvasive blood pressure measurement techniques compared to telemetry in cynomolgus monkeys and beagle dogs. J. Pharmacol. Toxicol. Methods 62 (1), 54–63.

Mitchell, D., et al., 1977. Pica: a species relevant behavioral assay of motion sickness in the rat. Physiol. Behav. 18 (1), 125–130.

Miyabe, T., et al., 2001. Chemical restraint by medetomidine and medetomidine–midazolam and its reversal by atipamezole in Japanese macaques (*Macaca fuscata*). Vet. Anaesth. Analg. 28 (3), 168–174.

Miyabe-Nishiwaki, T., et al., 2020. Evaluation of anaesthetic and cardiorespiratory effects after intramuscular administration of alfaxalone alone, alfaxalone-ketamine and alfaxalone-butorphanol-medetomidine in common marmosets (*Callithrix jacchus*). J. Med. Primatol. 49 (6), 291–299.

Miyabe-Nishiwaki, T., et al., 2021. Primate veterinarians' knowledge and attitudes regarding pain in macaques. J. Med. Primatol. 50 (5), 259–269.

Moeser, A.J., et al., 2008. Determination of minimum alveolar concentration of sevoflurane in juvenile swine. Res. Vet. Sci. 84 (2), 283–285.

Mogil, J.S., et al., 1999. Heritability of nociception I: responses of 11 inbred mouse strains on 12 measures of nociception. Pain 80 (1), 67–82.

Mogil, J.S., et al., 2005. Influence of nociception and stress-induced antinociception on genetic variation in isoflurane anesthetic potency among mouse strains. Anesthesiology 103 (4), 751–758.

Mogil, J.S., et al., 2006. Screening for pain phenotypes: analysis of three congenic mouse strains on a battery of nine nociceptive assays. Pain 126 (1–3), 24–34.

Mogil, J.S., et al., 2020. The development and use of facial grimace scales for pain measurement in animals. Neurosci. Biobehav. Rev. 116, 480–493.

Moldestad, O., et al., 2009. Tracheotomy improves experiment success rate in mice during urethane anesthesia and stereotaxic surgery. J. Neurosci. Methods 176 (2), 57–62.

Molina-Cimadevila, M.J., et al., 2014. Oral self-administration of buprenorphine in the diet for analgesia in mice. Lab. Anim. 48 (3), 0023677214532454–224.

Molina, A.M., et al., 2015. Analyses of anaesthesia with ketamine combined with different sedatives in rats. Vet. Med. 60 (7), 368–375.

Moll, X., et al., 2013. The effects on cardio-respiratory and acid-base variables of a constant rate infusion of alfaxalone-HPCD in sheep. Vet. J. 196 (2), 209–212.

Molony, V., et al., 1995. Assessment of acute and chronic pain after different methods of castration of calves. Appl. Anim. Behav. Sci. 46 (1–2), 33–48.

Monteiro Steagall, B.P., et al., 2013. Systematic review of nonsteroidal anti-inflammatory drug-induced adverse effects in dogs. J. Vet. Intern. Med. 27 (5), 1011–1019.

Morgan, C.J.A., Curran, H.V., 2012. Ketamine use: a review. Addiction 107 (1), 27–38.

Morgan, D., et al., 1999. Sensitivity to the discriminative stimulus and antinociceptive effects of μ opioids: role of strain of rat, stimulus intensity, and intrinsic efficacy at the μ opioid receptor. J. Pharmacol. Exp. Ther. 289 (2), 965–975.

Morozov, A., et al., 2021. Automatic recognition of macaque facial expressions for detection of affective states. eNeuro 8 (6).

Morris, T.H., 1995. Antibiotic therapeutics in laboratory animals. Lab. Anim. 29 (1), 16–36.

Morton, D.B., Griffiths, P.H., 1985. Guidelines on the recognition of pain, distress and discomfort in experimental animals and an hypothesis for assessment. Vet. Rec. 116 (16), 431–436.

Mosley, C.A.E., 2005. Anesthesia and analgesia in reptiles. Semin. Avian Exot. Pet Med. 14 (4), 243–262.

Moss, J.R., et al., 2014. A multicenter, randomized, double-blind placebo-controlled, single dose trial of the safety and efficacy of intravenous ibuprofen for treatment of pain in pediatric patients undergoing tonsillectomy. Paediatr. Anaesth. 24 (5), 483–489.

Mroszczak, E.J., et al., 1987. Ketorolac tromethamine absorption, distribution, metabolism, excretion, and pharmacokinetics in animals and humans. Drug Metab. Dispos. 15 (5), 618–626.

Mroszczak, E.J., et al., 1990. Ketorolac tromethamine pharmacokinetics and metabolism after intravenous, intramuscular, and oral administration in humans and animals. Pharmacotherapy 10 (6P2), 33S–39S.

Mulder, K.J., Mulder, J.B., 1979. Ketamine and xylazine anesthesia in the mouse. Vet. Med. Small Anim. Clin. 74 (4), 569–570.

Müller, B.R., et al., 2019. Facial expression of pain in Nellore and crossbred beef cattle. J. Vet. Behav. 34, 60–65.

Murayama, T., et al., 2005. Effect of continuous infusion of propofol on its concentration in blood with and without the liver in pigs. Transplant. Proc. 37 (10), 4567–4570.

Murphy, K.L., et al., 2010. Anaesthesia with a combination of ketamine and medetomidine in the rabbit: effect of premedication with buprenorphine. Vet. Anaesth. Analg. 37 (3), 222–229.

Murray, W.J., Fleming, P.J., 1972. Defluorination of methoxyflurane during anesthesia: comparison of man with other species. Anesthesiology 37 (6), 620–625.

Murrell, J.C., et al., 2005. Clinical investigation of remifentanil and propofol for the total intravenous anaesthesia of dogs. Vet. Rec. 156 (25), 804–808.

Murrell, J.C., et al., 2008. Comparative effects of halothane, isoflurane, sevoflurane and desflurane on the electroencephalogram of the rat. Lab. Anim. 42 (2), 161–170.

Musk, G.C., et al., 2005. Target-controlled infusion of propofol in dogs—evaluation of four targets for induction of anaesthesia. Vet. Rec. 157 (24), 766–770.

Muta, K., et al., 2021. Pharmacokinetics and effects on clinical and physiological parameters following a single bolus dose of propofol in common marmosets (*Callithrix jacchus*). J. Vet. Pharmacol. Ther. 44 (1), 18–27.

Nagel, M.L., et al., 1979. Comparison of the cardiopulmonary effects of etomidate and thiamylal in dogs. Am. J. Vet. Res. 40 (2), 193–196.

Nakamura, T., et al., 2017. Effects of a mixture of medetomidine, midazolam and butorphanol on anesthesia and blood biochemistry and the antagonizing action of atipamezole in hamsters. J. Vet. Med. Sci. 79 (7), 1230–1235.

Navarro, E., et al., 2020. Development of a facial expression scale using farrowing as a model of pain in sows. Animals 10 (11), 2113.

Ndawana, P.S., et al., 2015. Determination of the minimum infusion rate (MIR) of alfaxalone required to prevent purposeful movement of the extremities in response to a standardised noxious stimulus in goats. Vet. Anaesth. Analg. 42 (1), 65–71.

Nevalainen, T., et al., 1988. Evaluation of anaesthetic potency of medetomidine-ketamine combination in rats, guinea-pigs and rabbits. Acta Vet. Scand. Suppl. 85, 139–143.

Nickalls, R.W.D., Mapleson, W.W., 2003. Age-related iso-MAC charts for isoflurane, sevoflurane and desflurane in man. Br. J. Anaesth. 91 (2), 170–174.

Nilson, P.C., et al., 2005. Caudal thoracic air sac cannulation in zebra finches for isoflurane anesthesia. J. Neurosci. Methods 143 (2), 107–115.

Nogawa, H., et al., 2022. Pharmacological characterisation of electrocardiogram J-Tpeak interval in conscious Guinea pigs. Eur. J. Pharmacol., 175065.

Nolan, A., Reid, J., 1993a. Pharmacokinetics of propofol administered by infusion in dogs undergoing surgery. Br. J. Anaesth. 70 (5), 546–551.

Nolan, A., Reid, R., 1993b. Comparison of the postoperative analgesic and sedative effects of carprofen and papaveretum in the dog. Vet. Rec. 133 (10), 240–242.

Nolan, A., et al., 1987. Investigation of the antinociceptive activity of buprenorphine in sheep. Br. J. Pharmacol. 92 (3), 527–533.

Norris, M.L., Turner, W.D., 1983. An evaluation of tribromoethanol (TBE) as an anaesthetic agent in the Mongolian gerbil (*Meriones unguiculatus*). Lab. Anim. 17 (4), 324–329.

Norton, W.B., et al., 2016. Refinements for embryo implantation surgery in the mouse: comparison of injectable and inhalant anesthesias–tribromoethanol, ketamine and isoflurane–on pregnancy and pup survival. Lab. Anim. 50 (5), 335–343.

Norwich, K.H., 1977. Molecular Dynamics in Biosystems: The Kinetics of Tracers in Intact Organisms. Pergamon Press, Oxford; New York.

Nguyen, H.A., et al., 2020. Cognitive bias under adverse and rewarding conditions: a systematic review of rodent studies. Front. Behav. Neurosci. 14, 14.

O'Flaherty, D., 1994. Capnography. BMJ Books.

O'Keeffe, N.J., Healy, T.E.J., 1999. The role of new anesthetic agents. Pharmacol. Ther. 84 (3), 233–248.

Obernier, J.A., Baldwin, R.L., 2006. Establishing an appropriate period of acclimatization following transportation of laboratory animals. ILAR J. 47 (4), 364–369.

Oliver, V., et al., 2014. Psychometric assessment of the rat grimace scale and development of an analgesic intervention score. PLoS ONE 9 (5), e97882.

Oliver, V.L., et al., 2017. Evaluation of pain assessment techniques and analgesia efficacy in a female guinea pig (*Cavia porcellus*) model of surgical pain. J. Am. Assoc. Lab. Anim. Sci. 56 (4), 425–435.

Olson, M.E., et al., 1994. The parasympatholytic effects of atropine sulfate and glycopyrrolate in rats and rabbits. Can. J. Vet. Res. 58 (4), 254–271.

Ong, C.K.S., et al., 2010. Combining paracetamol (acetaminophen) with nonsteroidal antiinflammatory drugs: a qualitative systematic review of analgesic efficacy for acute postoperative pain. Anesth. Analg. 110 (4), 1170.

Oostrom, H., et al., 2013. A comparison between the v-gel supraglottic airway device and the cuffed endotracheal tube for airway management in spontaneously breathing cats during isoflurane anaesthesia. Vet. Anaesth. Analg. 40 (3), 265–271.

Orliaguet, G., et al., 2001. Minimum alveolar concentration of volatile anesthetics in rats during postnatal maturation. Anesthesiology 95 (3), 734–739.

Orr, H.E., et al., 2005. Assessment of ketamine and medetomidine anaesthesia in the domestic rabbit. Vet. Anaesth. Analg. 32 (5), 271–279.

Otto, K.A., et al., 2012. Electroencephalographic Narcotrend index, spectral edge frequency and median power frequency as guide to anaesthetic depth for cardiac surgery in laboratory sheep. Vet. J. 191 (3), 354–359.

Paasonen, J., et al., 2018. Functional connectivity under six anesthesia protocols and the awake condition in rat brain. Neuroimage 172, 9–20.

Pablo, L.S., 1993. Epidural morphine in goats after hindlimb orthopedic surgery. Vet. Surg. 22 (4), 307–310.

Pagliardini, S., et al., 2014. Ampakines enhance respiratory motor output in a murine model of Pompe disease. Am. J. Respir. Cell Mol. Biol. 53 (3), 326–335.

Pandit, J.J., Cook, T.M., 2013. National Institute for Clinical Excellence guidance on measuring depth of anaesthesia: limitations of EEG-based technology. Br. J. Anaesth. 110 (3), 325–328.

Panksepp, J., 2011. The basic emotional circuits of mammalian brains: do animals have affective lives? Neurosci. Biobehav. Rev. 35 (9), 1791–1804.

Papaioannou, V.E., Fox, J.G., 1993. Efficacy of tribromoethanol anesthesia in mice. Lab. Anim. Sci. 43 (2), 189–192.

Papich, M.G., 2008. An update on nonsteroidal anti-inflammatory drugs (NSAIDs) in small animals. Vet. Clin. N. Am. Small Anim. Pract. 38 (6), 1243–1266.

Park, C.M., et al., 1992. Improved techniques for successful neonatal rat surgery. Lab. Anim. Sci. 42 (5), 508–513.

Parr, L.A., et al., 2010. Brief communication: MaqFACS: a muscle-based facial movement coding system for the rhesus macaque. Am. J. Phys. Anthropol. 143 (4), 625–630.

Pascoe, P.J., Dyson, D.H., 1993. Analgesia after lateral thoracotomy in dogs epidural morphine vs. intercostal bupivacaine. Vet. Surg. 22 (2), 141–147.

Pascoe, P.J., et al., 2006. The effect of the duration of propofol administration on recovery from anesthesia in cats. Vet. Anaesth. Analg. 33 (1), 2–7.

Pasternak, G.W., 2014. Opioids and their receptors: are we there yet? Neuropharmacology 76, 198–203.

Pasternak, G.W., 2012. Preclinical pharmacology and opioid combinations. Pain Med. 13 (s1), S4–S11.

Paull, D.R., et al., 2007. The effect of a topical anaesthetic formulation, systemic flunixin and carprofen, singly or in combination, on cortisol and behavioural responses of merino lambs to mulesing. Aust. Vet. J. 85 (3), 98–106.

McNeil, P.E., 1992. Acute tubulo-interstitial nephritis in a dog after halothane anaesthesia and administration of flunixin meglumine and trimethoprim-sulphadiazine. Vet. Rec. 131 (7), 148–151.

Peeters, M.E., et al., 1988. Four methods for general anaesthesia in the rabbit: a comparative study. Lab. Anim. 22 (4), 355–360.

Penderis, J., Franklin, R.J., 2005. Effects of pre-versus post-anaesthetic buprenorphine on propofol-anaesthetized rats. Vet. Anaesth. Analg. 32 (5), 256–260.

Percie du Sert, N., et al., 2017. The IMPROVE guidelines (ischaemia models: procedural refinements of in vivo experiments). J. Cereb. Blood Flow Metab. 37 (11), 3488–3517.

Perez-Garcia, C.C., et al., 2003. A simple procedure to perform intravenous injections in the Mongolian gerbil (*Meriones unguiculatus*). Lab. Anim. 37 (1), 68–71.

Peterson, N.C., et al., 2017. To treat or not to treat: the effects of pain on experimental parameters. Comp. Med. 67 (6), 469–482.

Pfeiffer, N., et al., 2013. Cardiovascular effects of alfaxalone on hemodynamic function in pigs. Open Access Anim. Physiol., 15.

Philip, P., et al., 2006. The effects of coffee and napping on nighttime highway driving: a randomized trial. Ann. Intern. Med. 144 (11), 785–791.

Pinho, R.H., et al., 2020. Postoperative pain behaviours in rabbits following orthopaedic surgery and effect of observer presence. PLoS ONE 15 (10).

Pinho, R., et al., 2022. Validation of the rabbit pain behaviour scale (RPBS) to assess acute postoperative pain in rabbits (*Oryctolagus cuniculus*). PLoS ONE 17 (5), e0268973.

Piriou, V., et al., 2002. Pharmacological preconditioning: comparison of desflurane, sevoflurane, isoflurane and halothane in rabbit myocardium. Br. J. Anaesth. 89 (3), 486–491.

Plant, M., Lloyd, M., 2010. The ferret. In: The UFAW Handbook on the Care and Management of Laboratory and Other Research Animals, eighth ed. Wiley-Blackwell, pp. 418–432.

Pogatzki-Zahn, E.M., et al., 2007. Postoperative pain—clinical implications of basic research. Best Pract. Res. Clin. Anaesthesiol. 21 (1), 3–13.

Popilskis, S., et al., 1993. Efficacy of epidural morphine versus intravenous morphine for post-thoractotomy pain in dogs. Vet. Anaesth. Analg. 20 (1), 21–25.

Pounder, K.C., et al., 2018. Physiological and behavioural evaluation of common anaesthesia practices in the rainbow trout. Appl. Anim. Behav. Sci. 199, 94–102.

Pottie, R.G., et al., 2007. Effect of hypothermia on recovery from general anaesthesia in the dog. Aust. Vet. J. 85 (4), 158–162.

Prassinos, N.N., et al., 2005. A comparison of propofol, thiopental or ketamine as induction agents in goats. Vet. Anaesth. Analg. 32 (5), 289–296.

Preckel, B., Bolten, J., 2005. Pharmacology of modern volatile anaesthetics. Best Pract. Res. Clin. Anaesthesiol. 19 (3), 331–348.

Princi, T., et al., 2000. Experimental urethane anaesthesia prevents digoxin intoxication: electrocardiographic and histological study in rabbit. Pharmacol. Res. 42 (4), 355–359.

Prommer, E., 2006. Oxymorphone: a review. Support. Care Cancer 14 (2), 109–115.

Pugsley, M.K., 2002. The diverse molecular mechanisms responsible for the actions of opioids on the cardiovascular system. Pharmacol. Ther. 93 (1), 51–75.

Puig, N.R., et al., 2002. Effects of sevoflurane general anesthesia: immunological studies in mice. Int. Immunopharmacol. 2 (1), 95–104.

Pypendop, B.H., et al., 2014. Bioavailability of morphine, methadone, hydromorphone, and oxymorphone following buccal administration in cats. J. Vet. Pharmacol. Ther. 37 (3), 295–300.

Pypendop, B.H., et al., 2018. Comparison of two intravenous anesthetic infusion regimens for alfaxalone in cats. Vet. Anaesth. Analg. 45 (4), 459–466.

Raftery, A., 2013. Avian anaesthesia. In Pract. 35 (5), 272–278.

Ragbetli, M.C., et al., 2007. Effect of prenatal exposure to diclofenac sodium on Purkinje cell numbers in rat cerebellum: a stereological study. Brain Res. 1174, 130–135.

Raja, S.N., et al., 2020. The revised International Association for the Study of Pain definition of pain: concepts, challenges, and compromises. Pain 161 (9), 1976–1982.

Ramos-Cabrer, P., et al., 2005. Continuous noninvasive monitoring of transcutaneous blood gases for a stable and persistent BOLD contrast in fMRI studies in the rat. NMR Biomed. 18 (7), 440–446.

Rätsep, M.T., et al., 2013. Hemodynamic and behavioral differences after administration of meloxi-cam, buprenorphine, or tramadol as analgesics for telemeter implantation in mice. J. Am. Assoc. Lab. Anim. Sci. 52 (5), 560–566.

Readman, G.D., et al., 2013. Do fish perceive anaesthetics as aversive? PLoS ONE 8 (9), e73773.

Refinetti, R., Menaker, M., 1992. The circadian rhythm of body temperature. Physiol. Behav. 51 (3), 613–637.

Regan, M.J., Eger, E.I., 1967. Effect of hypothermia in dogs on anesthetizing and apneic doses of inhalation agents. Determination of the anesthetic index (Apnea/MAC). Anesthesiology 28 (4), 689–700.

Reid, J., Nolan, A.M., 1991. A comparison of the postoperative analgesic and sedative effects of flimixin and pap aver etum in the dog. J. Small Anim. Pract. 32 (12), 603–608.

Reid, J., et al., 2018. Measuring pain in dogs and cats using structured behavioural observation. Vet. J. 236, 72–79.

Reid, J., et al., 2013. Pain assessment in animals. In Pract. 35 (2), 51–56.

Reimann, H.M., Niendorf, T., 2020. The (un) conscious mouse as a model for human brain functions: key principles of anesthesia and their impact on translational neuroimaging. Front. Syst. Neurosci. 14, 8.

Rembert, M.S., Smith, J.A., Hosgood, G., 2004. A comparison of a forced-air warming system to traditional thermal support for rodent microenvironments. Lab. Anim. 38 (1), 55–63.

Riley, C., Andrzejowski, J., 2018. Inadvertent perioperative hypothermia. BJA Educ. 18 (8), 227.

Rhodes, S.A., 2009. Evaluation of Hypothermia for Anaesthesia in Neonatal Rats, Implications for Animal Welfare and Experimental Data (PhD thesis). University of Newcastle upon Tyne.

Richardson, C.A., Flecknell, P.A., 2005. Anaesthesia and post-operative analgesia following experimental surgery in laboratory rodents: are we making progress? Altern. Lab. Anim. 33 (2), 119–127.

Richter, S.H., et al., 2014. The effects of neonatal cryoanaesthesia-induced hypothermia on adult emotional behaviour and stress markers in C57BL/6 mice. Behav. Brain Res. 270, 300–306.

Rieg, T., et al., 2004. Kidney function in mice: thiobutabarbital versus alpha-chloralose anesthesia. Naunyn Schmiedebergs Arch. Pharmacol. 370 (4), 320–323.

Riendeau, D., et al., 2001. Etoricoxib (MK-0663): preclinical profile and comparison with other agents that selectively inhibit cyclooxygenase-2. J. Pharmacol. Exp. Ther. 296 (2), 558–566.

Rindfield, T., McBrian, S., 2012. Assisted ventilation without endotracheal intubation in rats. J. Invest. Surg. 25 (3), 197–199.

Risling, T.E., et al., 2012. Open-drop anesthesia for small laboratory animals. Can. Vet. J. 53 (3), 299.

Rivera, B., et al., 2005. A novel method for endotracheal intubation of mice and rats used in imaging studies. J. Am. Assoc. Lab. Anim. Sci. 44 (2), 52–55.

Riviere, J.E., Papich, M.G., 2001. Potential and problems of developing transdermal patches for veterinary applications. Adv. Drug Deliv. Rev. 50 (3), 175–203.

Riviere, J.E., et al., 1997. Interspecies allometric analysis of the comparative pharmacokinetics of 44 drugs across veterinary and laboratory animal species. J. Vet. Pharmacol. Ther. 20 (6), 453–463.

Robertson, S.A., et al., 1992. Cardiopulmonary, anesthetic, and postanesthetic effects of intravenous infusions of propofol in greyhounds and non-greyhounds. Am. J. Vet. Res. 53 (6), 1027–1032.

Robertson, S.A., et al., 2009. Antinociceptive and side-effects of hydromorphone after subcutaneous administration in cats. J. Feline Med. Surg. 11 (2), 76–81.

Robinson, F.P., Patterson, C.C., 1985. Changes in liver function tests after propofol ("Diprivan"). Postgrad. Med. J. 61 (Suppl 3), 160–161.

Rock, M.L., et al., 2014. The time-to-integrate-to-nest test as an indicator of wellbeing in laboratory mice. J. Am. Assoc. Lab. Anim. Sci. 53 (1), 24–28.

Rodriguez, P., et al., 2006. Transcutaneous arterial carbon dioxide pressure monitoring in critically ill adult patients. Intensive Care Med. 32 (2), 309–312.

Rodríguez, J.M., et al., 2012. Comparison of the cardiopulmonary parameters after induction of anaesthesia with alphaxalone or etomidate in dogs. Vet. Anaesth. Analg. 39 (4), 357–365.

Rollin, B.E., 2011. Animal pain: what it is and why it matters. J. Ethics 15 (4), 425–437.

Romanov, A., et al., 2014. Paradoxical increase in the bispectral index during deep anesthesia in New Zealand white rabbits. J. Am. Assoc. Lab. Anim. Sci. 53 (1), 74–80.

Rombough, P.J., 2007. Ontogenetic changes in the toxicity and efficacy of the anaesthetic MS222 (tricaine methanesulfonate) in zebrafish (*Danio rerio*) larvae. Comp. Biochem. Physiol. A Mol. Integr. Physiol. 148 (2), 463–469.

Ross, L.G., Ross, B., 2009. Anaesthetic and Sedative Techniques for Aquatic Animals. John Wiley & Sons.

Roughan, J.V., Flecknell, P.A., 2001. Behavioural effects of laparotomy and analgesic effects of ketoprofen and carprofen in rats. Pain 90 (1), 65–74.

Roughan, J.V., Flecknell, P.A., 2002. Buprenorphine: a reappraisal of its antinociceptive effects and therapeutic use in alleviating post-operative pain in animals. Lab. Anim. 36 (3), 322–343.

Roughan, J.V., Flecknell, P.A., 2003. Evaluation of a short duration behaviour-based post-operative pain scoring system in rats. Eur. J. Pain 7 (5), 397–406.

Roughan, J.V., Flecknell, P.A., 2004. Behaviour-based assessment of the duration of laparotomy-induced abdominal pain and the analgesic effects of carprofen and buprenorphine in rats. Behav. Pharmacol. 15 (7), 461.

Roughan, J.V., Flecknell, P.A., 2006. Training in behaviour-based post-operative pain scoring in rats—an evaluation based on improved recognition of analgesic requirements. Appl. Anim. Behav. Sci. 96 (3–4), 327–342.

Rousseau-Blass, F., et al., 2021. A pharmacokinetic-pharmacodynamic study of intravenous midazolam and flumazenil in adult New Zealand white—Californian rabbits (*Oryctolagus cuniculus*). J. Am. Assoc. Lab. Anim. Sci. 60 (3), 319–328.

Royal, J.M., et al., 2013. Assessment of postoperative analgesia after application of ultrasound-guided regional anesthesia for surgery in a swine femoral fracture model. J. Am. Assoc. Lab. Anim. Sci. 52 (3), 265–276.

Ruane-O'Hora, T., et al., 2009. The effect of ketamine and saffan on the beta-endorphin and ACTH response to hemorrhage in the minipig. Physiol. Res. 58 (6), 799–805.

Rubal, B.J., Buchanan, C., 1986. Supplemental chloralose anesthesia in morphine premedicated dogs. Lab. Anim. Sci. 36 (1), 59–64.

Rufiange, M., et al., 2020. Prewarming followed by active warming is superior to passive warming in preventing hypothermia for short procedures in adult rats (*Rattus norvegicus*) under isoflurane anesthesia. J. Am. Assoc. Lab. Anim. Sci. 59 (4), 377–383.

Ruíz-López, P., et al., 2020. Intraoperative nociception-antinociception monitors: a review from the veterinary perspective. Vet. Anaesth. Analg. 47 (2), 152–159.

Russell, W., Burch, R.L., 1959. The Principles of Humane Experimental Technique. Methuen & Co. Limited, London.

Rusyn, I., et al., 2014. Trichloroethylene: mechanistic, epidemiologic and other supporting evidence of carcinogenic hazard. Pharmacol. Ther. 141 (1), 55–68.

Sadar, M.J., et al., 2018. Pharmacokinetics of buprenorphine after intravenous and oral transmucosal administration in guinea pigs (*Cavia porcellus*). Am. J. Vet. Res. 79 (3), 260–266.

Sadler, K.E., et al., 2022. Innovations and advances in modelling and measuring pain in animals. Nat. Rev. Neurosci. 23 (2), 70–85.

Saha, D.C., et al., 2007. Comparison of cardiovascular effects of tiletamine-zolazepam, pentobarbital, and ketamine-xylazine in male rats. J. Am. Assoc. Lab. Anim. Sci. 46 (2), 74–80.

Saha, J.K., et al., 2005. Acute hyperglycemia induced by ketamine/xylazine anesthesia in rats: mechanisms and implications for preclinical models. Exp. Biol. Med. 230 (10), 777–784.

Sahbaie, P., et al., 2006. Transcutaneous blood gas CO_2 monitoring of induced ventilatory depression in mice. Anesth. Analg. 103 (3), 620–625.

Sakaguchi, M., et al., 1996. Anesthesia induced in pigs by use of a combination of medetomidine, butorphanol, and ketamine and its reversal by administration of atipamezole. Am. J. Vet. Res. 57 (4), 529–534.

Sandercock, D.A., et al., 2014. Avian reflex and electroencephalogram responses in different states of consciousness. Physiol. Behav. 133, 252–259.

Sanders, R.D., et al., 2013. Impact of anaesthetics and surgery on neurodevelopment: an update. Br. J. Anaesth. 110 (Suppl. 1(suppl. 1)), i53–i72.

Santos, M., et al., 2013. Effects of intramuscular alfaxalone alone or in combination with diazepam in swine. Vet. Anaesth. Analg. 40 (4), 399–402.

Santos, M., et al., 2016. Effects of intramuscular dexmedetomidine in combination with ketamine or alfaxalone in swine. Vet. Anaesth. Analg. 43 (1), 81–85.

Scheller, M.S., et al., 1988. MAC of sevoflurane in humans and the New Zealand white rabbit. Can. J. Anaesth. 35 (2), 153–156.

Schiene, K., et al., 2011. Antinociceptive and antihyperalgesic effects of tapentadol in animal models of inflammatory pain. J. Pharmacol. Exp. Ther. 339 (2), 537–544.

Schlapp, G., et al., 2015. Administration of the nonsteroidal anti-inflammatory drug tolfenamic acid at embryo transfer improves maintenance of pregnancy and embryo survival in recipient mice. J. Assist. Reprod. Genet., 1–5.

Schreiner, V., et al., 2020. Design and in vivo evaluation of a microparticulate depot formulation of buprenorphine for veterinary use. Sci. Rep. 10 (1), 1–14.

Schug, S.A., et al., 2020. APM:SE Working Group of the Australian and New Zealand College of Anaesthetists and Faculty of Pain Medicine. Acute Pain Management: Scientific Evidence, fifth ed. ANZCA & FPM, Melbourne.

Schwarte, L.A., Ince, C., 2003. Mechanical ventilation of mice. In: Ince, C. (Ed.), The Physiological Genomics of the Critically Ill Mouse. Kluwer Academic Publishers.

Schwarte, L.A., et al., 2000. Mechanical ventilation of mice. Basic Res. Cardiol. 95 (6), 510–520.

Schwenke, D.O., Cragg, P.A., 2004. Comparison of the depressive effects of four anesthetic regimens on ventilatory and cardiovascular variables in the guinea pig. Comp. Med. 54 (1), 77–85.

Scott, E.M., Buckland, R., 2006. A systematic review of intraoperative warming to prevent postoperative complications. AORN J. 83 (5), 1090–1113.

Sear, J.W., et al., 1985. Haematological and biochemical changes during anaesthesia with propofol ("Diprivan"). Postgrad. Med. J. 61 (Suppl. 3), 165–168.

Sebel, P.S., Lowdon, J.D., 1989. Propofol: a new intravenous anesthetic. Anesthesiology 71 (2), 260–277.

Severs, W.B., et al., 1981. Urethane anesthesia in rats. Pharmacology 22 (4), 209–226.

Schmitz, S., et al., 2016. Comparison of physiological parameters and anaesthesia specific observations during isoflurane, ketamine-xylazine or medetomidine-midazolam-fentanyl anaesthesia in male guinea pigs. PLoS ONE 11 (9), e0161258.

Schmitz, S., et al., 2017. Repeated anaesthesia with isoflurane and medetomidine-midazolam-fentanyl in guinea pigs and its influence on physiological parameters. PLoS ONE 12 (3), e0174423.

Shafford, H.L., et al., 2004. Intra-articular lidocaine plus bupivacaine in sheep undergoing stifle arthrotomy. Vet. Anaesth. Analg. 31 (1), 20–26.

Sharp, F.R., Hammel, H.T., 1974. The effects of chloralose-urethan anesthesia on temperature regulation in dogs. J. Appl. Physiol. 33 (2), 229–233.

Shavit, Y., et al., 1998. Effects of prenatal morphine exposure on NK cytotoxicity and responsiveness to LPS in rats. Pharmacol. Biochem. Behav. 59 (4), 835–841.

Sheffield, C.W., et al., 1994. Mild hypothermia during isoflurane anesthesia decreases resistance to *E. coli* dermal infection in guinea pigs. Acta Anaesthesiol. Scand. 38 (3), 201–205.

Shibuta, H., et al., 2019. Comparison of the anesthetic effect by the injection route of mixed anesthesia (medetomidine, midazolam and butorphanol) and the effect of this anesthetic agent on the respiratory function. J. Vet. Med. Sci. 82 (1), 35–42.

Shientag, L.J., et al., 2012. A therapeutic dose of ketoprofen causes acute gastrointestinal bleeding, erosions, and ulcers in rats. J. Am. Assoc. Lab. Anim. Sci. 51 (6), 832–841.

Shih, J., et al., 2012. Delayed environmental enrichment reverses sevoflurane-induced memory impairment in rats. Anesthesiology 116 (3), 586–602.

Shukla, M., et al., 2007. Comparative plasma pharmacokinetics of meloxicam in sheep and goats following intravenous administration. Comp. Biochem. Physiol. C Toxicol. Pharmacol. 145 (4), 528–532.

Shukla, R., Shukla, S.B., 1983. The effect of polyethylene glycol-200 on metabolic acidosis induced by chloralose anaesthesia. J. Vet. Pharmacol. Ther. 6 (2), 149–152.

Sikoski, P., et al., 2007. Comparison of heating devices for maintaining body temperature in anesthetized laboratory rabbits (*Oryctolagus cuniculus*). J. Am. Assoc. Lab. Anim. Sci. 46 (3), 61–63.

Silva, A., Antunes, L., 2012. Electroencephalogram-based anaesthetic depth monitoring in laboratory animals. Lab. Anim. 46 (2), 85–94.

Silva, A., et al., 2011. Performance of electroencephalogram-derived parameters in prediction of depth of anaesthesia in a rabbit model. Br. J. Anaesth. 106 (4), 540–547.

Silva, N.E.O.F., et al., 2020. Validation of the Unesp-Botucatu composite scale to assess acute postoperative abdominal pain in sheep (USAPS). PLoS ONE 15, e0239622.

Simons, S., Tibboel, D., 2006. Pain perception development and maturation. Semin. Fetal Neonatal Med. 11 (4), 227–231.

Siriarchavatana, P., et al., 2016. Anesthetic activity of alfaxalone compared with ketamine in mice. J. Am. Assoc. Lab. Anim. Sci. 55 (4), 426–430.

Sixtus, R.P., et al., 2021. Differential effects of four intramuscular sedatives on cardiorespiratory stability in juvenile guinea pigs (*Cavia porcellus*). PLoS ONE 16 (11), e025955.

Skolleborg, K.C., et al., 1990. Distribution of cardiac output during pentobarbital versus midazolam/fentanyl/fluanisone anaesthesia in the rat. Lab. Anim. 24 (3), 221–227.

Skues, M.A., et al., 1993. Patient-controlled analgesia in children. A comparison of two infusion techniques. Pediatr. Anesth. 3 (4), 223–228.

Sladky, K.K., Mans, C., 2012. Clinical anesthesia in reptiles. J. Exot. Pet Med. 21 (1), 17–31.

Slamberová, R., et al., 2005. Cross-generational effect of prenatal morphine exposure on neurobehavioral development of rat pups. Physiol. Res. 54 (6), 655–660.

Slingsby, L.S., Waterman-Pearson, A.E., 2000. Postoperative analgesia in the cat after ovariohysterectomy by use of carprofen, ketoprofen, meloxicam or tolfenamic acid. J. Small Anim. Pract. 41 (10), 447–450.

Smiler, K.L., et al., 1990. Tissue response to intramuscular and intraperitoneal injections of ketamine and xylazine in rats. Lab. Anim. Sci. 40 (1), 60–64.

Smith, G., 1991. Pain after surgery. Br. J. Anaesth. 67 (3), 233–234.

Smith, L.J., et al., 2006. A single dose of liposome-encapsulated hydromorphone provides extended analgesia in a rat model of neuropathic pain. Comp. Med. 56 (6), 487–492.

Smith, L.J., et al., 2013. Pharmacokinetics of ammonium sulfate gradient loaded liposome-encapsulated oxymorphone and hydromorphone in healthy dogs. Vet. Anaesth. Analg. 40 (5), 537–545.

Smith, R.P., et al., 2000. Pain and stress in the human fetus. Eur. J. Obstet. Gynecol. Reprod. Biol. 92 (1), 161–165.

Smith, B.J., et al., 2016. Pharmacokinetics and paw withdrawal pressure in female guinea pigs (*Cavia porcellus*) treated with sustained-release buprenorphine and buprenorphine hydrochloride. J. Am. Assoc. Lab. Anim. Sci. 55 (6), 789–793.

Sneddon, L.U., 2012. Clinical anesthesia and analgesia in fish. J. Exot. Pet Med. 21 (1), 32–43.

Sneddon, L.U., et al., 2014. Defining and assessing animal pain. Anim. Behav. 97, 201–212.

Sneddon, L.U., 2020. Can fish experience pain? In: The Welfare of Fish. Springer, pp. 229–249.

Sneyd, J.R., Rigby-Jones, A.E., 2010. New drugs and technologies, intravenous anaesthesia is on the move (again). Br. J. Anaesth. 105 (3), aeq190–254.

Sonner, J.M., 2002. Issues in the design and interpretation of minimum alveolar anesthetic concentration (MAC) studies. Anesth. Analg. 95 (3), 609–614.

Sonner, J.M., et al., 2000. Naturally occurring variability in anesthetic potency among inbred mouse strains. Anesth. Analg. 91 (3), 720–726.

Sotocinal, S.G., et al., 2011. The rat grimace scale: a partially automated method for quantifying pain in the laboratory rat via facial expressions. Mol. Pain 7. https://doi.org/10.1186/1744-8069-7-55.

Sousa, M.G., et al., 2011. Comparison between auricular and standard rectal thermometers for the measurement of body temperature in dogs. Can. Vet. J. 52 (4), 403–406.

Souza, M.J., et al., 2008. Pharmacokinetics of orally administered tramadol in domestic rabbits (*Oryctolagus cuniculus*). Am. J. Vet. Res. 69 (8), 979–982.

Speth, R.C., et al., 2001. Regarding the inadvisability of administering postoperative analgesics in the drinking water of rats (*Rattus norvegicus*). Contemp. Top. Lab. Anim. Sci. 40 (6), 15–17.

Sramek, M.K., et al., 2015. The safety of high-dose buprenorphine administered subcutaneously in cats. J. Vet. Pharmacol. Ther. 38 (5), 434–442.

Stark, R.D., 1985. A review of the safety and tolerance of propofol ("Diprivan"). Postgrad. Med. J. 61, 152–156.

Steagall, P.V., et al., 2015. A preliminary investigation of the thermal antinociceptive effects of codeine in cats. J. Feline Med. Surg. 17 (12), 1061–1064.

Steagall, P.V.M., Monteiro-Steagall, B.P., 2013. Multimodal analgesia for perioperative pain in three cats. J. Feline Med. Surg. 15 (8), 737–743.

Steagall, P.V., et al., 2021. Pain management in farm animals: focus on cattle, sheep and pigs. Animals 11 (6), 1483.

Steffens, S., et al., 2022. 3D-print design of a stereotaxic adaptor for the precision targeting of brain structures in infant mice. Eur. J. Neurosci. 55 (3), 725–732.

Steffey, E.P., et al., 1974. Anesthetic potency (MAC) of nitrous oxide in the dog, cat, and stump-tail monkey. J. Appl. Physiol. 36, 530–532.

Stegmann, G.F., Bester, L., 2001. Sedative-hypnotic effects of midazolam in goats after intravenous and intramuscular administration. Vet. Anaesth. Analg. 28 (1), 49–55.

Steiner, A.R., et al., 2020. Systematic review: anaesthetic protocols and management as confounders in rodent blood oxygen level dependent functional magnetic resonance imaging (BOLD fMRI)—part A: effects of changes in physiological parameters. Front. Neurosci., 1052.

Steiner, A.R., et al., 2021. Systematic review: anesthetic protocols and management as confounders in rodent blood oxygen level dependent functional magnetic resonance imaging (BOLD fMRI)—part B: effects of anesthetic agents, doses and timing. Animals 11 (1), 199.

Stevens, C.W., 2011. Analgesia in amphibians: preclinical studies and clinical applications. Vet. Clin. North Am. Exot. Anim. Pract. 14 (1), 33–44.

Steward, C.A., et al., 2005. Methodological considerations in rat brain BOLD contrast pharmacological MRI. Psychopharmacology (Berl) 180 (4), 687–704.

Stogner, S.W., Payne, D.K., 1992. Oxygen toxicity. Ann. Pharmacother. 26 (12), 1554–1562.

Stokes, E.L., et al., 2009. Reported analgesic and anaesthetic administration to rodents undergoing experimental surgical procedures. Lab. Anim. 43 (2), 149–154.

Storer, R.J., et al., 1997. A simple method, using 2-hydroxypropyl-beta-cyclodextrin, of administering alpha-chloralose at room temperature. J. Neurosci. Methods 77 (1), 49–53.

Stout, R.W., et al., 2001. Transcutaneous blood gas monitoring in the rat. Comp. Med. 51 (6), 524–533.

Stratmann, G., et al., 2009. Increasing the duration of isoflurane anesthesia decreases the minimum alveolar anesthetic concentration in 7-day-old but not in 60-day-old rats. Anesth. Analg. 109 (3), 801–806.

Sumikawa, S., et al., 2017. Effect of basic fibroblast growth factor on radiation-induced oral mucositis in male Syrian hamsters. Int. J. Radiat. Biol. 93 (12), 1343–1349.

Svendsen, O., et al., 2007. Nociception after intraperitoneal injection of a sodium pentobarbitone formulation with and without lidocaine in rats quantified by expression of neuronal c-fos in the spinal cord—a preliminary study. Lab. Anim. 41 (2), 197–203.

Svendsen, P., Ainsworth, M., Carter, A., 1990. Acid-base status and cardiovascular function in pigs anaesthetized with α-chloralose. Scand. J. Lab. Anim. Sci. 17 (3), 89–95.

Svorc, P., et al., 2018. Arterial pH and blood gas values in rats under three types of general anesthesia: a chronobiological study. Physiol. Res. 67 (5), 721–728.

Tahamtani, F.M., et al., 2021. Assessment of mobility and pain in broiler chickens with identifiable gait defects. Appl. Anim. Behav. Sci. 234, 105183.

Tang, W., et al., 2020. Alternative anesthesia of neonatal mice for global rAAV delivery in the brain with non-detectable behavioral interference in adults. Front. Behav. Neurosci. 14, 115.

Tappe-Theodor, A., et al., 2019. Pros and cons of clinically relevant methods to assess pain in rodents. Neurosci. Biobehav. Rev. 100, 335–343.

Tashiro, M., Tohei, A., 2022. Recommended doses of medetomidine-midazolam-butorphanol with atipamezole for preventing hypothermia in mice. J. Vet. Med. Sci. 84 (3), 445–453.

Tashiro, M., et al., 2020. Duration of thermal support for preventing hypothermia induced by anesthesia with medetomidine-midazolam-butorphanol in mice. J. Vet. Med. Sci. 82 (12), 1757–1762.

Tasbihgou, S.R., et al., 2018. Accidental awareness during general anaesthesia—a narrative review. Anaesthesia 73 (1), 112–122.

Taylor, D.K., 2019. Influence of pain and analgesia on cancer research studies. Comp. Med. 69 (6), 501–509.

Taylor, P.M., 1991. Anaesthesia in sheep and goats. In Pract. 13 (1), 31–36.

Taylor, P.M., Houlton, J.E.F., 1984. Post-operative analgesia in the dog: a comparison of morphine, buprenorphine and pentazocine. J. Small Anim. Pract. 25 (7), 437–451.

Ter Horst, E.N., et al., 2018. Sufentanil–medetomidine anaesthesia compared with fentanyl/fluanisone–midazolam is associated with fewer ventricular arrhythmias and death during experimental myocardial infarction in rats and limits infarct size following reperfusion. Lab. Anim. 52 (3), 271–279.

Thaete, L.G., et al., 2013. Impact of anaesthetics and analgesics on fetal growth in the mouse. Lab. Anim. 47 (3), 175–183.

Thal, S.C., Plesnila, N., 2007. Non-invasive intraoperative monitoring of blood pressure and arterial pCO2 during surgical anesthesia in mice. J. Neurosci. Methods 159 (2), 261–267.

Thawley, V., Waddell, L.S., 2013. Pulse oximetry and capnometry. Top. Companion Anim. Med. 28 (3), 124–128.

Theisen, M.M., et al., 2009. Ventral recumbency is crucial for fast and safe orotracheal intubation in laboratory swine. Lab. Anim. 43 (1), 96–101.

Thiede, A.J., et al., 2014. Pharmacokinetics of sustained-release and transdermal buprenorphine in Göttingen minipigs (*Sus scrofa* domestica). J. Am. Assoc. Lab. Anim. Sci. 53 (6), 692–699.

Thomas, A.A., et al., 2012. An alternative method of endotracheal intubation of common marmosets (*Callithrix jacchus*). Lab. Anim. 46 (1), 71–76.

Thomas, A.A., et al., 2016. Efficacy of intrathecal morphine in a model of surgical pain in rats. PLoS One 11 (10), e0163909.

Thomas, J., Lerche, P., 2022. Anaesthesia and Analgesia for Veterinary Technicians, sixth ed. Elsevier, New York.

Thomasson, B., et al., 1974. Spinal anaesthesia in the guinea-pig. Lab. Anim. 8 (2), 241–244.

Thompson, A.C., et al., 2004. Analgesic efficacy of orally administered buprenorphine in rats: methodologic considerations. Comp. Med. 51 (1), 43–48.

Thomson, L., Paton, J., 2014. Oxygen toxicity. Paediatr. Respir. Rev. 15 (2), 120–123.

Topic Popovic, N., et al., 2012. Tricaine methane-sulfonate (MS-222) application in fish anaesthesia. J. Appl. Ichthyol. 28 (4), 553–564.

Tordoff, M.G., et al., 2007. Forty mouse strain survey of water and sodium intake. Physiol. Behav. 91 (5), 620–631.

Tordoff, M.G., et al., 2008. Preferences of 14 rat strains for 17 taste compounds. Physiol. Behav. 95 (3), 308–332.

Torres, M.D., et al., 2012. Effects of an intravenous bolus of alfaxalone versus propofol on intraocular pressure in sheep. Vet. Rec. 170 (9), 226.

Tranquilli, W.J., et al., 1985. Anesthetic potency of nitrous oxide in young swine (*Sus scrofa*). Am. J. Vet. Res. 46 (1), 58–60.

Tremoleda, J.L., et al., 2012. Anaesthesia and physiological monitoring during in vivo imaging of laboratory rodents: considerations on experimental outcomes and animal welfare. EJNMMI Res. 2 (1), 1–23.

Tschoner, T., 2021. Methods for pain assessment in calves and their use for the evaluation of pain during different procedures—a review. Animals 11 (5), 1235.

Tubbs, J.T., et al., 2011. Effects of buprenorphine, meloxicam, and flunixin meglumine as postoperative analgesia in mice. J. Am. Assoc. Lab. Anim. Sci. 50 (2), 185–347.

Turner, P.V., Albassam, M.A., 2005. Susceptibility of rats to corneal lesions after injectable anesthesia. Comp. Med. 55 (2), 175–182.

Turner, P.V., et al., 2006. Pharmacokinetics of meloxicam in rabbits after single and repeat oral dosing. Comp. Med. 56 (1), 63–67.

Tuttle, A.H., et al., 2018. A deep neural network to assess spontaneous pain from mouse facial expressions. Mol. Pain 14, 1744806918763658.

Tzabazis, A., et al., 2004. EEG-controlled closed-loop dosing of propofol in rats. Br. J. Anaesth. 92 (4), 564–569.

Tzannes, S., et al., 2000. The use of sevoflurane in a 2:1 mixture of nitrous oxide and oxygen for rapid mask induction of anaesthesia in the cat. J. Feline Med. Surg. 2 (2), 83–90.

Ungerer, M.J., 1978. A comparison between the bain and magill anaesthetic systems during spontaneous breathing. Can. Anaesth. Soc. J. 25 (2), 122–124.

Uzun, M., et al., 2015. The investigation of airway management capacity of v-gel and cobra-PLA in anaesthetised rabbits. Acta Cir. Bras. 30 (1), 80–86.

Vachon, P., 2014. Hargreaves does not evaluate nociception following a surgical laparotomy in Xenopus leavis frogs. Res. Vet. Sci. 97 (2), 470–473.

Vainio, O.M., et al., 1992. Cardiovascular effects of a ketamine-medetomidine combination that produces deep sedation in Yucatan mini swine. Lab. Anim. Sci. 42 (6), 582–588.

Valk, B.I., Struys, M.M., 2021. Etomidate and its analogs: a review of pharmacokinetics and pharmacodynamics. Clin. Pharmacokinet. 60 (10), 1253–1269.

van Camp, N., et al., 2003. Simultaneous electroencephalographic recording and functional magnetic resonance imaging during pentylenetetrazol-induced seizures in rat. Neuroimage 19 (3), 627–636.

Van der Linden, A., et al., 2007. Current status of functional MRI on small animals: application to physiology, pathophysiology, and cognition. NMR Biomed. 20 (5), 522–545.

van der Vijver, R.J., et al., 2013. Perioperative pain relief by a COX-2 inhibitor affects ileal repair and provides a model for anastomotic leakage in the intestine. Surg. Innov. 20 (2), 113–118.

Van Pelt, L.F., 1977. Ketamine and xylazine for surgical anesthesia in rats. J. Am. Vet. Med. Assoc. 171 (9), 842–844.

Van Vliet, B.N., et al., 2000. Direct and indirect methods used to study arterial blood pressure. J. Pharmacol. Toxicol. Methods 44 (2), 361–373.

Vanacker, B., et al., 1987. Changes in intraocular pressure associated with the administration of propofol. Br. J. Anaesth. 59 (12), 1514–1517.

Varga, M., 2017. Airway management in the rabbit. J. Exot. Pet Med. 26 (1), 29–35.

Varughese, S., Ahmed, R., 2021. Environmental and occupational considerations of anesthesia: a narrative review and update. Anesth. Analg. 133 (4), 826.

Velasco Gallego, M.L., et al., 2021. Effects of isoflurane and sevoflurane alone and in combination with butorphanol or medetomidine on the bispectral index in chickens. BMC Vet. Res. 17 (1), 1–11.

Vergneau-Grosset, C., Benedetti, I.C.C., 2022. Fish sedation and anesthesia. Vet. Clin. North Am. Exot. Anim. Pract. 25 (1), 13–29.

Verstegen, J., Fargetton, X., Donnay, I., Ectors, F., 1990. Comparison of the clinical utility of medetomidine/ketamine and xylazine/ketamine combinations for the ovariectomy of cats. Vet. Rec. 127 (17), 424–426.

Viberg, H., et al., 2014. Paracetamol (acetaminophen) administration during neonatal brain development affects cognitive function and alters its analgesic and anxiolytic response in adult male mice. Toxicol. Sci. 138 (1), 139–147.

Vijn, P.C., Sneyd, J.R., 1998. I.v. anaesthesia and EEG burst suppression in rats: bolus injections and closed-loop infusions. Br. J. Anaesth. 81 (3), 415–421.

Viñuela-Fernández, I., et al., 2007. Pain mechanisms and their implication for the management of pain in farm and companion animals. Vet. J. 174 (2), 227–239.

Virtanen, R., 1988. Pharmacological profiles of medetomidine and its antagonist, atipamezole. Acta Vet. Scand. Suppl. 85, 29–37.

Virtanen, R., MacDonald, E., 1985. Comparison of the effects of detomidine and xylazine on some alpha 2-adrenoceptor-mediated responses in the central and peripheral nervous systems. Eur. J. Pharmacol. 115 (2–3), 277–284.

Virtanen, R., et al., 1988a. Highly selective and specific antagonism of central and peripheral alpha 2-adrenoceptors by atipamezole. Arch. Int. Pharmacodyn. Ther. 297, 190–204.

Virtanen, R., Savola, J.M., Saano, V., et al., 1988b. Characterization of the selectivity, specificity and potency of medetomidine as an alpha 2-adrenoceptor agonist. Eur. J. Pharmacol. 150 (1–2), 9–14.

Viscardi, A.V., Turner, P.V., 2018. Efficacy of buprenorphine for management of surgical castration pain in piglets. BMC Vet. Res. 14 (1), 1–12.

Viscardi, A.V., et al., 2021. Analgesic comparison of flunixin meglumine or meloxicam for soft-tissue surgery in sheep: a pilot study. Animals 11 (2), 423.

Vishwakarma, R.K., et al., 2013. Total intravenous anaesthesia (TIVA) with propofol in sheep: a clinical and haematobiochemical study. Indian J. Vet. Surg. 34 (1), 32–34.

Visser, E., Schug, S.A., 2006. The role of ketamine in pain management. Biomed. Pharmacother. 60 (7), 341–348.

Vivien, B., et al., 1999. Minimum alveolar anesthetic concentration of volatile anesthetics in normal and cardiomyopathic hamsters. Anesth. Analg. 88 (3), 489–493.

Voipio, H.M., et al., 1990. Evaluation of anesthetic potency of medetomidine-ketamine combination in mice. In: IX ICLAS Symposium Proceedings.

Vullo, C., et al., 2014. Pharmacokinetics of tramadol and its major metabolite after intramuscular administration in piglets. J. Vet. Pharmacol. Ther. 37 (6), 603–606.

Vuong, C., et al., 2013. The effects of opioids and opioid analogs on animal and human endocrine systems. Endocr. Rev. 31 (1), 98–132.

Wagner, J.G., 1974. A safe method for rapidly achieving plasma concentration plateaus. Clin. Pharmacol. Ther. 16 (4), 691–700.

Walker, L.A., Buscemi-Bergin, M., 1983. Renal hemodynamics in conscious rats: effects of anesthesia, surgery, and recovery. Am. J. Physiol. Renal Physiol. 245 (1), F67–F74.

Walsh, V.P., et al., 2012. A comparison of two different ketamine and diazepam combinations with an alphaxalone and medetomidine combination for induction of anaesthesia in sheep. N. Z. Vet. J. 60 (2), 136–141.

Walters, E.T., 2018. Nociceptive biology of molluscs and arthropods: evolutionary clues about functions and mechanisms potentially related to pain. Front. Physiol. 9, 1049.

Warne, L.N., et al., 2015. A review of the pharmacology and clinical application of alfaxalone in cats. Vet. J. 203 (2), 141–148.

Waterman, A.E., 1988. Use of propofol in sheep. Vet. Rec. 122 (11), 260.

Waterman, A.E., et al., 1991. Analgesic activity and respiratory effects of butorphanol in sheep. Res. Vet. Sci. 51 (1), 19–23.

Watkins, S.B., Hall, L.W., Clarke, K.W., 1987. Propofol as an intravenous anaesthetic agent in dogs. Vet. Rec. 120 (14), 326–329.

Weary, D.M., et al., 2006. Identifying and preventing pain in animals. Appl. Anim. Behav. Sci. 100 (1–2), 64-76.

Weber, R., et al., 2006. A fully noninvasive and robust experimental protocol for longitudinal fMRI studies in the rat. Neuroimage 29 (4), 1303–1310.

Weinert, D., Waterhouse, J., 2007. The circadian rhythm of core temperature: effects of physical activity and aging. Physiol. Behav. 90 (2–3), 246–256.

Weiskopf, R.B., Bogetz, M.S., 1984. Minimum alveolar concentrations (MAC) of halothane and nitrous oxide in swine. Anesth. Analg. 63 (5), 529–532.

Welberg, L.A., et al., 2006. Ketamine/xylazine/acepromazine anesthesia and postoperative recovery in rats. J. Am. Assoc. Lab. Anim. Sci. 45 (2), 13–20.

Wellington, D., et al., 2013. Comparison of ketamine-xylazine and ketamine-dexmedetomidine anesthesia and intraperitoneal tolerance in rats. J. Am. Assoc. Lab. Anim. Sci. 52 (4), 481–487.

Wells, S., et al., 2009. Urethral obstruction by seminal coagulum is associated with medetomidine-ketamine anesthesia in male mice on C57BL/6J and mixed genetic backgrounds. J. Am. Assoc. Lab. Anim. Sci. 48 (3), 296–299.

Welsh, E.M., et al., 1997. Beneficial effects of administering carprofen before surgery in dogs. Vet. Rec. 141 (10), 251–253.

Wemyss-Holden, S.A., et al., 1999. The laryngeal mask airway in experimental pig anaesthesia. Lab. Anim. 33 (1), 30–34.

West, S.E., et al., 2020. Intraperitoneal alfaxalone and alfaxalone–dexmedetomidine anesthesia in Sprague–Dawley rats (*Rattus norvegicus*). J. Am. Assoc. Lab. Anim. Sci. 59 (5), 531–538.

Whelan, G. and Flecknell, P.A., 1992. The assessment of depth of anaesthesia in animals and man. Lab. Anim. 26 (3), 153–162.

Whelan, G., Flecknell, P.A., 1995. Anaesthesia of laboratory rabbits using etorphine/methotrime-prazine and midazolam. Lab. Anim. 29 (1), 83–89.

Whelan, G., et al., 1999. Anaesthesia of the common marmoset (*Callithrix jacchus*) using continuous intravenous infusion of alphaxalone/alphadalone. Lab. Anim. 33 (1), 24–29.

White, G.L., Holmes, D.D., 1976. A comparison of ketamine and the combination ketamine-xylazine for effective surgical anesthesia in the rabbit. Lab. Anim. Sci. 26 (5), 804–806.

White, M.C., Wolf, A.R., 2004. Pain and stress in the human fetus. Best Pract. Res. Clin. Anaesthesiol. 18 (2), 205–220.

White, P.F., et al., 1982. Ketamine—its pharmacology and therapeutic uses. Anesthesiology 56 (2), 119–136.

White, K.L., et al., 2017. A clinical evaluation of the pharmacokinetics and pharmacodynamics of intravenous alfaxalone in cyclodextrin in male and female rats following a loading dose and constant rate infusion. Vet. Anaesth. Analg. 44 (4), 865–875.

White, K., et al., 2022. Alfaxalone Population Pharmacokinetics in the Rat: Model Application for PK/PD Design in Inbred and Outbred Strains and Sexes. Authorea, https://doi.org/10.22541/au.165339543.34703499/v1.

Whittaker, A.L., et al., 2014. The assessment of general well-being using spontaneous burrowing behaviour in a short-term model of chemotherapy-induced mucositis in the rat. Lab. Anim. 49 (1), 30–39.

Whittaker, A.L., et al., 2021. Identification of animal-based welfare indicators in captive reptiles: a delphi consultation survey. Animals 11 (7), 2010.

Wiklund, L., Thoren, L., 1985. Intraoperative blood component and fluid therapy. Acta Anaesthesiol. Scand. 29 (s82), 1–8.

Wilding, L.A., et al., 2017. Benefits of 21% oxygen compared with 100% oxygen for delivery of isoflurane to mice (*Mus musculus*) and rats (*Rattus norvegicus*). J. Am. Assoc. Lab. Anim. Sci. 56 (2), 148–154.

Williams, C.J., et al., 2019. Analgesia for non-mammalian vertebrates. Curr. Opin. Physio. 11, 75–84.

Wixson, S.K., et al., 1987. A comparison of pentobarbital, fentanyl-droperidol, ketamine-xylazine and ketamine-diazepam anesthesia in adult male rats. Lab. Anim. Sci. 37 (6), 726–730.

Wood, M., Woad, A.J.J., 1984. Contrasting effects of halothane, isoflurane, and Enflurane on in vivo drug metabolism in the rat. Anesth. Analg. 63 (8), 709.

Woolf, C.J., Chong, M.-S., 1993. Preemptive analgesia-treating postoperative pain by preventing the establishment of central sensitization. Anesth. Analg. 77 (2), 362.

Woolf, C.J., Wall, P.D., 1986. Morphine-sensitive and morphine-insensitive actions of C-fibre input on the rat spinal cord. Neurosci. Lett. 64 (2), 221–225.

Wright-Williams, S.L., et al., 2007. Effects of vasectomy surgery and meloxicam treatment on fae-cal corticosterone levels and behaviour in two strains of laboratory mouse. Pain 130 (1–2), 108–118.

Wu, C.L., Raja, S.N., 2011. Treatment of acute postoperative pain. Lancet 377 (9784), 2215–2225.

Yaksh, T.L., et al., 1988. Spinal pharmacology of agents which alter pain transmission and muscle tone. In: Local-spinal Therapy of Spasticity. Springer Berlin Heidelberg, Berlin, Heidelberg, pp. 19–36.

Yeung, K.R., et al., 2014. Comparison of indirect and direct blood pressure measurements in ba-boons during ketamine anaesthesia. J. Med. Primatol. 43 (4), 217–224.

Young, J., Kapoor, V., 2010. Principles of anaesthetic vaporizers. Anaesth. Intensive Care Med. 11 (4), 140–143.

Yoshida, K., et al., 2015. Prediction formulas for individual opioid analgesic requirements based on genetic polymorphism analyses. PLoS ONE 10 (1), e0116885–13.

Ypsilantis, P., et al., 2005. A comparative study of invasive and oscillometric methods of arterial blood pressure measurement in the anesthetized rabbit. Res. Vet. Sci. 78 (3), 269–275.

Ypsilantis, P., et al., 2007. Organ toxicity and mortality in propofol-sedated rabbits under prolonged mechanical ventilation. Anesth. Analg. 105 (1), 155–166.

Ypsilantis, P., et al., 2011. Attenuation of propofol tolerance conferred by remifentanil co-administration does not reduce propofol toxicity in rabbits under prolonged mechanical venti-lation. J. Surg. Res. 168 (2), 253–261.

Yu, A., et al., 2020. Preliminary investigation to address pain and haemorrhage following the spay-ing of female cattle. Animals 10 (2), 249.

Zacny, J.P., et al., 1998. Comparing the subjective, psychomotor and physiological effects of in-travenous pentazocine and morphine in normal volunteers. J. Pharmacol. Exp. Ther. 286 (3), 1197–1207.

Zehnder, A., 2008. Intraosseous catheter placement in small mammals. Lab. Anim. 37 (8), 351–352.

Zeller, W., et al., 1998. Adverse effects of tribromoethanol as used in the production of transgenic mice. Lab. Anim. 32 (4), 407–413.

Zhang, E.Q., et al., 2017. Heating pad performance and efficacy of 2 durations of warming after isoflurane anesthesia of Sprague–Dawley Rats (*Rattus norvegicus*). J. Am. Assoc. Lab. Anim. Sci. 56 (6), 786–791.

Zhang, Y.J., et al., 2020. 2020 the preclinical pharmacological study on HX0969W, a novel water-soluble pro-drug of propofol, in rats. PeerJ 8, e8922.

Zhang, X.Y., et al., 2022. Systematic review and meta-analysis of studies in which burrowing be-haviour was assessed in rodent models of disease-associated persistent pain. Pain, 10–1097.

Zhou, Y., et al., 2013. Efficacy comparison of the novel water-soluble propofol prodrug HX0969w and fospropofol in mice and rats. Br. J. Anaesth. 111 (5), 825–832.

Zhu, M., et al., 2004. On the role of anesthesia on the body/brain temperature differential in rats. J. Therm. Biol. 29 (7–8), 599–603.

Zullian, C., et al., 2016. Plasma concentrations of buprenorphine following a single subcutaneous administration of a sustained release formulation of buprenorphine in sheep. Can. J. Vet. Res. 80 (3), 250–253.

Zuurbier, C.J., et al., 2014. Optimizing anesthetic regimen for surgery in mice through minimiza-tion of hemodynamic, metabolic, and inflammatory perturbations. Exp. Biol. Med. 239 (6), 737–746.

Index

Note: Page numbers followed by *f* indicate figures and *t* indicate tables.

Printed and bound by CPI Group (UK) Ltd, Croydon, CR0 4YY

08/06/2025

01896869-0005